Responding to Patients in Crisis

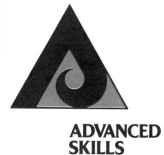

**ADVANCED
SKILLS**

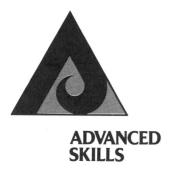

**ADVANCED
SKILLS**

Responding to Patients in Crisis

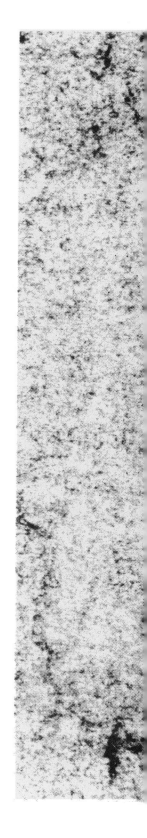

S Springhouse Corporation
Springhouse, Pennsylvania

Staff

Executive Director, Editorial
Stanley Loeb

Senior Publisher
Matthew Cahill

Art Director
John Hubbard

Senior Editor
Stephen Daly

Clinical Project Director
Patricia Dwyer Schull, RN, MSN

Editors
Neal Fandek, Kathy Goldberg, Elizabeth Mauro, Elizabeth Weinstein

Clinical Editors
Sherri Inez Becker, RN, CCRN; Tina R. Dietrich, RN, BSN, CCRN; Mary Jane McDevitt, RN, BS

Copy Editors
Cynthia C. Breuninger *(supervisor)*, Priscilla DeWitt, Traci A. Ginnona, Jennifer Mintzer, Dorothy Oren, Nancy Papsin, Doris Weinstock

Designers
Stephanie Peters *(associate art director)*, Matie Patterson *(senior designer)*, Lynn Foulk, Joseph Laufer

Illustrators
Dan Fione, Jean Gardner, Linda Gist, Bob Jackson, Robert Neumann, Judy Newhouse, Mary Stangl

Art Production
Anet Oakes, Ann Raphun, Robert Wieder

Typography
David Kosten *(director)*, Diane Paluba *(manager)*, Elizabeth Bergman, Joyce Rossi Biletz, Phyllis Marron, Robin Mayer, Valerie Rosenberger

Manufacturing
Deborah Meiris *(director)*, T.A. Landis *(manager)*

Production Coordination
Patricia W. McCloskey

Editorial Assistants
Maree DeRosa, Beverly Lane, Mary Madden

AS6-010993

Library of Congress Cataloging-in-Publication Data
Responding to patients in crisis.
  p. cm. – (Advanced skills)
  Includes bibliographical references and index.
  1. Emergency nursing.   I. Springhouse
Corporation.   II. Series.
  [DNLM: 1. Emergency Nursing. 2. Critical
  Care. WY 154 R434 1993]
RT120.E4R47 1993
610.73'61 – dc20
DNLM/DLC   93-1937
ISBN 0-87434-557-X   CIP

Contents

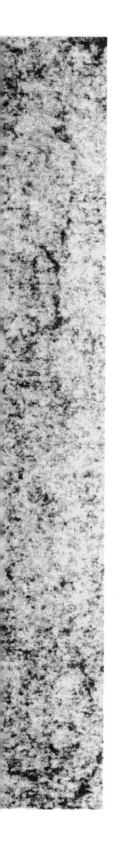

Advisory board

At the time of publication, the advisors
held the following positions.

Cecelia Gatson Grindel, RN, PhD
Nurse Researcher
Lehigh Valley Hospital
Allentown, Pa.

Judith Ski Lower, RN, MSN, CCRN, CNRN
Nurse Manager, Neurology Critical Care Unit
Johns Hopkins Hospital
Baltimore

Kathleen M. Malloch, RN, BSN, MBA, CNA
Vice President, Patient Care Services
Del Webb Memorial Hospital
Sun City West, Ariz.

Marguerite K. Schlag, RN, MSN, EdD
Director, Nursing Education and Development
Robert Wood Johnson University Hospital
New Brunswick, N.J.

Karen L. Then, RN, MN
Assistant Professor, Faculty of Nursing
University of Calgary, Alberta

Contributors

At the time of publication, the contributors held the following positions.

Shana Marie Bollinger, RN, AA
Clinical Nurse
Johns Hopkins University
Oncology Center
Baltimore

Anne E. Braun, RN,C, MSN, CCRN, CEN
Instructor, Critical Care Nursing
Crozer-Chester Medical Center
Upland, Pa.

Marian J. Hoffman, RN, MSN, CNSN
Clinical Nurse Specialist
Education Nurse Specialist
Lehigh Valley Hospital
Allentown, Pa.

Bonnie Kosman, RN, MSN, CDE
Nursing Supervisor
Lehigh Valley Home Care
Allentown, Pa.

Tammy Ann McCourt, RN, BSN, CCRN
Senior Partner, Neurotrauma Unit
University of Maryland
Baltimore

Barbara A. Moyer, RN, MSN
Education Nurse Specialist
Lehigh Valley Hospital
Allentown, Pa.

Deborah Panozzo Nelson, RN, MS, CCRN
Cardiovascular Clinical Specialist
EMS Nursing Education
LaGrange, Ill.

Gerarda Savinski-Bozinko, RN, BSN, CCRN
Clinical Educator
Crozer-Chester Medical Center
Upland, Pa.

Virginia Huddleston Secor, RN, MSN, CCRN
Adjunct Faculty
Vanderbilt University
Nashville

Brenda K. Shelton, RN, MS, CCRN, OCN
Critical Care Clinical Nurse Specialist
Johns Hopkins University
Oncology Center
Baltimore

Daniele Shollenberger, RN, MSN
Education Nurse Specialist
Lehigh Valley Hospital
Allentown, Pa.

Gwendolyn A. Smith, RN, CCRN
Clinical Coordinator, Burn Treatment Center
Crozer-Chester Medical Center
Upland, Pa.

Pamela Becker Weilitz, RN, MSN
Manager
Barnes Hospital
Washington University Medical Center
St. Louis

FOREWORD

Responding effectively to a patient in a life-threatening crisis may be the ultimate test of your nursing skills. Such a crisis can occur anywhere — in a hospital, an extended care facility, a doctor's office, or a patient's home. You'll have little time to act and, at times, you may have to intervene alone. To manage a crisis effectively, your response must be almost reflexive. Yet you also need a firm grasp of new equipment technology, a thorough knowledge of the underlying pathophysiology, and the ability to anticipate — and meet — the patient's acute needs. You must be able to identify warning signs and interpret laboratory data promptly — early detection may be the only way to stop your patient from slipping into an irreversible decline. You must know which steps to take immediately, then follow up with interventions designed to stabilize your patient and then restore his well-being.

Where can you turn to obtain the detailed, comprehensive information you need? *Responding to Patients in Crisis* fits the bill precisely. The latest book in the Advanced Skills series, it zeroes in on both the immediate interventions that can save your patient's life and the continuing care that will keep him stabilized.

The book consists of seven chapters, each focusing on crises within a body system. The first chapter covers cardiovascular crises, including cardiogenic shock, hypertensive crisis, myocardial infarction, and cardiac arrest. Chapter 2 guides you through respiratory crises, such as pulmonary embolism, adult respiratory distress syndrome, and pulmonary edema. Chapter 3 explores such neurologic crises as head injury, cerebral aneurysm, arteriovenous malformation, and status epilepticus.

Chapter 4 tells what to do if your patient has a gastrointestinal (GI) crisis, such as ruptured esophageal varices, perforated ulcer, GI hemorrhage, or hepatic failure. Chapter 5 covers metabolic and endocrine crises, including diabetic ketoacidosis, thyroid storm, and adrenal crisis. Hematologic crises — disseminated intravascular coagulation (DIC) and sickle-cell crisis — are the focus of Chapter 6. Finally, Chapter 7 covers multisystem crises, describing how to manage anaphylactic shock and other disorders.

For convenience and easy reference, all the chapters follow the same format. A brief introduction defines the crisis and describes its causes, pathophysiology, and potential complications. Next comes a section on assessment, which emphasizes how to set priorities. After describing the emergency interventions you must take, the chapter details the ongoing treatment and nursing care that the patient will need once he emerges from the crisis.

As you use this book, you'll come upon logos—graphic devices that signal key information. The *Pathophysiology* logo, for instance, alerts you to descriptions and illustrations of how crises develop. The *Assessment insight* logo accents clues that will help you pinpoint your patient's chief problem. The *Emergency interventions* logo calls your attention to the steps you must take to resolve a crisis. The *Complications* logo flags potential complications to stay alert for during and after a crisis. Finally, the *Clinical preview* logo presents a detailed case study of a patient in crisis, showing how the nurse's clinical findings helped determine appropriate interventions for resolving the situation.

Throughout this book, you'll find many helpful illustrations, tables, and charts that will boost your knowledge of pathophysiology, make your assessments more accurate, and clarify difficult technical topics. For instance, Chapter 1 includes a chart that presents hemodynamic values in cardiogenic shock as well as illustrations of the procedure used in percutaneous transluminal coronary angioplasty. In Chapter 6, you'll find tables listing diagnostic findings in sickle-cell crisis and DIC. A chart in Chapter 7 details assessment findings in organ failure.

Following the last chapter is a list of other books and articles on crises recommended by the authors. Next, you'll find the *Advanced skilltest*, a multiple-choice self-test that lets you assess what you've learned and determine which areas of crisis care you need to review. The answers, along with complete rationales, immediately follow the test.

The needs of patients in crisis are varied and complex. From initial diagnosis to effective treatment to the patient's recovery, you'll find that *Responding to Patients in Crisis* tells you what you need to know. With its emphasis on follow-through nursing care, this concise book will prove an essential addition to your personal library. If you're already familiar with the basics of crisis care, use it to update your knowledge. If you're new to this aspect of care, consider this book a crucial aid to meeting nursing's greatest challenge—saving patients' lives. I can't recommend *Responding to Patients in Crisis* highly enough.

Anne E. Braun, RN,C, MSN, CCRN, CEN

Instructor, Critical Care Nursing
Crozer-Chester Medical Center
Upland, Pa.

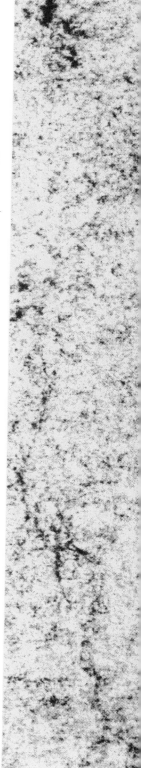

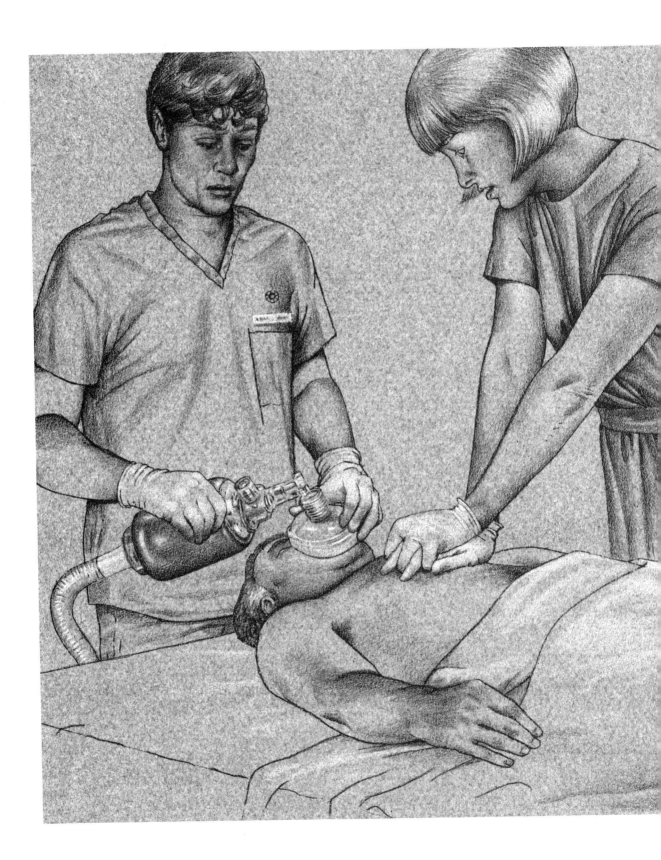

CHAPTER 1

Cardiovascular crises

Because a cardiovascular crisis can be quickly fatal, it demands immediate assessment and intervention. Each second counts, and your patient's life may well depend on your decisions. Consequently, you must respond rapidly yet effectively, and be prepared to perform life-support measures to avert brain damage or death.

This chapter can help you skillfully manage a cardiovascular crisis. It not only describes the steps you must take to safeguard your patient's well-being but also reviews the causes and pathophysiology of the crisis—information that will help you understand the basis for your nursing actions.

For each of the six cardiovascular crises discussed in the chapter, you'll find out how to perform an emergency assessment and which interventions you should take immediately. You'll also review the ongoing medical and nursing care your patient must receive after his initial treatment.

Hypertensive crisis

This crisis is characterized by a rapid, sharp rise in blood pressure. The speed and severity of the increase in blood pressure can compromise your patient's cerebral, renal, and cardiovascular functions. Hypertensive crisis can lead to death unless treated promptly. (See *Responding to hypertensive crisis.*)

In most patients, blood pressure is considered excessively elevated when mean systolic pressure exceeds 180 mm Hg and mean diastolic pressure exceeds 120 mm Hg. However, keep in mind that hypertensive crisis isn't a particular blood pressure reading but a clinical state. (See *Classifying blood pressure.*)

Causes

Hypertensive crisis can result from:
• untreated or inadequately treated essential hypertension
• renal disease, such as acute or chronic glo-

EMERGENCY INTERVENTIONS

Responding to hypertensive crisis

Without prompt treatment, hypertensive crisis can lead to rapid death from brain damage or cerebrovascular accident (CVA) or to a more gradual death from renal impairment.

Reduce blood pressure
• Your first priority is to reduce blood pressure—quickly but cautiously. As ordered, give nitroprusside, hydralazine, or diazoxide (vasodilators), trimethaphan (a ganglionic blocking agent), or phentolamine (an alpha-adrenergic blocking agent). These drugs can increase heart rate, stroke volume, cardiac work load, and cardiac output. Usually, you'll administer these medications I.V., titrating the dosage to the patient's response.
—Nitroprusside acts directly on arteriolar smooth muscle. Within seconds, it decreases peripheral resistance and arterial pressure and increases venous capacity. It also reduces preload and afterload, decreasing myocardial oxygen demand.
—Hydralazine acts directly on arteriolar smooth muscle, acting within 15 minutes when given I.V. or within 30 minutes when given I.M.
—Diazoxide acts within 3 to 5 minutes to dilate arteriolar smooth muscle, reducing peripheral vascular resistance and blood pressure. Expect the doctor to order repeated, low-dose I.V. injections of diazoxide to reduce blood pressure more gradually than a single large bolus and to minimize the risk of CVA or myocardial infarction (MI).
—Trimethaphan blocks sympathetic and parasympathetic impulses and induces arteriolar and venous dilation within 1 to 2 minutes. The extent of the resulting blood pressure drop depends largely on the patient's position. To maximize drug effects, raise the head of his bed no more than 10 degrees.
—Phentolamine induces vasodilation within seconds. It's especially useful for hypertensive crisis associated with excessive catecholamine release secondary to pheochromocytoma or monoamine oxidase inhibitor interactions.
—As ordered, give other drugs to reduce preload, afterload, and blood pressure, such as I.V. nitroglycerin, I.M. reserpine, I.V. methyldopa, or I.V. labetalol (first by bolus, then by continuous infusion).

Monitor blood pressure
• When antihypertensive drug therapy begins, monitor the patient's blood pressure closely. These drugs have a rapid onset and may cause extreme vasodilation. Assess blood pressure every 5 minutes for the first 15 minutes, every 15 minutes for the next hour, then every hour until it's stable.
• When administering drugs I.V., increase the infusion rate gradually until the patient's blood pressure begins to drop. When the patient's blood pressure stabilizes at the desired level, the doctor will start the transition from I.V. to oral drug administration.
• Throughout drug therapy, continue to assess the patient frequently for hypotension and signs and symptoms of heart failure, MI, and CVA. Monitor his hemodynamic indicators—preferably with an arterial line—to evaluate the effectiveness of antihypertensive therapy.

merulonephritis, pyelonephritis, and renal vascular disease
• eclampsia
• intracerebral hemorrhage
• acute left ventricular failure
• polycythemia
• pituitary tumors
• coarctation of the aorta
• adrenocortical hyperfunction
• monoamine oxidase (MAO) inhibitor interactions.

Pathophysiology

Two distinct but usually concurrent mechanisms occur in hypertensive crisis—dilation of cerebral arterioles and damage to the arteriolar wall. With normal fluctuations in blood pressure, the brain maintains adequate perfusion through autoregulation: When blood pressure drops, the cerebral arterioles dilate; when it rises, these arterioles constrict to maintain constant cerebral blood flow.

However, in hypertensive crisis, blood pressure climbs so high that the arterioles, already constricted, can no longer withstand the pressure and dilate suddenly. With the brain hyperperfused under such high pressure, fluid moves into the interstitial spaces, causing cerebral edema, hemorrhage (or both) and, possibly, hypertensive encephalopathy. (See *How hypertension damages blood vessels,* page 4.)

Excessive mean arterial pressure (MAP) can cause necrotizing arteriolitis (arteriolar inflammation) within hours. The inflamed, damaged vessels affect target organs in the following pattern:
• In the eyes, the retinal arteries become severely constricted, leading to retinopathy.
• In the kidneys, severe arteriolar constriction impairs circulation and may cause renal failure. During hypertensive crisis, arteriolar changes are accelerated, and accelerated (or malignant) hypertension ensues.
• In the heart, excessively high pressure in the aorta at the end of diastole impedes systolic ejection. With intra-aortic pressure so high, the left ventricle must generate more wall tension or work harder to open the aortic valve when systole begins. This high afterload increases oxygen demand and the heart's work load. And

---

Classifying blood pressure

The Joint National Committee on the Detection, Evaluation, and Treatment of High Blood Pressure recently revised its guidelines for classifying hypertension. The terms *mild, moderate,* and *severe* have been replaced with *normal* (systolic pressure below 130 mm Hg and diastolic pressure below 85 mm Hg), *high normal* (130 to 139 mm Hg systolic and 85 to 89 mm Hg diastolic), and *four stages* of hypertension, in order of increasing severity. They are:
• stage 1: 140 to 159 mm Hg systolic and 90 to 99 mm Hg diastolic
• stage 2: 160 to 179 mm Hg systolic and 100 to 109 mm Hg diastolic
• stage 3: 180 to 209 mm Hg systolic and 110 to 119 mm Hg diastolic
• stage 4: more than 210 mm Hg systolic and more than 120 mm Hg diastolic.

Diuretics and beta blockers represent the drugs of choice for initial therapy. Alternative drugs, reserved for patients for whom diuretics and beta blockers are contraindicated, include angiotensin-converting enzyme inhibitors, alpha blockers, alpha-beta blockers, and calcium channel blockers.

---

the imbalance between oxygen demand and supply may cause myocardial ischemia, leading to myocardial infarction (MI), pulmonary edema, or both.

Complications

These depend on whether the patient has accelerated hypertension or hypertensive encephalopathy. For a patient with accelerated hypertension who receives treatment and avoids renal damage, the prospects for long-term survival are good. Without treatment, however, death can occur within months from cerebrovascular accident, MI, or renal failure.

If the patient has hypertensive encephalopathy and doesn't receive treatment, cerebral damage may lead to death. However, with prompt treatment, hypertensive encephalopathy can be halted and perhaps even reversed.

PATHOPHYSIOLOGY

How hypertension damages blood vessels

Vascular injury from hypertension begins with alternating areas of dilation and constriction in the arterioles.

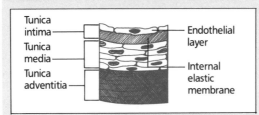

Tunica intima — Endothelial layer
Tunica media
Tunica adventitia — Internal elastic membrane

Chronic hypertension injures the endothelial layer of the arterial wall, which promotes platelet adhesion and aggregation in the injured area.

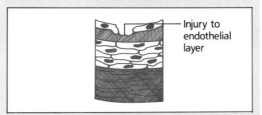

Injury to endothelial layer

Independently, angiotensin induces endothelial wall contraction, allowing plasma to leak through interendothelial spaces.

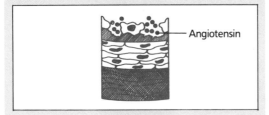

Angiotensin

Eventually, plasma constituents deposited in the vessel wall cause medial necrosis, as shown here.

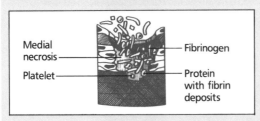

Medial necrosis — Fibrinogen
Platelet — Protein with fibrin deposits

Assessment
History
Some patients in hypertensive crisis are asymptomatic and discover their condition during a routine blood pressure check. However, hypertensive crisis may cause obvious symptoms— severe headache, nausea, dizziness, shortness of breath, anginal pain, and visual disturbances. (See *Detecting hypertensive crisis.*)

Ask the patient if he's ever been told he has high blood pressure. Find out if he's ever taken antihypertensive drugs. Commonly, the patient will report that he used to have hypertension but stopped taking his medication when his blood pressure dropped.

If the patient has a history of hypertension, find out how closely he complied with therapy, whether therapy was effective, and whether he had any associated complications. If he has no history of hypertension, try to uncover possible causes of hypertensive crisis. For instance, ask if he's had similar symptoms before. If so, did he consult a doctor? What was his medical diagnosis and treatment, if any? Has he had any major acute or chronic illnesses requiring hospitalization? If so, what was the course of the illness? How was it treated? Did he have any complications?

Find out which drugs the patient is taking; certain drugs, such as cough medicines and analgesics, may raise blood pressure or make antihypertensive therapy less effective. Does he use alcohol, tobacco, or caffeine? Does he take any prescription, over-the-counter, or recreational drugs? Document drug use carefully.

Ask the female patient about her pregnancy history, and find out if she has begun menopause. Does she use oral contraceptives or estrogen? Has she ever had pregnancy-induced hypertension?

With any patient, inquire about cardiovascular and other risk factors for hypertension, such as a history of heart or blood vessel disease, diabetes mellitus, hyperlipidemia, congenital heart defects, rheumatic fever, or syncope. Ask the patient if he has a history of renal disease or obesity. Note whether he's overweight.

Physical examination

Measuring blood pressure by sphygmomanometer is an essential step in assessing hypertensive crisis. The changes associated with hypertensive crisis typically occur when diastolic pressure reaches at least 120 mm Hg.

Next, assess for damage to target organs by evaluating the patient for retinal changes and examining the cardiovascular, neurologic, and renal systems.

Funduscopic examination. Check for arteriolar narrowing, arteriovenous compression, hemorrhages, exudates, and papilledema — possible signs of hypertensive crisis. Grade hypertensive retinopathy from I to IV, representing the mildest form to the most severe:
• grade I — arterial narrowing or spasm
• grade II — arteriovenous nicking
• grade III — hemorrhages and exudates, indicating accelerated hypertension
• grade IV — papilledema, indicating malignant hypertension.

Cardiovascular examination. Note tachycardia, precordial heave, murmur of aortic insufficiency, a third heart sound (S_3, usually accompanying congestive heart failure), a fourth heart sound (S_4, signifying a rigid left ventricle), and arrhythmias. Also note dependent edema, lateral displacement of the point of maximal impulse (indicating cardiomegaly, which can trigger or result from hypertensive crisis), a bruit auscultated over the flanks or anteriorly over the renal vasculature, and weak peripheral pulses.

Neurologic examination. Assess the patient for an altered level of consciousness (LOC), as indicated by confusion, somnolence, or stupor. Check for visual and focal deficits, nystagmus, localized muscle weakness, and seizures.

Renal examination. Assess the patient for oliguria and azotemia.

Diagnostic tests

The doctor will order diagnostic tests to identify the cause of hypertension and evaluate the effects of hypertensive crisis on target organs.

Detecting hypertensive crisis

A patient with hypertensive crisis may exhibit any of these classic signs and symptoms.

Headache
The patient typically complains of severe suboccipital or occipital headache, which may subside when he moves from a supine to an upright position (from the decrease in cerebrospinal fluid pressure).

Other neurologic effects
Dizziness, syncope, numbness, weakness, and blurred vision may result from vasoconstriction and arterial damage.

Cardiovascular effects
The patient may complain of anginal pain and palpitations. These symptoms stem from an imbalance in oxygen supply and demand, caused by increased afterload.

Renal effects
Expect peripheral edema from increased sodium and water retention. Fatigue, weakness, nocturia, and excessive urine sediment also may signal renal involvement.

Epistaxis
This safety mechanism relieves severe hypertension and may help prevent cerebral edema and hemorrhage.

Blood tests should be performed before urine and renal testing.

Complete blood count. Typically, this shows polycythemia.

Hematocrit. Decreased hematocrit may signal renal failure.

Serum potassium. This level will decrease if primary aldosteronism causes the hypertension.

Blood urea nitrogen (BUN) and creatinine clearance test. These tests help detect renal causes of hypertension.

Serum glucose. This level will be elevated if hypertension results from diabetes mellitus, Cushing's syndrome, or pheochromocytoma.

Serum uric acid. This test may reveal hyperuricemia associated with hypertension.

Urinary vanillylmandelic acid. This level may be elevated in pheochromocytoma.

Urinalysis. This test may reveal proteinuria and hematuria if renal dysfunction causes the hypertension.

Renal arteriography. This study may identify renal artery stenosis as the cause of hypertension.

Excretory urography. This test may indicate renal disease (although it can't pinpoint the underlying cause).

Chest X-ray. This identifies cardiomegaly.

Electrocardiography (ECG). This test may indicate left ventricular hypertrophy or ischemia from hypertension.

Ongoing treatment

After emergency treatment, interventions aim to limit target organ damage by reducing systolic pressure below 160 mm Hg and diastolic pressure below 95 mm Hg. Once the patient's blood pressure is stabilized, he'll require long-term oral drug therapy tailored to his needs and responses. (See *Guide to common antihypertensive drugs.*)

Drug treatment

Antihypertensive drug therapy commonly involves a *stepped-care approach.* For example, in *step 1,* the doctor prescribes less than a full dose of a thiazide-like diuretic or a beta blocker, such as atenolol, metoprolol, or propranolol. Then he proceeds to a full dose, if necessary and desirable. If this regimen doesn't achieve blood pressure control, he moves to the next step.

In *step 2,* the doctor may add a small dose of an adrenergic-inhibiting agent—for example, clonidine, guanabenz, methyldopa, reserpine, or a beta blocker. Or he adds a small dose of a thiazide-like diuretic. He may make additional substitutions at this point, such as adding an angiotensin-converting enzyme (ACE) inhibitor or a calcium channel blocker. If these measures don't control blood pressure, therapy proceeds to the next step.

In *step 3,* the doctor may add a vasodilator (such as hydralazine or minoxidil) or a calcium channel blocker, or may increase all dosages to the maximum. If the patient responds poorly, the doctor moves to *step 4,* adding a second or third agent, or a diuretic.

Once drug therapy begins, assess the patient for both desired and adverse effects. Ask him if he's experiencing any adverse effects. Urge him to comply with therapy to maintain blood pressure control. If he has modifiable cardiovascular risk factors, such as hyperlipidemia or smoking, encourage him to minimize these. Suggest nonpharmacologic ways to enhance the effectiveness of antihypertensive drugs, such as exercise, stress management techniques, and weight loss.

Surgery

Essential hypertension doesn't warrant surgery. However, surgery may be used when hypertension occurs secondary to a confirmed disorder and isn't adequately controlled by medical measures. (See *Causes of secondary hypertension,* pages 9 and 10.)

Surgery may be needed for impending renal failure with bilateral renovascular disease, marked renal artery stenosis, pheochromocytoma, and poor tolerance for antihypertensive drugs. Patients with renal artery stenosis who are poor surgical risks may benefit from percutaneous transluminal dilatation using an inflatable, balloon-tipped catheter.

Ongoing nursing interventions

Direct your efforts toward ensuring compliance with therapy—a challenge for many hypertensive patients.

Guide to common antihypertensive drugs

DRUG	DESCRIPTION AND ACTION	COMMON ADVERSE EFFECTS
Adrenergic blockers		
Atenolol (Tenormin)	Beta$_1$-selective blocker without membrane-stabilizing or intrinsic sympathomimetic activities; lacks selectivity in high doses	Bradycardia, dizziness, postural hypotension, cold extremities, fatigue
Clonidine (Catapres)	Centrally acting alpha-adrenergic blocker that decreases sympathetic cardioaccelerator and vasoconstrictor outflow from the central nervous system	Dry mouth, sedation, drowsiness, headaches, rebound hypertension
Guanabenz (Wytensin)	See *clonidine*.	Dry mouth, sedation, drowsiness, fatigue, impotence, dizziness
Methyldopa (Aldomet)	Central action uncertain; an alpha-adrenergic blocker with net effect of reduced peripheral resistance	Lassitude, drowsiness, dry mouth, mild orthostatic hypotension, positive Coombs' test (with high doses), positive rheumatoid and lupus erythematosus factors, impotence
Metoprolol (Lopressor)	Beta$_1$-selective blocker, specifically of receptors in cardiac muscle; also inhibits beta$_2$-adrenergic receptors in bronchial and vascular muscle in higher doses	Fatigue, dizziness, depression, bradycardia
Nadolol (Corgard)	Nonselective beta-adrenergic blocker for available beta-receptor sites; has little direct myocardial depressant activity	Bradycardia, dizziness, fatigue, bronchospasm
Penbutolol (Levatol)	Nonselective beta-adrenergic blocker; action may stem from peripheral antiadrenergic effects that lead to decreased cardiac output	Bradycardia, dizziness, pulmonary edema
Prazosin (Minipress)	Alpha-adrenergic blocker with net effect of reduced peripheral resistance	Syncope with first dose, postural hypotension, palpitations, dizziness, lack of energy, weakness
Propranolol (Inderal)	Nonselective beta-adrenergic blocker that competes with beta-adrenergic stimulators for available receptor sites	Fatigue, dizziness, vivid dreams, depression, impotence; masks symptoms of hypoglycemia
Terazosin (Hytrin)	See *prazosin*.	Dizziness, orthostatic hypotension, blurred vision, nausea, peripheral edema, weight gain, impotence
Timolol (Blocadren)	Nonselective beta-adrenergic blocker that lacks significant intrinsic sympathomimetic and direct myocardial depressant activity	Fatigue, headaches, bradycardia, dizziness, pruritus, dyspnea
Angiotensin-converting enzyme (ACE) inhibitors		
Captopril (Capoten)	Prevents conversion of angiotensin I to angiotensin II, which interrupts the renin-angiotensin-aldosterone system	Cutaneous rash, taste impairment, proteinuria, leukopenia
Enalapril (Vasotec)	See *captopril*.	Headaches, dizziness, fatigue, agranulocytosis, hypotension, angioedema
Lisinopril (Prinivil, Zestril)	See *captopril*.	Headaches, dizziness, fatigue, depression, hypotension
Calcium channel blockers		
Nicardipine (Cardene)	Inhibits transmembrane flux of calcium into cardiac and smooth-muscle cells; acts specifically on vascular muscle	Constipation, dizziness, nervousness, tachycardia

(continued)

Guide to common antihypertensive drugs (continued)

DRUG	DESCRIPTION AND ACTION	COMMON ADVERSE EFFECTS
Calcium channel blockers (continued)		
Verapamil (Calan SR, Isoptin SR)	Sustained-release calcium channel blocker; reduces total peripheral resistance, causing vasodilation and subsequent blood pressure reduction	Constipation, dizziness, hypotension
Diuretics		
Bumetanide (Bumex)	Primarily inhibits reabsorption of sodium chloride and water in the ascending loop of Henle; also exerts a weak diuretic effect in the proximal tubules	Hyperglycemia, hyperuricemia, hypochloremia, hyponatremia, hypokalemia, fluid and electrolyte imbalance
Chlorothiazide (Diuril)	Increases renal excretion of sodium chloride and water, mainly by inhibiting sodium reabsorption in the early distal tubules; initial antihypertensive effect caused by volume reduction and lowered cardiac output	Hyponatremia, hypokalemia, hyperuricemia, hypercalcemia, hyperglycemia
Chlorthalidone (Hygroton, Thalitone)	See chlorothiazide.	Hyperglycemia, hyperuricemia, hypercalcemia, hyponatremia, hypokalemia
Furosemide (Lasix)	Primarily inhibits reabsorption of sodium chloride and water in the ascending loop of Henle; also exerts a weak diuretic effect in the proximal and distal tubules	Hyperglycemia, hyperuricemia, hypochloremia, hyponatremia, hypokalemia, fluid and electrolyte imbalance, mild diarrhea, deafness (in large doses)
Hydrochlorothiazide (Esidrix, HydroDIURIL, Oretic)	See chlorothiazide.	Hyperglycemia, hyperuricemia, hypercalcemia, hyponatremia, hypokalemia
Metolazone (Diulo, Zaroxolyn)	Primarily inhibits sodium reabsorption at the cortical diluting site and in the proximal convoluted tubules	Hyperglycemia, hyperuricemia, hypercalcemia, hyponatremia, hypokalemia, azotemia
Spironolactone (Aldactone)	Antagonizes aldosterone in the distal tubules, increasing excretion of sodium and water but sparing potassium	Gynecomastia, menstrual irregularity, amenorrhea, postmenopausal bleeding, hyperkalemia
Triamterene (Dyrenium)	Has a diuretic effect on the distal renal tubules to inhibit the reabsorption of sodium in exchange for potassium	Blood dyscrasia, photosensitivity, rash, hyperkalemia
Vasodilators		
Hydralazine (Apresoline)	Peripheral vasodilator that directly relaxes vascular smooth muscle	Postural hypotension, headaches, tachycardia, nausea, vomiting, palpitations, fatigue, lupuslike syndrome (incidence less than 1%; occurs with high doses and prolonged therapy)
Minoxidil (Loniten)	Extremely potent peripheral vasodilator given to patients resistant to traditional antihypertensive therapy	Hypertrichosis, fluid retention, weight gain, precipitation of angina, cardiac tamponade, electrocardiogram changes, tachycardia

• Teach the patient about his disorder. Inform him that his blood pressure exceeds normal limits. Emphasize that he needs long-term treatment and follow-up care, even if his symptoms disappear. Warn him that although treatment can control hypertension, it won't cure it. Stress that he can help ensure an excellent prognosis by following the prescribed treatment regimen.

• Encourage the patient to participate in his care. Urge him to obtain a blood pressure kit,

Causes of secondary hypertension

This chart presents some common causes of secondary hypertension. Other conditions that can lead to hypertension include pregnancy, increased intracranial pressure, advanced collagen disease, and use of such drugs as oral contraceptives, estrogens, corticosteroids, sympathetic stimulators, monoamine oxidase inhibitors, appetite suppressants, and antihistamines. *Note:* Once the cause is treated, secondary hypertension usually disappears.

CAUSE	SIGNS AND SYMPTOMS	DIAGNOSTIC TESTS	TREATMENT
Renovascular hypertension (RVH) The leading cause of secondary hypertension, RVH affects children and adolescents more frequently than adults. It usually results from renal artery stenosis caused by atherosclerosis or arterial wall fibromuscular dysplasia. Renal ischemia results, causing reduced kidney perfusion, which triggers the renin-angiotensin-aldosterone system.	Few signs or symptoms. Suspect RVH in a patient with hypertension before age 25 (especially with diastolic pressure greater than or equal to 110 mm Hg); sudden onset of labile or uncontrollable hypertension; hypertension onset before age 45 in a woman not taking oral contraceptives; hypertension onset soon after age 50; rapid acceleration of previously well-controlled hypertension; hypertensive retinopathy; or a systolic or diastolic bruit in the upper abdomen or flank.	• Rapid-sequence excretory urography • Plasma renin activity (PRA) test • Renal vein renin concentration • Renal angiography • Renal scan • Pharmacologic angiotensin blockade test	• Dietary sodium and calorie restriction • Diuretics • Antihypertensive medications • Renal artery revascularization • Renal artery bypass graft • Percutaneous transluminal renal angioplasty • Nephrectomy (occasionally)
Coarctation of the aorta This aortic narrowing, most common at the lower end of the aortic arch, usually has a congenital cause.	Lower blood pressure in the legs than in the arms, pulsating intercostal arteries (from enlargement of arteries carrying collateral blood flow around the coarctation), and diminished or absent femoral pulses	• Chest X-ray • Aortography	• Surgical repair
Pheochromocytoma This disorder stems from a chromaffin tumor, usually in the adrenal medulla but occasionally elsewhere. The tumor produces and secretes excessive epinephrine and norepinephrine, which leads to hypertension and other effects. When the tumor secretes continuously, blood pressure remains persistently high.	With intermittent secretion of epinephrine and norepinephrine, signs and symptoms include sudden hypertensive episodes, severe headache with palpitations, accelerated metabolism, excessive sweating, heat intolerance, and anxiety	• Vanillylmandelic acid test • Urine catecholamine test • Computed tomography (CT) scan	• Tumor removal
Hyperaldosteronism This condition may result from primary aldosteronism (Conn's syndrome) caused by adrenal tumor or hyperplasia; from secondary aldosteronism stemming from conditions that stimulate aldosterone production; or from pseudoaldosteronism resulting from excessive licorice intake. Excessive aldosterone secretion by the adrenal cortex leads to excessive sodium reabsorption, which increases intravascular fluid volume and thus blood pressure.	High normal blood pressure, muscle weakness, polyuria, nocturia, polydipsia, tetany, paresthesia, and headache	• Serum aldosterone test • Urine aldosterone test • PRA test • CT scan	• Tumor removal • Spironolactone therapy • Treatment of the underlying cause

(continued)

Causes of secondary hypertension (continued)

CAUSE	SIGNS AND SYMPTOMS	DIAGNOSTIC TESTS	TREATMENT
Cushing's syndrome This condition results from an adrenal cortex tumor or hyperplasia causing excessive glucocorticoid secretion.	Central or girdle obesity, buffalo hump, purplish abdominal striae, hirsutism, moon face, edema, and high normal blood pressure	• Plasma cortisol test • Urine 17-hydroxycorticosteroid test • PRA test • Dexamethasone suppression test	• Tumor removal
Renal parenchymal disease This condition usually stems from an immune system response to infection, such as chronic glomerulonephritis or pyelonephritis. Inflammatory changes take place in the renal glomeruli and interstitia; consequently, the kidneys can't excrete sodium, which stimulates the renin-angiotensin-aldosterone system.	Edema, oliguria, orthopnea, dyspnea, and hypertension	• Excretory urography • Renal angiography	• Specific to the cause

and teach him how to use it to check his blood pressure periodically.
• Encourage the patient to keep a record of his home blood pressure readings and to bring the records to all doctor appointments.
• If necessary and appropriate, arrange for a home health nurse to make periodic follow-up visits to monitor the patient's blood pressure and evaluate his blood pressure measurement technique.
• Evaluate orthostatic effects on blood pressure by taking two or more blood pressure readings—one with the patient supine, the second with him in an upright position (such as high Fowler's). Compare blood pressure on the left and right sides by taking measurements in both arms.

Myocardial infarction

MI occurs when a portion of the myocardium is deprived of oxygenated coronary blood flow, resulting in cellular ischemia, tissue injury, necrosis (cell death), and loss of tissue function. Depending on the degree of imbalance between oxygen supply and demand, tissue changes may progress quickly from ischemia to acute injury. Interventions must begin at once to minimize cardiac damage and avert death. (See *Responding to MI.*)

Most infarctions are *transmural,* with tissue changes affecting the full myocardial thickness from epicardium to endocardium. *Subendocardial* infarctions involve the endocardium and some portion of the myocardium. (A newer method of classifying MIs distinguishes those that cause Q-wave changes on an ECG from those that don't.)

Causes

MI results from significant occlusion of the coronary arteries, which disrupts the balance of oxygen supply and demand. The occlusion typically results from a combination of factors, such as coronary artery disease (CAD), thrombosis, and coronary artery spasm.

In *CAD,* the intimal layer of the coronary artery wall becomes narrowed or obstructed, for example, from fatty deposits, fibrosis, calcification, or hemorrhage. Eventually, a fibrous plaque forms, impeding blood flow through the artery and limiting myocardial perfusion. A 75% occlusion, determined by angiography, is a probable cause of MI.

Thrombosis may result from rupture of an atherosclerotic plaque, hemorrhage into the

EMERGENCY INTERVENTIONS

Responding to MI

If your patient has suffered a myocardial infarction (MI), you must intervene promptly to minimize cardiac damage and avert death. Focus your emergency interventions on relieving pain, reducing myocardial oxygen consumption, and maintaining cardiac output. Medical therapy aims to optimize cardiac output by manipulating preload and afterload.

Specific measures depend on the patient's signs and symptoms and any complications he has developed. However, all patients with acute MI need bed rest to reduce oxygen demand, supplemental oxygen, and I.V. line insertion to provide access for emergency medications. Until the appropriate drugs are administered, infuse dextrose 5% in water at a keep-vein-open rate.

Manage pain
Pain management is the first priority. Pain stimulates sympathetic nervous system (SNS) activity, leading to an even greater oxygen demand. Morphine, the preferred analgesic, depresses central nervous system activity, in turn reducing both anxiety and the heart's metabolic demands. The drug also dilates veins to decrease preload. Expect to administer morphine I.V. at prescribed intervals until chest pain subsides. If morphine is ineffective, the doctor will increase the dosage or order an alternative drug.

As ordered, give I.V. nitroglycerin to dilate coronary arteries and reduce preload. Titrate the dosage to achieve effective pain control. Because nitroglycerin dilates vessels, it may lead to hypotension, so be sure to monitor the patient's blood pressure carefully.

Caution: Don't administer nitroglycerin and morphine to a patient with a right ventricular MI because these drugs may depress an already low pulmonary artery wedge pressure (PAWP), causing a further drop in cardiac output. If PAWP is low, expect to administer fluids, such as isotonic 0.9% sodium chloride solution, to boost diastolic filling in an attempt to improve cardiac output.

Reduce oxygen consumption
To reduce oxygen consumption and help manage pain, administer other prescribed drugs, such as nitrates, calcium channel blockers, beta-adrenergic blockers, or angiotensin-converting enzyme (ACE) inhibitors.

Calcium channel blockers, including nifedipine, diltiazem, and verapamil, block calcium influx into the cells, dilating coronary arteries and decreasing contractility. If your patient is receiving a calcium channel blocker, stay alert for signs of congestive heart failure from reduced contractility.

Beta-adrenergic blockers, such as propranolol and timolol, block SNS stimulation, causing reductions in heart rate, contractility, and oxygen demand. Some beta blockers are $beta_1$-selective, acting primarily on the heart, whereas others are nonselective, acting on both the heart and peripheral blood vessels.

ACE inhibitors, such as captopril and enalapril, inhibit the enzyme that converts angiotensin I to angiotensin II, a potent vasoconstrictor. Thus, these drugs cause arterial dilation, which decreases afterload and oxygen demand.

Prepare for thrombolytic therapy
If appropriate, prepare the patient for thrombolytic therapy as ordered. Candidates for thrombolytic therapy include patients with acute ST-segment elevation and chest pain that has lasted no more than 6 hours. Timely use of thrombolytic agents can restore myocardial perfusion and prevent further damage from MI by dissolving thrombi or digesting the fibrin network. When effective, these drugs relieve chest pain, restore the ST segment to baseline, and induce reperfusion arrhythmias within 30 to 45 minutes.

Contraindications for thrombolytic therapy include surgery within the past 2 months, active bleeding, a history of cerebrovascular accident, intracranial neoplasm, arteriovenous malformation, aneurysm, or uncontrolled hypertension.

plaque, or intimal erosion over the fibrous plaque cap. Such conditions establish a perfect medium for platelet aggregation, which leads to mechanical obstruction of the artery.

Coronary artery spasm also leads to mechanical obstruction of coronary arteries. The cause of the spasm is unknown.

Less common causes of MI include:
• arteritis, for example, from luetic (syphilitic) or granulomatous lesions, polyarteritis nodosa, lupus erythematosus, rheumatoid arthritis, and ankylosing spondylitis
• coronary artery trauma, for example, from laceration or iatrogenic injury
• hematologic abnormalities, including polycythemia vera, thrombocytosis, disseminated intravascular coagulation, and thrombocytopenic purpura
• disproportional myocardial demand, as occurs in aortic valvular disease, thyrotoxicosis, prolonged hypotension, carbon monoxide poisoning, use of amphetamines or cocaine, or pulmonary hypertension.

Predisposing factors. The risk for CAD—and thus MI—increases with age; a history of hypertension or diabetes mellitus; elevated levels of serum triglycerides, low-density lipoproteins, or cholesterol; decreased levels of serum high-density lipoproteins; excessive saturated fat intake; obesity; a family history of CAD; a sedentary life-style; smoking; stress; and, possibly, type A personality (suggested by an aggressive, competitive attitude).

Pathophysiology
With too little oxygen for the heart's needs, myocardial metabolism shifts from aerobic to anaerobic. This leads to production of lactic acid, which stimulates pain receptors. Anaerobic metabolism must last at least 25 minutes before necrosis occurs. Necrosis is responsible for many of the life-threatening events associated with MI, such as inadequate cardiac output, depressed contractility, and arrhythmias.

Because the coronary arteries lie on the epicardial surface and perfuse inward, the endocardium is at greatest risk when oxygen supply diminishes. The extent of injury, which starts in the subendocardium and extends toward the epicardium, depends on such factors as the duration of ischemia, how quickly the occlusion developed, which coronary artery is involved, how much myocardial tissue the involved artery supplies, the extent of collateral blood flow, and the presence of concurrent spasm.

Most MIs involve the left ventricle because this heart chamber is under the greatest pressure, does most of the heart's work, and uses most of its oxygen. Only 10% of MIs involve the right ventricle.

The specific infarction site depends on the location of the coronary artery occlusion. In the left ventricle, common infarction sites include the anterior wall, inferior wall, septum, lateral wall, apex, and posterior wall. (See *Coronary arteries and MI sites.*)

Although infarction can occur solely in the right ventricle, a right ventricular MI is usually associated with an inferior or posterior left ventricular MI because the right coronary artery and its posterior descending branch perfuse these areas. (Up to 45% of inferior-wall MIs have some right ventricular involvement.) Doctors now evaluate the right ventricle more closely in patients with MI because of the high incidence of pulmonary disease in MI patients, which raises right ventricular afterload, increasing oxygen demand and jeopardizing right ventricular cells. Right ventricular MI can significantly depress cardiac output, resulting in heart failure or cardiogenic shock. (See *Adapting your care to the infarction site,* page 14.)

Complications
The most serious complications of MI result from the severe drop in cardiac output, which impairs peripheral perfusion of the capillary bed. Life-threatening complications include arrhythmias, heart failure, cardiogenic shock, rupture of the papillary muscle or ventricular septum, ventricular aneurysm, embolism, and infarction extension. Pericarditis, another potential complication, is less serious. (See *Recognizing hazards of MI,* page 15.)

Coronary arteries and MI sites

The primary area of myocardial infarction (MI) and the resulting structural damage depend on which major coronary arteries are occluded and how well the collateral circulation perfuses the affected area.

Coronary artery disease stimulates development of collateral circulation, possibly through release of vasodilators. Collateral circulation is especially well developed in patients with a 75% or greater reduction in the lumen of the coronary artery. During recovery from acute MI, nearly 40% of patients develop collateral circulation.

Collateral circulation seems to reduce myocardial necrosis in patients with coronary artery occlusion. In those with extensive collateral vessel development, collateral vessels can perfuse the area even if the artery is totally occluded—as long as no stress is placed on the heart.

The chart below correlates the major regions and structures supplied by coronary arteries with the areas of infarction associated with obstruction of these arteries.

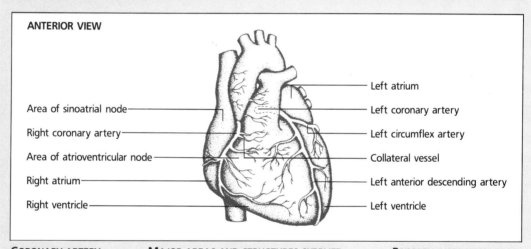

ANTERIOR VIEW

Area of sinoatrial node — Left atrium

Right coronary artery — Left coronary artery

Area of atrioventricular node — Left circumflex artery

Right atrium — Collateral vessel

Right ventricle — Left anterior descending artery

Left ventricle

CORONARY ARTERY	MAJOR AREAS AND STRUCTURES SUPPLIED	PRIMARY INFARCTION AREA
Right	• Sinoatrial (SA) node • Atrioventricular (AV) node • Bundle of His • Right atrium and right ventricle • Inferior and diaphragmatic surface of left ventricle • Posterior third of septum • Posteroinferior division of left bundle branch	• Inferior wall • Inferoposterior wall • Right ventricle
Left	• Massive left ventricular area	• Left ventricle
Left anterior descending	• Anterior wall of left ventricle • Anterior two-thirds of septum • Bundle of His • Right bundle branch • Anterosuperior division of left bundle branch • Posteroinferior division of left bundle branch	• Anterior wall • Septum • Anterolateral wall • Inferioapical wall • Apex
Left circumflex	• SA node • AV node • Inferior and diaphragmatic surface of left ventricle • Lateral wall of left ventricle • Left atrium • Posteroinferior division of left bundle branch	• Lateral wall • Inferolateral wall • Posterior wall • Inferoposterior wall

Adapting your care to the infarction site

When you suspect your patient has had a myocardial infarction (MI), one of your first priorities is to relieve his chest pain. How you do this depends partly on the site of the MI. Although morphine and nitroglycerin are indicated for the patient with left ventricular MI, these drugs may cause further harm if MI involves the right ventricle.

Consider the case of Samuel Garrison, age 52, who is brought to the hospital after suffering chest pain while at home.

Assessing the problem

You quickly examine Mr. Garrison and see that his jugular vein is distended. His blood pressure measures 95/56 mm Hg and his cardiac rhythm is a normal sinus rhythm of 90 beats/minute. His respiratory rate is 18 breaths/minute and his breath sounds are clear.

One hour later, Mr. Garrison complains that his chest pain has returned. The pain persists even after you give him two sublingual nitroglycerin tablets. You immediately notify the doctor, obtain an electrocardiogram (ECG), and take his vital signs again. His vital signs reveal a disturbing trend. Systolic blood pressure has dropped to 76 mm Hg, the heart rate has increased to 100 beats/minute, and the respiratory rate has increased to 24 breaths/minute. The 12-lead ECG shows changes consistent with inferior-wall MI—elevated ST segments in leads II, III, and aV$_F$ of the left ventricle.

When Mr. Garrison inhales, you notice that his jugular vein distends even more—typical of right

ventricular MI. When you check for pulsus paradoxus, you find a systolic blood pressure of only 60 mm Hg during inspiration. To investigate further, you record a right-sided ECG, which reveals more evidence of a right ventricular MI: ST-segment elevation in the right-sided leads V$_4$ and V$_5$.

Changing your care goals

Now that you've identified right ventricular MI, you change your care goals to reflect the doctor's new treatment goals: improving right ventricular stroke volume and restoring left ventricular filling pressures.

As ordered, you administer I.V. fluids to help Mr. Garrison achieve optimal preload. However, you do this cautiously, monitoring his pulmonary artery pressures to gauge the effects of fluid on his hemodynamic status. To maintain his cardiac output, you administer dopamine, a positive inotropic agent. And you avoid interventions that reduce preload, such as placing Mr. Garrison in high Fowler's position or administering diuretics, nitroglycerin, or morphine.

Ensuring the patient's well-being

You continue to monitor the patient, assessing his ECG readings, vital signs, and hemodynamic pressures. Because GI disturbances and liver enlargement often complicate a right ventricular MI, you check Mr. Garrison regularly to detect these problems early and avert serious consequences.

Assessment

History

The patient's history supplies the most definitive data for diagnosing MI; typically, diagnostic studies are used only to support history findings. So focus your history taking on gathering clues that help identify MI. Find out if the patient has a history of cardiac or respiratory disease, cardiac surgery, chest trauma, or intestinal disease. Also determine if he has a family history of cardiac disease, drinks alcohol

excessively, uses any illicit drugs, and which medications he is taking.

Approximately 80% of patients with acute MI complain of chest discomfort—probably from stimulation of nerve endings in the ischemic or injured myocardium. However, MI is just one of over 100 possible causes of chest discomfort. To rule out pulmonary, GI, musculoskeletal, and other causes of chest pain, you'll need to evaluate the patient's complaint carefully. (See *Evaluating chest pain,* page 16.)

COMPLICATIONS

Recognizing hazards of MI

Myocardial infarction (MI) can cause a wide range of severe and life-threatening complications.

Arrhythmias
After an MI, arrhythmias can arise from ischemia or from damage to the sinoatrial node (the heart's intrinsic pacemaker) or the heart's conduction system. Monitor the patient's electrocardiogram (ECG) for abnormal heart rhythms, including premature ventricular contractions, ventricular tachycardia, ventricular fibrillation, heart block, bradycardia, and tachycardia.

Heart failure
Right ventricular, left ventricular, or biventricular heart failure may arise from depressed myocardial contractility. You can identify this complication from reduced cardiac output and changes in pulmonary artery pressures, such as increased pulmonary artery systolic and diastolic pressures and elevated pulmonary artery wedge pressure (PAWP). The chest X-ray may also help assess heart failure.

Cardiogenic shock
An extreme form of heart failure, cardiogenic shock occurs when perfusion is so poor that the heart's metabolic demands can't be met and myocardial contractility is depressed. Suspect this complication if your patient has deteriorating hemodynamic pressures, hypotension, reduced urine output, an S_3 heart sound, and sluggish capillary refill.

Mitral insufficiency
If the MI involves the papillary muscles, which hold the mitral valve in place, these muscles may become dysfunctional or rupture, leading to heart failure or cardiogenic shock. Mitral insufficiency secondary to acute MI is a surgical emergency necessitating valve replacement.

Suspect this complication if you auscultate a holosystolic murmur, if the patient has pronounced dyspnea, and if his pulmonary artery pressure and PAWP increase (with large v waves appearing on the pressure waveform). Echocardiography typically shows valve dysfunction.

Septal rupture
If the septum sustains damage from an MI, it weakens and may rupture, causing acute heart failure and possibly cardiogenic shock. Surgical correction is required to maintain cardiac output. To detect this complication, auscultate for a loud murmur. Increasing pulmonary artery pressure and PAWP and elevated oxygen saturation of the right ventricle confirm the diagnosis.

Ventricular aneurysm
When infarcted or necrotic tissue weakens, an outpouching of muscle mass forms. This mass contracts paradoxically, limiting cardiac output. Suspect this complication if a 12-lead ECG shows persistent ST-segment elevation.

Embolism
Rupture of atherosclerotic plaque, intimal erosion, and platelet erosion contribute to the risk of embolism after MI. Cerebral and pulmonary emboli carry the greatest threat of death. Embolism can be identified by ventilation-perfusion scan mismatch and angiography.

Ventricular rupture
Spontaneous rupture of the weakened heart muscle leads to cardiac arrest. This complication usually is identified during an autopsy.

Suspect acute MI as the cause of your patient's chest discomfort if he reports any of the following symptoms:
• dull, aching, gnawing, crushing, squeezing, or pressurelike pain (possible feelings of tightness, pressure, or a clenched-fist effect)
• pain in the midsternal area or pain that radiates to the left arm or left jaw (sometimes, however, pain felt more diffusely across the entire chest)
• pain brought on by exertion
• pain that starts gradually, builds in intensity, and is constant rather than episodic
• associated signs and symptoms, including

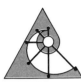

Evaluating chest pain

If your patient complains of chest pain, you can use the following approach to help pinpoint the cause of the symptom, determine how serious it is, and gauge how aggressively to intervene.

Quality
Have the patient describe the pain. What does it feel like? Has he had it before? If so, what did he do for it?

Region
Have the patient point to the area where he feels the pain. Is it localized, diffuse, or does it radiate?

Severity
Have the patient rate his pain on a scale of 1 to 10, with 10 representing intolerable pain. Does it prevent the patient from resting?

Setting
Ask the patient when the pain typically starts. Does it occur with rest? With exertion? After meals?

Time
Ask if the chest pain comes on suddenly or gradually. How long does it typically last? Is it constant or episodic?

Aggravators
Ask the patient what worsens his pain—for example, meals, certain foods, exertion, palpation, certain positions, or deep breathing.

Alleviators
Find out if certain actions help relieve the chest pain. Does it subside when the patient rests, changes position, or takes nitrates or antacids? Does he use any home remedies?

Associated signs or symptoms
Does the patient have any other signs or symptoms when he feels chest pain? Any shortness of breath? Nausea? Cough or hemoptysis? Fever?

shortness of breath, nausea, vomiting, and diaphoresis.

Ask the patient to rate the pain on a scale of 1 to 10, with 10 denoting excruciating pain. However, severe chest pain doesn't necessarily indicate an MI. In fact, anginal pain may be more severe than pain from an acute MI. Nonetheless, the patient's description of pain severity does help guide interventions.

Also keep in mind that roughly 20% of patients with acute MI don't experience any discomfort. Most of these patients are diabetic or elderly and have neuropathies that limit the sensation of discomfort.

Physical examination
Physical findings in a patient with MI vary widely, depending on the location and size of the infarction and, more important, how well the patient is compensating and maintaining cardiac output. Because most clinical indicators reflect decreased cardiac output, focus your examination on assessing the adequacy of cardiac output.

Palpation. Determine how palpation affects the patient's discomfort. Firmly touch the area where the patient locates his discomfort. If palpation improves or worsens the discomfort, you can rule out MI and other cardiac causes.

Positional changes. Have the patient turn onto his right side, then his left side. Then instruct him to sit up. If any of these positional changes alters his discomfort, suspect a noncardiac origin.

Respiration. Have the patient take a deep breath. If this alters his discomfort, you can probably assume he doesn't have MI. (However, if he has pericarditis as a complication of MI, a deep breath will exacerbate the discomfort.)

General appearance. Evaluate your patient's general appearance and demeanor. If he seems acutely ill, anxious, and apprehensive, suspect an MI.

Vital signs. Although vital signs may be within normal limits even in acute MI, repeat measurements may detect suspicious trends. For instance, catecholamines, substances released from the sympathetic nervous system (SNS), may trigger discomfort and anxiety and will elevate all vital signs. Cardiac output is also maintained: The heart rate and blood pressure increase in an attempt to boost perfusion, and the respiratory rate rises to maintain oxygenation. If compensation fails, expect decreased blood pressure, extreme tachypnea, and an extremely increased heart rate, possibly accompanied by arrhythmias. Fever typically occurs 24 to 48 hours after MI as an inflammatory response to tissue injury.

Color. The patient with MI typically has pale, cool, moist skin. Unless he's in shock, don't expect ashen or gray skin. Also assess his capillary refill; sluggish refill is one of the first signs of decreased perfusion.

Peripheral pulses. Assess the quality and amplitude of peripheral pulses. With MI, pulse quality may diminish slightly. However, unless the patient is in shock, his pulses won't be thready or fleeting. Keep in mind that pulse amplitude reflects stroke volume (the volume ejected with each heartbeat).

Urine output. Urine output indirectly reflects cardiac output. A urine output below 400 ml/ 24 hours suggests decreased cardiac output.

Mentation changes. If cerebral perfusion is impaired, expect restlessness, agitation, and demanding behavior. Eventually, the patient becomes lethargic.

Heart sounds. Auscultate for S_4, which may occur late in diastole just before the first heart sound (S_1). Reflecting atrial kick into a stiff, noncompliant left ventricle, S_4 typically sounds like *lub-dub*.

You also may detect an acute systolic murmur if papillary muscle dysfunction has developed as a complication of MI. Pericarditis, another complication, produces an audible friction rub.

Other signs. If heart failure is complicating MI, you may auscultate S_3 and adventitious breath sounds (such as wheezes, crackles, or rhonchi). You also may detect jugular vein distention.

Diagnostic tests
Tests used to support the diagnosis of MI include the 12-lead ECG, cardiac enzyme analysis, and radionuclide imaging (such as thallium scans).

12-lead ECG. This study visualizes the heart's electrical activity from 12 different angles. It is most useful in identifying cardiac conduction changes resulting from myocardial ischemia, injury, and infarction. However, many factors can affect ECG accuracy—how long ago the MI occurred, conduction defects (such as left bundle-branch block), use of a pacemaker, acute pericarditis, ventricular aneurysm, and electrolyte changes.

Transmural acute MI causes such classic ECG changes as ST-segment elevation, pathologic Q waves, and inverted T waves. (See *ECG characteristics in transmural acute MI*, page 18.)

Cardiac enzyme analysis. Certain enzymes and their isoenzymes spill into the plasma 30 to 60 minutes after myocardial injury, increasing their serum concentration.

Creatine kinase (CK), essential to energy production, reflects normal tissue catabolism. Elevated serum CK levels indicate trauma to cells with high CK content.

CK may be separated into three isoenzymes with distinct molecular structures: CK-BB, found mainly in brain tissue; CK-MM, found mainly in skeletal muscle; and CK-MB, found mainly in cardiac muscle but present in smaller amounts in skeletal muscle. To help diagnose MI, the doctor typically orders CK enzyme fractionation and measurement of CK isoenzymes to locate the site of tissue destruction.

The pattern of enzyme levels is especially important when looking for evidence of MI. CK-MB rises dramatically 4 to 8 hours after the onset of MI, peaks at 18 to 24 hours, and may stay elevated for up to 72 hours.

ECG characteristics in transmural acute MI

In transmural acute myocardial infarction (MI), the 12-lead electrocardiogram (ECG) shows certain classic features.

Baseline ECG complex
Note the brisk downstroke of the QRS complex in a normal ECG waveform, which then returns to baseline.

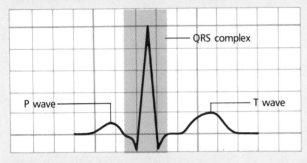

Hours after blood flow obstruction
For 6 to 12 hours after a transmural acute MI, the ST segment remains elevated instead of returning briskly to baseline. Consider ST-segment elevation significant if it persists for at least 2 mm (represented by two small boxes) and appears in at least two of the 12 ECG leads (those that view the injured epicardial area).

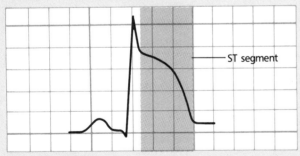

Hours to days later
Although still elevated, the ST segment now starts to return to baseline (see above right). However, the Q wave becomes abnormal, widening to more than 0.02 second and deepening to more than 25% of the R wave. An abnormal Q wave indicates the electrical death of myocardial cells, which can no longer transmit electrical impulses. Also, the T wave now is inverted. Symmetrical T-wave inversion or a depressed ST segment reflects ischemia.

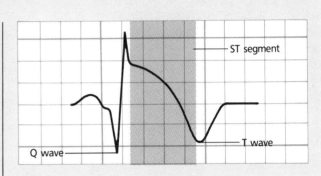

Days to weeks later
The ST segment continues its return to baseline.

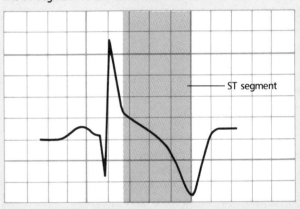

Weeks to months later
All ECG features have returned to normal except the Q wave. Once the Q wave becomes abnormal, it will remain abnormal in only a small percentage of patients.

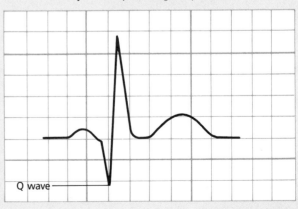

Lactate dehydrogenase (LDH) is present in nearly all body tissues. Cellular damage causes an increase in total serum LDH. However, five tissue-specific isoenzymes can be identified and measured. Two of them, LDH_1 and LDH_2, appear mainly in the heart. The myocardial LDH level rises later than the CK level (12 to 48 hours after infarction starts), peaks in 2 to 5 days, and falls to normal in 7 to 10 days (unless tissue necrosis persists). In acute MI, the concentration of LDH_1 exceeds LDH_2 within 12 to 48 hours after symptom onset. This reversal of the normal isoenzyme pattern typifies myocardial damage.

Levels of *serum aspartate aminotransferase* (AST, formerly known as SGOT) rise 6 to 10 hours after onset of chest pain from MI. They peak in 24 to 48 hours and drop to normal in 4 to 5 days. The degree of elevation depends on the number of damaged cells and the interval between the onset of infarction and the time the sample is drawn. (See *Elevation patterns for cardiac enzymes.*)

Radionuclide imaging. Advances in nuclear medicine now permit more reliable detection of myocardial damage when the patient history, ECG, or cardiac enzyme tests are inconclusive. The *technetium-99m pyrophosphate scan* (also called the PYP scan, MI scan, or hot-spot imaging) shows the location and size of newly damaged myocardial tissue from a recent MI. It's most useful when done 12 hours to 10 days after symptom onset.

A radioactive isotope, technetium is absorbed by injured cells, forming a "hot spot." The size of the spot corresponds to the injury size. The results of isotope uptake are graded subjectively from 1 + to 4 +, according to the size of the spot. Small MIs or subendocardial MIs may not be detected, yielding a false-negative result.

Thallium ("cold-spot") imaging may be used as an adjunct to diagnosis. This test detects areas of ischemia and infarction in the myocardium. A radioactive isotope, thallium concentrates in normal myocardial tissue but not in infarcted or ischemic tissue. On the scan, areas of heavy isotope uptake appear light while areas of poor uptake (cold spots)

Elevation patterns for cardiac enzymes

After myocardial infarction (MI), creatine kinase (CK) is the first enzyme to rise and is the most specific enzyme indicator of myocardial cell damage. Other serum enzymes that will show an increase after MI are aspartate aminotransferase (AST), formerly SGOT, 12 to 48 hours after the MI, and lactate dehydrogenase (LDH), usually 12 to 72 hours after the MI.

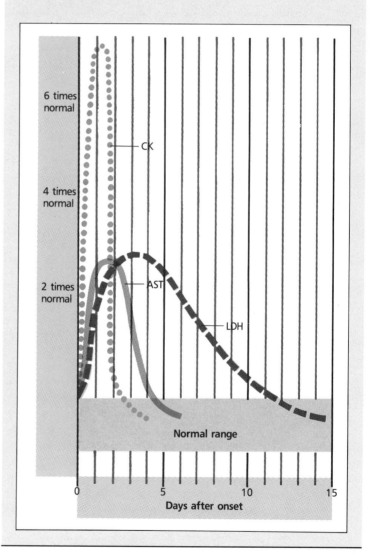

Using the Forrester classification system

Hemodynamic complications are common after myocardial infarction. The Forrester classification system classifies these complications by degree of severity and acts as a guide for drug treatment and other interventions. Included in this system are the cardiac index, pulmonary artery wedge pressure, and treatment appropriate to each classification.

CLASSIFICATION	CARDIAC INDEX (minute/m²)	PULMONARY ARTERY WEDGE PRESSURE	TREATMENT
Subset I No heart failure	Greater than 2.2 liters	Lower than 18 mm Hg	Administer sedatives.
Subset II Pulmonary congestion	Greater than 2.2 liters	Higher than 18 mm Hg	*Normal blood pressure*: Administer diuretics. *Elevated blood pressure*: Administer vasodilators.
Subset III Hypoperfusion of blood	Less than 2.2 liters	Lower than 18 mm Hg	*Elevated heart rate*: Add volume. *Decreased heart rate*: Pacemaker therapy.
Subset IV Congestion and hypoperfusion of lungs and vital organs	Less than 2.2 liters	Higher than 18 mm Hg	*Normal blood pressure*: Administer vasodilators. *Decreased blood pressure*: Administer inotropic agents.

appear dark, signaling poor perfusion, which may indicate abnormal tissue.

Other studies. *Magnetic resonance imaging* (MRI) identifies infarcted areas and assesses myocardial wall motion through the use of a powerful magnetic field. *Positron emission tomography* (PET) tracks short-lived positron-emitting radioactive compounds and generates a computer image to identify MI. PET measures the emissions of injected isotopes and converts them into a tomographic image. MRI and PET are still largely investigational in evaluating MI.

Echocardiography, which records ultrasonic waves reflected from the heart, helps evaluate cardiac function or wall motion after MI. *Multiple-gated acquisition (MUGA) scanning* helps determine the extent of muscle impairment and damage after MI. This technique involves injection of a radiopharmaceutical that attaches to red blood cells (RBCs); a scintillation camera then records RBC movement.

Cardiac catheterization and *coronary an-* *giography* help evaluate ventricular dysfunction and coronary artery patency after MI.

Ongoing treatment
After initial interventions help stabilize the patient, ongoing treatment involves monitoring hemodynamic indicators to identify complications promptly. The Forrester classification system uses classifications of MI to identify appropriate drug therapy and other interventions. (See *Using the Forrester classification system.*)

If drug therapy fails to improve perfusion, the doctor may insert an intra-aortic balloon pump to assist the failing heart. For optimal effectiveness, this treatment must begin within 2 hours after all pharmacologic alternatives are tried.

The doctor may use various techniques to help restore myocardial perfusion. Thrombolytic agents dissolve clots and prevent ischemic myocardial tissue from becoming infarcted. (See *Thrombolytic therapy for MI.*)

Thrombolytic therapy for MI

The timely use of thrombolytic agents after myocardial infarction (MI) can help dissolve thrombi, restore myocardial perfusion, and prevent extensive necrosis.

DRUG	INDICATIONS	DOSAGE	SPECIAL CONSIDERATIONS
Alteplase (Activase)	Lysis of coronary artery thrombi after acute MI	*Adults (over 65 kg):* 60 mg I.V. in the first hour, of which 6-10 mg is given by I.V. bolus over first 1 to 2 minutes, then 20 mg/hour by infusion for another 2 hours, for a total dose of 100 mg. *Adults (65 kg or less):* 1.25 mg/kg with 60% given in the first hour (10% of the first hour's dose given over the first 1 to 2 minutes).	• Expect to begin alteplase infusion within 6 hours after MI onset. Expect to give heparin during or after alteplase administration as part of treatment regimen. • Prepare solution with sterile water for injection. Do not mix other drugs with alteplase. Use 18G needle for preparing solution—aim water stream at lyophilized cake. Expect a slight foaming to occur. Do not use vial if vacuum is absent. • You may dilute drug with 0.9% sodium chloride solution or dextrose 5% in water (D_5W). Reconstituted or diluted solutions remain stable for up to 8 hours at room temperature. • Expect altered results in coagulation and fibrinolytic tests. Aprotinin (150 to 200 units/ml) in the blood sample may attenuate this effect. • Monitor the patient for bleeding. Excessive I.V. dose can cause bleeding from punctures and recent wounds and in GI, genitourinary, and intracranial sites. Avoid I.M. injections, venipuncture, and arterial puncture during alteplase therapy. Use pressure dressings or ice packs on recent puncture sites to prevent bleeding. • Monitor electrocardiogram for transient arrhythmias associated with perfusion.
Anistreplase (Eminase)	Lysis of coronary artery thrombi after acute MI	*Adults:* 30 units I.V. by direct injection over 2 to 5 minutes.	• Contraindicated in patients with active internal bleeding, history of cerebrovascular accident, recent (within the past 2 months) intraspinal or intracranial surgery or trauma, aneurysm, arteriovenous malformation, intracranial neoplasm, uncontrolled hypertension, or known bleeding diathesis. • Consider risk versus benefit in patients with recent (within 10 days) major surgery, trauma, GI or genitourinary bleeding and in patients with cerebrovascular disease or hypertension. • Unlike other thrombolytics that must be infused, anistreplase is given by direct injection over 2 to 5 minutes. • Reconstitute the drug by slowly adding 5 ml of sterile water for injection. • Do not mix the drug with other medications; do not dilute the solution after reconstitution. • If the drug is not administered within 30 minutes of reconstitution, discard the vial. • Carefully monitor the patient for bleeding, the most common adverse reaction, which may occur internally and at external puncture sites. • Teach the patient signs of internal bleeding. Tell him to report these immediately. Advise the patient about proper dental care to avoid excess gum trauma.

(continued)

Thrombolytic therapy for MI *(continued)*

DRUG	INDICATIONS	DOSAGE	SPECIAL CONSIDERATIONS
Streptokinase (Kabikinase, Streptase)	Lysis of coronary artery thrombi after acute MI	*Adults:* 1,500,000 IU by I.V. infusion over 60 minutes; or intracoronary loading dose of 15,000 to 20,000 IU via coronary artery catheter, then a maintenance dose of 2,000 to 4,000 IU/minute for 60 minutes as an infusion.	• Streptokinase increases thrombin time, activated partial thromboplastin time (APTT), and prothrombin time (PT). It sometimes reduces hematocrit moderately. • Reconstitute vial with 5 ml 0.9% sodium chloride solution, and further dilute to 45 ml; roll gently to mix. (Do not shake.) Use immediately; refrigerate remainder and discard after 24 hours. Store powder at room temperature. • Rate of I.V. infusion depends on thrombin time and streptokinase resistance; higher loading dose may be necessary in patients with recent streptococcal infection or streptokinase treatment. • Monitor the patient for spontaneous bleeding, prolonged systemic hypocoagulability, bleeding or oozing from percutaneous trauma site, transient blood pressure lowering or elevation, atrial or ventricular arrhythmias, periorbital edema, gum bleeding, nausea, urticaria, ecchymosis, phlebitis at injection site, hypersensitivity, fever, musculoskeletal pain, minor breathing difficulty, bronchospasm, angioneurotic edema, and hematuria. • Do not stop therapy for minor allergic reactions that are treatable with antihistamines or corticosteroids. • If minor bleeding proves controllable with pressure, do not lower dose so that more plasminogen is available for conversion to plasmin. • Streptokinase antibodies can persist for 6 months or longer after initial dose, so urokinase may be appropriate if further thrombolytic therapy becomes necessary. • Using streptokinase with anticoagulants may cause hemorrhage. You may need to stop anticoagulant therapy before starting streptokinase. • Aminocaproic acid inhibits streptokinase-induced plasminogen activation.
Urokinase (Abbokinase, Abbokinase Open-Cath)	Lysis of coronary artery thrombosis	*Adults:* 6,000 IU/minute of urokinase intra-arterially via coronary artery catheter until artery opens maximally, usually within 15 to 30 minutes. Drug administration may prove necessary for up to 2 hours. Average total dose amounts to 500,000 IU.	• Urokinase increases thrombin time, APTT, and PT and sometimes reduces hematocrit. • To reconstitute I.V. solution, add 5.2 ml sterile water for injection; dilute further with 0.9% sodium chloride solution or D₅W before infusion. Don't use bacteriostatic water, which contains preservatives. A catheter-clearing product is available in a single-dose vial containing 5,000 IU urokinase with the proper diluent. Discard unused portion; product contains no preservatives. • Monitor the patient for spontaneous bleeding, prolonged systemic hypocoagulability, bleeding or oozing from percutaneous trauma sites, low hematocrit, transient lowering or elevation of blood pressure, atrial or ventricular arrhythmias, periorbital edema, bleeding gums, nausea, urticaria, ecchymosis, phlebitis at injection site, hypersensitivity, anaphylaxis, musculoskeletal pain, bronchospasm, and hematuria. • Concomitant use with anticoagulants may cause hemorrhage; if this occurs, stop anticoagulant administration and allow effects to diminish. You may need to reverse effects of oral anticoagulant therapy before starting urokinase. • To prevent bleeding, don't use urokinase with aspirin, indomethacin, phenylbutazone, or other drugs that affect platelet activity.

Other techniques include coronary artery bypass graft (CABG) surgery, laser angioplasty, percutaneous transluminal atherectomy, and percutaneous transluminal coronary angioplasty (PTCA). The doctor will choose the technique best suited to the patient's needs.

Surgery

CABG. This procedure directly revascularizes the myocardium, creating an alternate route for blood to perfuse the heart. A grafted saphenous vein or an internal mammary artery is used to bypass the occluded artery. The graft is anastomosed proximally to the aorta and distally to the coronary artery and the occlusion. During the procedure, the patient is placed on cardiopulmonary bypass, which diverts blood from the heart to the machine so that the heart can be stopped during revascularization. Cardiopulmonary bypass shunts blood to the oxygenator through cannulas placed in the inferior and superior vena cava, then returns oxygenated blood via a cannula in the ascending aortic arch.

CABG surgery may pose risks for a patient with a low ejection fraction. The lower the preoperative ejection fraction, the greater the perioperative risk of death from cardiogenic shock. The normal ejection fraction is 67%. Typically, a patient with an ejection fraction below 13% isn't a candidate for this procedure.

Laser angioplasty. Although experimental, laser angioplasty is gaining wider use as an alternative to CABG surgery. Like traditional angioplasty, it involves threading a catheter over the occluded arterial site. The laser then directs high beams of light to vaporize plaque and thrombi. (See *Laser angioplasty.*)

A procedure combining traditional balloon angioplasty with laser angioplasty is also under investigation. The laser is used during balloon inflation to create a smooth, patent lumen.

Percutaneous transluminal atherectomy. In this promising technique, a tiny rotating blade encased in a catheter slices or pulverizes plaque. The plaque is then pushed into the catheter tip and removed.

Laser angioplasty

Laser angioplasty has yet to be perfected, but several methods have been effective in relieving stenosis and opening occlusions that cannot be opened with balloon angioplasty alone. The hot-tipped laser is used to create a channel wide enough to admit a balloon catheter, which widens the channel even further. The direct-energy laser beam burns or perforates any plaque obstructing the vessel.

A hot-tipped laser moves through a stenosed region.

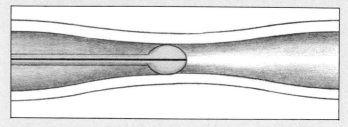

A direct-energy laser beam ablates the plaque.

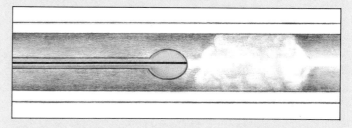

When the channel is opened, the balloon is positioned and then inflated.

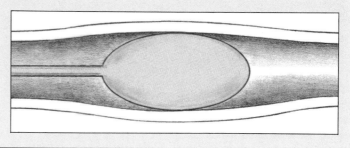

Other treatments
PTCA. This nonsurgical procedure, which dilates occluded coronary arteries, is performed

Understanding PTCA

Percutaneous transluminal coronary angioplasty (PTCA) offers some patients with localized disease a nonsurgical alternative to coronary artery bypass graft surgery. In this procedure, a tiny balloon catheter is used to dilate a coronary artery that has been narrowed by an atherosclerotic plaque.

The procedure for PTCA resembles that for cardiac catheterization. The doctor threads a guiding catheter through a femoral or brachial artery, then backward into the ascending aorta and into the ostium of the right or left coronary artery.

The doctor advances a guide wire from the balloon catheter through the coronary artery until its tip is beyond the portion narrowed by plaque formation.

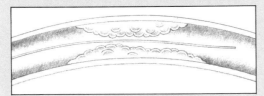

The doctor then advances the balloon catheter over the guide wire until the balloon is wedged into the narrowing.

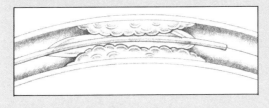

Once in position, the balloon is inflated with a mixture of contrast material and 0.9% sodium chloride solution. The inflated balloon opens the narrowed artery by splitting and compressing the plaque and slightly stretching the artery wall.

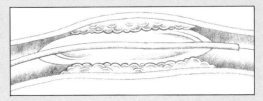

After the balloon reaches 3 to 6.5 atmospheres of pressure, it's deflated. The balloon is then repeatedly inflated until distal perfusion pressure falls about 30%. The catheter and balloon are then removed from the artery.

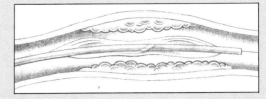

PTCA has widened the narrow part of the artery, improving blood flow to the heart.

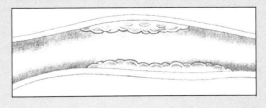

in the cardiac catheterization laboratory with the patient under local anesthesia. Guided by fluoroscopy, the doctor threads a balloon-tipped catheter into a coronary artery with a proximal, accessible, noncalcified atherosclerotic lesion. As the balloon inflates, the plaque is compressed against the vessel wall, permitting coronary blood to flow more freely. (See *Understanding PTCA.*)

The mechanism by which PTCA restores perfusion isn't fully understood. However, the "controlled vessel injury" presumably leads to such coronary artery changes as splitting and redistribution of plaque, and stretching of the artery wall. After the fibrous cap of the vessel breaks, the exposed matter beneath it is removed by phagocytosis. As the vessel heals, endothelialization and clotting occur simultaneously, enlarging the diameter of the occluded artery segment and improving blood flow.

Emergency PTCA may be performed during an acute anginal episode or in the early stages of an MI. During the procedure, the doctor may inject a thrombolytic agent into the affected vessel.

Most patients chosen for PTCA have unstable angina that hasn't responded to conventional drug or surgical therapy. Even those with multivessel disease may be candidates. However, disease of the left main coronary artery contraindicates PTCA because of the risk of complete occlusion of the entire anterior and lateral walls.

Before the procedure, expect to administer prophylactic antibiotics, aspirin, nifedipine, heparin, dipyridamole, low-molecular-weight dextran, and nitroglycerin.

If such complications as acute MI or arterial dissection develop during PTCA, the patient must be taken to the operating room immediately for CABG surgery. Therefore, if your patient is scheduled for PTCA, make sure he also signs a consent form for CABG surgery (if your hospital requires this).

Ongoing nursing interventions

Ongoing care for the patient who's had an MI emphasizes cardiac rehabilitation and patient teaching. Be sure to monitor the patient for complications.

Cardiac rehabilitation

• Start the patient on a program of cardiac rehabilitation to regain cardiovascular fitness while minimizing the risk of another cardiac event when he has been hemodynamically stable and pain-free for 24 hours.
• Increase the patient's activity level progressively according to metabolic equivalents of a task (METs), which measure an activity's stress on the cardiovascular and pulmonary systems. One MET equals 3.5 ml of oxygen consumption per kilogram of body weight per minute. Your role in this program will primarily be to monitor the patient.
• Continuously monitor the patient's heart rate, heart rhythm, and ST-segment changes during activity. Subjective symptoms and blood pres-

sure changes are assessed before and after the activity. A heart rate increase of more than 10 beats/minute over baseline, a decrease in systolic blood pressure, or development of symptoms represents an undesirable response to a given activity level.
• Test the patient's stamina before discharge. He should be able to climb one flight of stairs and walk 30′ (9 m) successfully. He'll also undergo a stress test so that the health care team can formulate a more precise exercise regimen.
• Observe the patient during activities to make sure he doesn't attempt too much too soon.

Patient teaching

• Teach the patient about the suspected cause of his condition, the disease process, prescribed drugs and other therapeutic measures, required dietary changes, and ways to reduce his risk factors for MI.
• Tell him what to anticipate during rehabilitation. Mention that he'll begin a controlled program of monitored, progressively increasing activity to prevent the harmful effects of prolonged bed rest while maintaining a balance between oxygen supply and demand.
• Teach the patient's family about the rehabilitation process. Prepare them for the patient's emotional reaction to his condition, which may include anxiety, denial, anger, depression, and aggression. Make sure family members understand why the patient must change his lifestyle, and urge them to support these changes.

Cardiogenic shock

A state of profoundly impaired tissue perfusion and reduced cardiac output, cardiogenic shock impairs the supply of blood, oxygen, nutrients, and electrolytes to body cells. As cardiac output reaches a perilous low blood flow to the capillary bed—the site of gas exchange with cells—is bypassed. This leads to abnormal cellular metabolism, then cellular injury.

Cardiogenic shock has a mortality approaching 85%. Among survivors, the long-

Responding to cardiogenic shock

Preventing further damage to the patient's heart is your overall priority in cardiogenic shock. This means you must take measures to increase his myocardial oxygen supply, boost his cardiac output, and reduce his left ventricular work load. Immediate interventions depend on the severity of shock and the patient's signs and symptoms.
• First, assess his ABCs (airway, breathing, and circulation). If these are adequate, elevate the head of the bed to reduce discomfort if he's in respiratory distress. Start an I.V. line at a keep-vein-open rate.
• As appropriate, arrange for patient transfer to the intensive care unit for vasoactive drug therapy and possible use of a mechanical assist device.
• If the patient has chest discomfort, administer morphine, as prescribed, to relieve pain and anxiety. Insert an indwelling urinary catheter to allow precise measurement of hourly urine output—an indirect indicator of cardiac output. Prepare for insertion of hemodynamic monitoring lines.
• To help support the failing heart, initiate oxygen therapy, as ordered, based on the patient's arterial blood gas values. Some patients may require mechanical ventilation. However, be aware that posi-

tive-pressure ventilation may further decrease cardiac output.
• To reduce the heart's work load, enforce bed rest and administer prescribed afterload-reducing agents, such as vasodilators. Withhold negative inotropic drugs, such as beta blockers or calcium channel blockers, because they may depress contractility and worsen the existing problem. Notify the doctor any time a medication is withheld.
• To improve contractility, administer prescribed positive inotropic drugs, such as digitalis glycosides, dopamine, dobutamine, and amrinone.
• To optimize the patient's volume status, verify that he's hypervolemic by assessing for adventitious breath sounds, skin turgor, excessive jugular vein distention, sacral edema, and a positive hepatojugular reflex. Administer diuretics as ordered. Also give venodilators, such as nitrates and morphine, as ordered.
• To dilate the patient's vessels, administer prescribed vasodilators.
• Assess for desired and adverse effects of all administered drugs.
• Monitor the patient's hemodynamic values.

term prognosis is poor. Immediate, expert intervention is the patient's only hope for averting death. (See *Responding to cardiogenic shock.*)

Causes

Cardiogenic shock can result from any condition that significantly impairs ventricular pumping. It usually arises when at least 40% of the ventricle is dysfunctional. Although the left ventricle is involved in most cases, right ventricular dysfunction can also induce cardiogenic shock.

Ventricular impairment typically stems from CAD. By impairing myocardial perfusion, CAD causes tissue ischemia and, ultimately, necrosis or MI. Myocardial necrosis reduces cardiac output by compromising contractility. The greater the extent of tissue damage from the MI, the

greater the risk of cardiogenic shock. Infarcted tissue may accumulate, contributing to the total amount of dysfunctional heart muscle. Thus, a patient with several old, small infarctions may have a significant amount of dysfunctional muscle, placing him at high risk for cardiogenic shock.

Anterior-wall infarction is more likely to trigger cardiogenic shock than inferior-wall infarction because the damaged area is the heart's main pumping muscle. Right ventricular MI also can cause cardiogenic shock by impairing perfusion to the lungs and left side of the heart, reducing left ventricular output.

Other causes of cardiogenic shock include end-stage cardiomyopathy, a ruptured interventricular septum, an atrial thrombus that impedes intracardiac blood flow, valvular heart disease (such as aortic stenosis and mitral regurgitation), cardiac tamponade, massive pulmonary embolism, arrhythmias, papillary muscle dysfunction, and myocarditis. Cardiogenic shock also may follow cardiac arrest or prolonged cardiac surgery.

Pathophysiology

The primary pathophysiologic changes in cardiogenic shock stem from a profound decrease in left ventricular output—regardless of which ventricle is failing. The drop in cardiac output triggers a series of compensatory mechanisms aimed at maintaining perfusion of the capillary bed. The primary compensatory mechanism is sympathetic stimulation, which increases the heart rate, left ventricular filling pressure, and systemic vascular resistance in an attempt to promote perfusion. (See *Compensatory responses that boost cardiac output.*)

Initially, these responses maintain perfusion. However, if cardiac output doesn't improve, a vicious cycle ensues: Myocardial damage further diminishes cardiac output, decreases coronary artery perfusion, and worsens myocardial hypoxia, leading to more injury to the myocardium. Once this cycle begins, only rapid, expert medical and nursing care can help to break it.

When compensation fails, capillary bed perfusion is bypassed and cellular ischemia ensues. Metabolism changes from aerobic to anaerobic—the only available means of generating energy. Production of lactic acid during anaerobic metabolism results in acidosis. As blood pH falls, enzymes are released that destroy cell membrane integrity, causing irreversible cell damage. The stages of cell damage correspond with the severity and duration of shock.

Acidosis leads to arterial dilation, which causes a sharp fall in blood pressure—a late sign of shock. Poor blood flow, depleted cellular energy stores, and high lactic acid levels impair contractility so severely that the heart simply stops pumping.

Complications

Multisystem organ failure—progressive failure of two or more organ systems—is the major complication of cardiogenic shock and the final common pathway to death. Typically, the respiratory, renal, and hematologic systems are in-

PATHOPHYSIOLOGY

Compensatory responses that boost cardiac output

As cardiac output drops in cardiogenic shock, a series of compensatory sympathetic nervous system (SNS) responses occurs.

Enhanced contractility

Stretch receptors or baroreceptors in the left atrium sense the drop in incoming volume and initiate enhanced myocardial contractility. Receptors in the vena cava and right atrium respond to the drop in volume by causing constriction of veins. Serving as the body's own autotransfusion mechanism, vasoconstriction displaces about 500 ml of blood from the venous system to the arterial tree.

Vasoconstriction

As renal perfusion drops, stretch receptors or baroreceptors in the kidneys trigger release of renin, causing intense vasoconstriction. This vasoconstriction is an attempt at maintaining perfusion.

SNS-triggered responses

When stretch receptors or baroreceptors in the aortic arch sense a drop in cardiac output, the glossopharyngeal nerve sends a message to the medulla and SNS stimulation occurs. This triggers the following events:
• The heart rate increases by 20%.
• Arteries and veins constrict.
• The coronary and carotid arteries dilate, as do vessels supplying large muscles.
• The thirst center in the hypothalamus is activated.
• Glycogen is released from the liver and converted to glucose.

These early compensatory responses, which attempt to maintain perfusion, produce early cardiogenic shock. When compensation fails, late signs of shock develop, such as a heart rate above 120 beats/minute, lowered blood pressure, urine output above 30 ml/hour, and acidosis.

volved. Profound respiratory hypoperfusion causes adult respiratory distress syndrome; renal hypoperfusion leads to tubular necrosis; and hematologic effects result in disseminated intravascular coagulation.

The patient also risks infection—not just from multisystem organ failure itself but also from alterations in the immune response, decreased blood supply to the GI tract, and invasive lines used for interventions. Death occurs when vital organs can't overcome the catastrophic effects of profound hypoperfusion.

Assessment

History

Cardiogenic shock must be detected in its early stage to prevent death. Pay special attention to history data that point to an increased risk of cardiogenic shock. To help determine your patient's risk, ask yourself the following questions: Does he have any risk factors, such as a history of MI? Has he had more than one MI? Were the MIs complicated or uncomplicated? Does he have a history of cardiomyopathy, CAD, embolism, valvular heart disease, or arrhythmias? Has he undergone cardiac surgery?

Because cardiogenic shock most commonly follows an MI, investigate any complaint of chest pain carefully to help identify the MI early and ensure prompt intervention.

Physical examination

Physical findings depend on the stage of shock. To recognize cardiogenic shock promptly, you must identify the compensatory changes that occur in the early stages of shock.

Early shock. Stimulation of the sympathetic nervous system causes various changes that may seem insignificant when considered alone but point to shock when correlated with each other and the patient's history.
• *Increased heart rate.* Typically, the heart rate rises about 20% in early cardiogenic shock.
• *Arterial and venous constriction.* Look for signs of vasoconstriction—pallor, sluggish capillary refill, and reduced peripheral pulse quality. Pulse amplitude will increase from a normal +2 or +3 to +4. At this stage, the patient's

pulses won't be weak or thready (+1).
• *Coronary artery dilation.* This compensatory mechanism promotes myocardial perfusion, making arrhythmias unlikely at this stage.
• *Carotid artery dilation.* This compensatory mechanism increases oxygen flow to the brain and may cause such mentation changes as a heightened awareness or a feeling of impending doom, fearfulness, restlessness, or anxiety. The patient may also exhibit demanding behavior at this stage. These effects also may reflect the arousal-enhancing effect of epinephrine, released by central nervous system stimulation.
• *Dilation of vessels supplying large muscles.* This response increases the patient's strength. In fact, you may need to institute safety precautions because he may be able to remove restraining devices at this time, which could lead to injury.
• *Thirst stimulation.* Note any patient complaints of thirst. Low cardiac output triggers stimulation of the thirst center in an attempt to enhance fluid volume, and thus boost perfusion, through increased fluid intake.

Late shock. When compensatory mechanisms are depleted, the patient displays the classic clinical profile of shock. Assessment findings now reflect impaired perfusion to the capillary bed, cell damage, anaerobic metabolism, and acidosis. At this stage, the patient has little chance for survival, even if perfusion is restored.

Look for signs of reduced cardiac output. In late shock, the heart rate typically measures less than 100 beats/minute. When auscultating heart sounds, you may hear S_3, signifying ventricular gallop from increased ventricular filling pressure. As the respiratory rate increases, you may hear crackles or wheezes when you auscultate the lungs—possibly from narrowed airways and increased fluid in the lungs.

Expect reduced blood pressure, such as a MAP below 60 mm Hg and systolic pressure below 90 mm Hg (or at least 30 mm Hg lower than baseline). Pulse pressure narrows, and peripheral pulses become weak and thready. You may detect arrhythmias on the ECG monitor. The skin is cold and clammy.

Assess for other characteristic changes, such as urine output below 30 ml/hour. The patient may become less responsive and exhibit mentation changes. Inspect his skin, which will appear ashen, gray, or even cyanotic, with mottled extremities. Expect slow capillary refill. Look for weak or floppy muscles.

Diagnostic tests

To help evaluate the adequacy of perfusion, measure cardiac output, and identify the severity of shock, the doctor may order arterial blood gas (ABG) analysis, serum lactic acid and enzyme measurements, and hemodynamic monitoring. Serial testing helps determine the patient's prognosis. As with physical findings, diagnostic results vary with the stage of shock. (To help track the severity of shock, you may plot laboratory values and hemodynamic findings on a flow sheet.)

ABG analysis. ABG values reveal the degree of hypoxia and the severity of acidosis. Early in shock, during compensation, blood pH remains normal (7.34 to 7.45). The partial pressure of arterial carbon dioxide ($PaCO_2$) measures 35 to 45 mm Hg, and the partial pressure of arterial oxygen (PaO_2) ranges from 80 to 100 mm Hg. Expect a bicarbonate (HCO_3^-) level of 22 to 26 mEq/liter and an arterial oxygen saturation (SaO_2) value above 97%.

As acidosis develops, the pH value will move toward the acidic side (above 7.35 but below 7.39) — evidence that the respiratory system is compensating for acidosis effectively by eliminating more carbon dioxide (an acid). Other ABG values will also reflect compensated metabolic acidosis: $PaCO_2$ of 37 mm Hg, PaO_2 of 64 mm Hg, HCO_3^- of 22 mEq/liter, and SaO_2 of 96%.

However, as shock progresses and compensation starts to fail, ABG values will reveal acute metabolic acidosis. The pH drops below 7.35, $PaCO_2$ falls to 28 mm Hg, PaO_2 drops to 50 mm Hg, HCO_3^- decreases to 12 mEq/liter, and SaO_2 falls to 80%. These results indicate partial respiratory compensation: Although the respiratory system is still trying to eliminate acid (reflected by reduced $PaCO_2$), it can no longer keep pH within normal limits. De-creased SaO_2 reflects an abnormally high extraction of oxygen from the blood.

Beware of a falling HCO_3^- level accompanied by an adequate but reduced PaO_2 (above 50 mm Hg) and signs and symptoms of reduced perfusion. These findings reflect poor circulation.

Serum lactic acid levels. The serum lactic acid level rises with acidosis. In shock, expect a serum lactic acid level above 2 mEq/liter. As the lactic acid concentration rises, the patient's survival odds decline. (A patient who enters the hospital in shock with a serum lactic acid level above 10 mEq/liter has virtually no chance for survival because of extensive cell damage.)

Serum enzyme levels (CK, AST, LDH, and their isoenzymes). These tests may be used to confirm MI, the leading cause of cardiogenic shock. However, they're not specific to cardiogenic shock.

Hemodynamic monitoring. Essential to managing shock, hemodynamic monitoring helps determine the severity of shock and evaluates the patient's response to treatment. Expect the doctor to insert a pulmonary artery catheter to measure cardiac output, cardiac index, and the contributing factors of preload (reflected by pulmonary artery wedge pressure [PAWP] and right atrial pressure), afterload (reflected by systemic vascular resistance and pulmonary vascular resistance), and contractility (reflected by left ventricular stroke work and stroke volume). (See *Understanding hemodynamic terms,* page 30, and *Hemodynamic values in cardiogenic shock,* page 31.)

Ongoing treatment

For the patient in cardiogenic shock, ongoing treatment focuses on relieving signs and symptoms and reducing the severity of shock. Treatment goals include improving ventricular function and cardiac output, boosting myocardial oxygen supply, decreasing myocardial oxygen demand, and correcting hypoxia and metabolic acidosis.

Understanding hemodynamic terms

To ensure quality care for the patient with a cardiovascular crisis, you must be familiar with hemodynamic evaluation terms.

Cardiac output refers to the volume of blood ejected by the heart each minute. Normally, it measures 4 to 6 liters/minute. If your patient has a pulmonary artery catheter equipped with a thermistor, you can use the thermodilution technique to determine cardiac output. You also can determine cardiac output indirectly from your patient's mixed venous oxygen saturation. Otherwise, calculate cardiac output using mean arterial pressure (MAP), central venous pressure (CVP), and systemic vascular resistance (SVR). Follow this formula:

$$\text{Cardiac output} = \frac{\text{MAP} - \text{CVP}}{\text{SVR}}$$

Cardiac index takes body size into account. By calculating this parameter, you can determine if your patient's cardiac output meets his needs. Cardiac index normally ranges from 2.5 to 4.2 liters/minute/m². Many monitoring systems calculate cardiac index after the nurse inputs the patient's height and weight. Use this formula to calculate cardiac index:

$$\text{Cardiac index} = \frac{\text{cardiac output}}{\text{body surface area (m}^2\text{)}}$$

Preload indicators

Preload, which refers to ventricular volume plus pressure at the end of diastole, determines the length of muscle fibers when contraction begins. This length, in turn, determines contractile force and the velocity of muscle fiber shortening.

Central venous pressure (CVP) reflects right atrial pressure and thus helps gauge right ventricular preload. Normal CVP measures 4 to 12 cm H_2O, or 1 to 6 mm Hg.

Pulmonary artery diastolic pressure (PADP) reflects left ventricular preload. PADP approximates left ventricular pressures in a patient who doesn't have pulmonary or mitral valve disease. Normal PADP measures 8 to 15 mm Hg.

Pulmonary artery wedge pressure (PAWP) also reflects left ventricular preload. PAWP is more accurate than PADP if the patient has pulmonary or mitral valve disease. Normal PAWP is 4 to 12 mm Hg; a value greater than 28 mm Hg usually constitutes pulmonary edema.

Afterload indicators

Afterload is the impedance, or resistance, the ventricle works against to eject blood during systole. Impedance depends on arterial blood pressure, valve characteristics, ventricular radius, and wall thickness.

SVR helps gauge left ventricular afterload. Normal SVR is 900 to 1,200 dynes/second/cm⁻⁵ or absolute units. An indirect measurement, it's commonly calculated by the hemodynamic monitoring system. Or you may calculate it using this formula:

$$\text{SVR} = \frac{\text{MAP} - \text{CVP}}{\text{cardiac output}} \times \text{a constant of 80}$$

Pulmonary vascular resistance (PVR), which reflects right ventricular afterload, is the total resistance to blood flow in the pulmonary circulation. Normal PVR is 20 to 120 dynes/second/cm⁻⁵ or absolute units. PVR is derived from other hemodynamic measurements, including pulmonary artery pressure (PAP). To calculate PVR, use this formula:

$$\text{PVR} = \frac{\text{mean PAP} - \text{PAWP}}{\text{cardiac output}} \times \text{a constant of 80}$$

Contractility indicators

Contractility refers to ventricular contractility.

Stroke volume is the difference between volume at the end of diastole and left ventricular volume at the end of systole—in other words, the volume ejected with each heartbeat. Normal stroke volume is approximately 70 ml. Stroke volume is a derived parameter. You can calculate it using this formula:

$$\text{Stroke volume} = \frac{\text{cardiac output}}{\text{heart rate}}$$

Stroke volume index, which relates stroke volume to body size, produces a more accurate measurement than stroke volume. Normal stroke volume index is 40 ml/beat/m². To calculate stroke volume index, divide the cardiac index by the heart rate.

Left ventricular stroke work (LVSW) reflects myocardial contractility. The normal range is 35 to 85 g/m²/beat. To calculate LVSW, use this formula:

$$\text{LVSW} = \frac{\text{cardiac output} \times \text{MAP}}{\text{heart rate}} \times \text{a constant of 13.6}$$

Drug treatment

The doctor will tailor drug therapy to the patient's hemodynamic profile. Because the patient has reduced cardiac output, primary drug therapy will involve afterload-reducing agents. Nitroprusside, the major afterload-reducing agent used in critical care settings, is a potent vasodilator. With a greater effect on arteries than on veins, it reduces afterload more than preload. Expect to give nitroprusside by continuous I.V. infusion, usually starting at 0.5 mcg/kg/minute, and to titrate the dosage until the patient's afterload indicators improve.

Be aware that nitroprusside's vasodilating properties will contribute to declining blood pressure. If the patient is already hypotensive, this could further compromise his peripheral perfusion. If your patient has abnormally high afterload indicators, the doctor probably will combine nitroprusside with dopamine. While nitroprusside lowers afterload and reduces impedance to ventricular ejection, dopamine acts to maintain peripheral perfusion.

During combination therapy, titrate the nitroprusside dosage slowly, as ordered. Usually, you can give up to 3 mcg/kg/minute while maintaining the patient's systolic blood pressure at 90 mm Hg or higher. (However, some doctors use a MAP of 60 mm Hg rather than a systolic value as the goal.)

Dopamine provides both inotropic and pressor effects in I.V. dosages of up to 10 mcg/kg/minute. It may be used alone in a hypotensive patient with acceptable afterload indicators. However, if systolic blood pressure remains below 90 mm Hg or MAP measures less than 60 mm Hg despite high-dose I.V. dopamine, the doctor may consider giving epinephrine or norepinephrine to elevate the patient's blood pressure.

For a patient with high preload, you may need to administer nitroglycerin. Primarily a venodilator, this drug reduces venous return, and thus preload, to a more acceptable level. Although it acts mainly on veins, it also dilates arteries and thus will decrease blood pressure. When giving nitroglycerin by continuous I.V. drip, titrate the dosage, as ordered, based on the desired preload value while maintaining a systolic blood pressure of at least 90 mm Hg.

Hemodynamic values in cardiogenic shock

This chart compares normal hemodynamic values to the hemodynamic values seen in patients with cardiogenic shock. Note that these values should be interpreted as general guidelines; each patient's trends will be distinct.

MEASUREMENT	NORMAL VALUE	VALUE IN CARDIOGENIC SHOCK
Systolic blood pressure	120 mm Hg	Low
Pulse pressure	40 mm Hg	Narrow
Cardiac output	4 to 6 liters/minute	Less than 2.5 liters/minute
Cardiac index	2.5 to 4.2 liters/minute/m²	Less than 2.0 liters/minute/m²
Stroke volume	70 ml	Low
Heart rate	60 to 100 beats/minute	More than 100 beats/minute
Pulmonary artery diastolic pressure	8 to 15 mm Hg	High
Pulmonary artery wedge pressure	4 to 12 mm Hg	More than 30 mm Hg
Central venous pressure	4 to 12 cm H_2O or 1 to 6 mm Hg (depending on device)	High
Systemic vascular resistance	900 to 1,200 absolute units	More than 1,400 absolute units
Pulmonary vascular resistance	20 to 120 absolute units	More than 120 absolute units
Left ventricular stroke work index	35 to 85 g/m²/beat	High

As ordered and appropriate, administer sodium bicarbonate to correct acute metabolic acidosis. Use ABG values as a guide. Typically, a pH above 7.30 in a patient with cardiogenic shock warrants sodium bicarbonate administration.

Surgery

If severe CAD causes cardiogenic shock, the patient may benefit more from prompt surgical revascularization (within 24 hours of MI onset) than from drug therapy or an intra-aortic bal-

Devices used to treat cardiogenic shock

To improve the recovery odds for a patient with cardiogenic shock, the doctor may use an intra-aortic balloon pump (IABP) or a ventricular assist device (VAD).

Intra-aortic balloon pump
Placed in the descending thoracic aorta, the IABP pumps or propels blood in counterpoint to the heart's cycle of systole and diastole. After the balloon's catheter is connected to a pump console, the balloon is inflated and deflated automatically according to the patient's electrocardiogram or arterial waveform. Inflated during diastole, the balloon increases aortic diastolic pressure, which enhances coronary artery and peripheral perfusion.

The balloon is deflated immediately before systole, allowing the aortic valve to open under less pressure. This results in less work, less afterload, and less oxygen consumption.

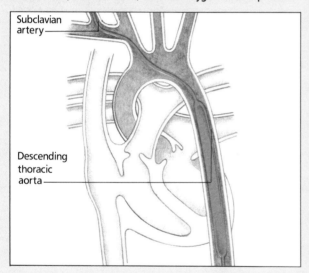

Subclavian artery

Descending thoracic aorta

Ventricular assist device
A VAD may be used temporarily to pump the heart's blood. Types of VADs include the left ventricular assist device, right ventricular assist device, and biventricular assist device. Battery operated, the VAD diverts blood from the ventricular apex to the ascending aorta via surgically implanted outflow and inflow lines. VADs allow the failing heart to rest while recovering. They almost completely control stroke volume, reducing left ventricular work load while maintaining adequate perfusion.

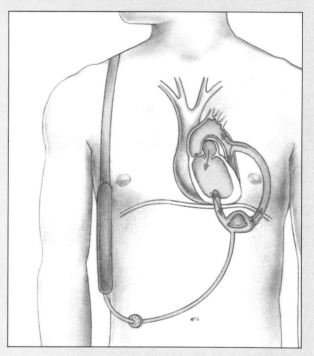

loon pump (IABP). If cardiogenic shock stems from papillary muscle rupture, the patient's mitral valve must be surgically replaced to reverse shock.

Other treatments
Some patients may require a mechanical device that reduces ventricular afterload and supports the failing heart. For instance, if the patient's hemodynamic profile doesn't improve suffi-ciently after 2 hours of aggressive drug therapy, the doctor may insert an IABP. Candidates for such a device include those with a PAWP exceeding 30 mm Hg and a cardiac index below 2 liters/minute/m^2 who don't respond to conventional treatment. (See *Devices used to treat cardiogenic shock*.)

Ongoing nursing interventions
After stabilization, monitor your patient closely. Additional nursing responsibilities depend on

the patient's signs and symptoms and on the specific treatment he has received.
• Closely assess the patient's hemodynamic profile every hour or as indicated, including his hemodynamic values, urine output, peripheral pulse quality, and capillary refill. If you detect deteriorating hemodynamic values—rising PAWP, falling cardiac output and cardiac index, and increasing systemic vascular resistance—report this to the doctor immediately.
• Monitor the ECG for such changes as ST-segment elevation and arrhythmias. Also assess the patient's mental status and examine his skin for color, temperature, and moistness.
• Titrate drug dosages and fluids to the patient's condition and hemodynamic profile, as ordered. Be sure to assess for both desired and adverse drug effects.
• If the patient has had an IABP implanted, assess for therapeutic response and for proper balloon inflation-deflation timing. Take measures to detect and prevent IABP complications. For instance, never flex the affected leg at the hip because this may displace or fracture the balloon catheter inserted in the leg. Assess the patient's pedal and radial pulses and skin color and temperature to make sure his leg circulation is adequate. Check the dressing on the catheter insertion site for bleeding. Also assess regularly for hematoma and signs of infection, and culture any drainage.
• Monitor ABG values as often as the patient's condition warrants and with every change in supplemental oxygenation. Pay special attention to the pH level, noting any trend toward acidosis. Adjust the oxygen flow rate based on ABG values. Monitor complete blood count and electrolyte levels.

Cardiac tamponade

This cardiovascular crisis occurs when excessive fluid accumulates within the pericardial space, leading to compression of the heart. Ultimately, both stroke volume and cardiac output decrease. To prevent grave consequences, the health care team must intervene quickly. (See *Responding to cardiac tamponade*, page 34.)

Cardiac tamponade may be acute or chronic. If fluid accumulates rapidly, as little as 150 ml can create a crisis. With slower accumulation (as in pericardial effusion associated with cancer), symptoms may not arise until 1 to 2 liters gather because the fibrous pericardial wall can stretch to accommodate the gradual increase.

Causes
Cardiac tamponade may result from pericarditis of almost any origin. Common causes of acute cardiac tamponade include acute pericarditis from bacterial infections, tuberculosis, uremia, and connective tissue disorders (including rheumatoid arthritis, systemic lupus erythematosus, rheumatic fever, vasculitis, and scleroderma). Hemopericardium (bleeding into the pericardial cavity)—another cause of acute tamponade—may stem from ventricular rupture after MI, rupture of an aortic aneurysm into the pericardial sac, a vascular pericardial tumor, penetrating or nonpenetrating chest wall trauma, or thoracic surgery. After cardiac surgery, inadequate mediastinal drainage may lead to acute tamponade. (See *When heart surgery causes cardiac tamponade*, page 35.)

Chronic cardiac tamponade may be caused by infection (such as tuberculosis or a parasitic infection), uremia, neoplasm, myxedema, high cholesterol levels, radiation therapy, Dressler's syndrome, or postpericardiotomy syndrome.

Pathophysiology
Compression of the heart from accumulated fluid increases intrapericardial pressure and impedes venous return. As a result, central venous filling pressure rises and ventricular filling diminishes, causing a low-flow state in the heart. Stroke volume and cardiac output from the left ventricle then diminish, even though the heart beats faster and vasoconstriction increases.

The amount of fluid and how fast it accumulates determine the severity of cardiac tamponade. With rapid accumulation of 100 ml of fluid, as occurs in hemorrhage, trauma, or surgery, the heart can't fully expand or stretch during diastole. The patient quickly becomes

Responding to cardiac tamponade

If your patient has signs and symptoms of acute cardiac tamponade, he may progress rapidly to cardiac arrest unless pericardial fluid is removed. Your main responsibility is maintaining his cardiac output until intrapericardial pressure is relieved.

Administering oxygen and aspirating fluid
• Administer oxygen to enhance tissue perfusion. The doctor will probably insert a central venous pressure line to monitor hemodynamic pressures. Check these pressures closely and assess the patient's blood pressure, pulse, and respirations every 5 to 10 minutes to help gauge cardiac output.
• Assist the doctor during pericardiocentesis (needle aspiration of pericardial fluid). This procedure is usually done in acute tamponade if the patient's systolic pressure drops more than 30 mm Hg from baseline. Aspirating as little as 25 ml of pericardial fluid dramatically improves arterial pressure and cardiac output.

Performing thoracotomy
• If acute cardiac tamponade is a complication of cardiac surgery, be prepared to assist with emergency thoracotomy. In extreme cases, emergency thoracotomy is done at the bedside in the intensive care unit.
• Gather a prepared thoracotomy tray and an emergency resuscitation cart with internal defibrillator paddles. Make sure all equipment is turned on and operational. Monitor the patient's blood pressure and hemodynamic indicators. As ordered, maintain volume infusion, vasopressor administration, or both to support failing cardiac output.
• During thoracotomy, assist the doctor as needed while monitoring the patient's response.

• After the procedure, monitor the patient's vital signs, which should improve immediately. Also monitor hemodynamic indicators and arterial blood gas values, and auscultate for heart and lung sounds. Administer pain medications, as needed and prescribed. Maintain the chest drainage system and monitor for such complications as hemorrhage and arrhythmias.

Maintaining hemodynamic support
• The doctor may order intravascular volume expanders and vasoactive drugs to maintain hemodynamic support. He usually orders colloids to maximize left ventricular filling and stroke volume, although initially he may order 0.9% sodium chloride solution or lactated Ringer's solution. As ordered, give the first 500 ml of colloid or I.V. solution over a 10-minute period; then infuse at a rate of 100 to 500 ml/hour, depending on the patient's hemodynamic response.
• Administer other drugs as ordered. Isoproterenol is useful in cardiac tamponade because it increases contractility. Arterial vasodilators, such as hydralazine and nitroprusside, reduce afterload and systemic vascular resistance and may be used to augment cardiac output. Depending on the cause of tamponade, the doctor also may order such drugs as vitamin K, antibiotics, or protamine, to promote clotting.
• If the patient has chronic tamponade, ensure hemodynamic stabilization and prepare him for diagnostic studies, as ordered. Assess him regularly for warning signs of a drop in cardiac output. The doctor will tailor specific treatment to the cause of the disorder.

symptomatic as the heart is compressed and circulation begins to fail.

If fluid accumulates more gradually, as in a neoplasm or uremia, the pericardial sac stretches gradually, accommodating as much as 2,500 ml before symptoms arise. Typically, pericardial effusion occurs when pericardial fluid volume exceeds 20 ml.

Complications
Left untreated, cardiac tamponade can progress quickly to cardiogenic shock and death as cardiac output and ventricular filling diminish.

Assessment
History
Cardiac tamponade usually has an insidious onset. However, once signs and symptoms ap-

When heart surgery causes cardiac tamponade

Inadequate mediastinal drainage may lead to acute cardiac tamponade after heart surgery. As fluid accumulates in the pericardial space, it compresses the heart. Ultimately, both stroke volume and cardiac output decrease.

That's what happened to Lucille Devine, age 65. She was admitted for surgery to treat triple-vessel coronary artery disease and cardiomyopathy. Before surgery, her ejection fraction was a low 30%.

During triple-bypass coronary artery graft surgery, the surgeon used one internal mammary graft and two saphenous vein grafts. Before cardiopulmonary bypass was stopped, however, Mrs. Devine needed dopamine and nitroprusside.

Assessing for postoperative problems

Two hours after Mrs. Devine returned from surgery, she developed sinus tachycardia. Her nurse, Kristine Mallory, measured her heart rate at 160 beats/minute. On inspection, Kristine noted that the patient's jugular vein was markedly distended. She measured 300 ml/hour of bloody fluid draining from the mediastinal tube.

When Kristine reviewed Mrs. Devine's laboratory results, she noted a hematocrit of 19%. The patient was still under the effects of anesthesia, but she opened her eyes when Kristine called her name. Occasionally, she triggered the ventilator.

When assessing Mrs. Devine's hemodynamic profile, Kristine noted the following values:

- *Cardiac index:* 1.6 liters/minute/m²
- *Systemic vascular resistance* (SVR): 680 dynes/second/cm⁻⁵ or absolute units
- *Mean arterial pressure* (MAP): 40 mm Hg
- *Right atrial pressure* (RAP): 17 mm Hg
- *Pulmonary artery diastolic pressure* (PADP): 16 mm Hg
- *Pulmonary artery wedge pressure* (PAWP): 18 mm Hg
- *Mixed venous oxygen saturation* ($S\bar{v}O_2$): 55%.

For Kristine, these findings added up to a suspicion of cardiac tamponade—especially the diastolic equalization of pressures.

Taking the right steps

Knowing that cardiac tamponade is a life-threatening crisis, Kristine notified the doctor immediately. He performed a median sternotomy at the bedside, aspirating 125 ml of blood from the pericardial sac. The procedure immediately improved Mrs. Devine's hemodynamic profile, as Kristine saw when she noted the new values:

- *Cardiac index:* 1.89 liters/minute/m²
- *SVR:* 900 dynes/second/cm⁻⁵ or absolute units
- *MAP:* 80 mm Hg
- *RAP:* 10 to 12 mm Hg
- *PADP:* 12 mm Hg
- *PAWP:* 13 mm Hg
- *$S\bar{v}O_2$:* 68%

Kristine then prepared Mrs. Devine for emergency surgery to identify and control bleeding sites.

---

pear, the patient may progress rapidly to circulatory collapse.

Review the patient's history for a precipitating disorder. Stay alert for characteristic complaints. For instance, in acute tamponade, the patient typically reports sudden onset of dyspnea and chest pain. He also may report retrosternal pain or a feeling of fullness in the head. In chronic tamponade, expect vague complaints, such as malaise, chest discomfort, anorexia, and dyspnea.

Physical examination

Assess your patient's general appearance and demeanor, including his position. With acute tamponade, he may have to sit upright and lean forward to breathe. He may be orthopneic, diaphoretic, and pale and may seem extremely anxious.

Look for the cardinal signs of cardiac tamponade—jugular vein distention (indicating rising venous pressure), decreasing systolic blood pressure with narrowing pulse pressure, muffled heart sounds, extreme tachycardia, and weak peripheral pulses.

Jugular vein distention. Inspect the patient's neck for a distended jugular vein, present in roughly 95% of patients with cardiac tamponade. However, be aware that this sign won't appear if the patient is hypovolemic.

Decreasing systolic blood pressure with narrowing pulse pressure. Measure your patient's blood pressure, correlating the reading with the inspiratory phase of respiration. Cardiac tamponade typically causes pulsus paradoxus—an abnormal decrease in systolic pressure (more than 10 mm Hg) during inspiration. This sign results from impaired peripheral perfusion, a consequence of cardiac decompensation. As the patient inhales, venous return, ventricular filling, and pulmonary blood flow increase, as does the capacity of the pulmonary vascular space. As a result, pulmonary venous return to the left side of the heart declines, reducing left ventricular filling and stroke volume.

Muffled heart sounds. You may have trouble auscultating your patient's heart sounds because fluid sequestration in the pericardial sac increases the distance between the heart and the chest wall.

Extreme tachycardia. In tamponade, expect an increased heart rate as the body desperately tries to improve stroke volume.

Weak peripheral pulses. Palpate peripheral pulses, which commonly are weak in cardiac tamponade.

Diagnostic tests
No single test confirms cardiac tamponade. In patients with acute tamponade and rapid hemodynamic deterioration, the doctor may make the diagnosis from history and physical findings. However, various tests help evaluate the disorder.

Chest X-ray. The cardiac silhouette may be enlarged or normal, depending on how fast the fluid has accumulated and whether the pericardial sac can accommodate the fluid. Other X-ray findings that may indicate tamponade include a slightly widened mediastinum, clear lung fields, and smoothed-out cardiac borders.

ECG. Persistent, diffuse ST-segment elevation suggests acute pericarditis. Electrical alternans (alternating variations in ECG waveform amplitude) is a classic finding in cardiac tamponade. In this abnormal pattern, the P wave, QRS complex, and T wave amplitude or polarity alternate with every other beat.

Echocardiography. This study may not be done if the doctor suspects acute tamponade. However, if cardiac decompensation hasn't occurred, the doctor may order echocardiography to differentiate tamponade from constrictive pericarditis and cardiac muscle dysfunction.

Hemodynamic profile. In cardiac tamponade, expect a persistently low cardiac output (less than 5 liters/minute) or cardiac index (less than 2.2 liters/minute/m^2); hypotension (MAP below 60 mm Hg); a heart rate above 110 beats/minute; narrowed pulse pressure; and similar right and left atrial pressures.

Pulmonary artery systolic pressure is usually normal, and pulmonary artery diastolic pressure (PADP) and right atrial pressure (RAP) are equal. PAWP is elevated and closely approximates PADP and RAP. Systemic vascular resistance increases with progressive reductions in stroke volume. As perfusion declines, mixed venous oxygen saturation ($S\bar{v}O_2$) diminishes.

Ongoing treatment
After emergency pericardiocentesis, when the patient is receiving hemodynamic support, he'll require close monitoring for recurrence of cardiac tamponade and signs suggesting the need for further surgery. (See *Assisting with pericardiocentesis.*)

Surgical intervention will depend on the cause of tamponade and the patient's general condition. For instance, an indwelling pericardial catheter may be inserted to drain or instill medications. A pericardial window, or pericardiectomy, may be done to prevent fluid accumulation.

Assisting with pericardiocentesis

To assist with emergency pericardiocentesis, follow these essential steps:
• Gather a prepared pericardiocentesis tray, a 12-lead electrocardiogram (ECG) machine, and an emergency resuscitation cart with a defibrillator.
• Position the head of the patient's bed at a 45- to 60-degree angle.
• Connect the precordial ECG lead to the hub of the aspiration needle with an alligator clamp and connecting wire.
• Monitor the ECG while the doctor inserts the intracardiac needle (see illustration). If the needle touches the myocardium, ST-segment elevation or premature ventricular contractions will occur.
• If a specimen is needed, have a specimen container ready.
• If the patient has a large amount of fluid in the pericardial sac, the doctor may insert a drain or a through-the-needle catheter to drain the fluid. He may leave the drain or catheter in place until the effusion stops or corrective surgery is performed. If infection occurs, you may instill prescribed antibiotics through the drain, clamp it, and drain the drugs later.
• After the procedure, monitor the patient's vital signs and hemodynamic indicators. Infuse prescribed I.V. solutions or vasopressors, as necessary, to maintain blood pressure. As cardiac compression is relieved, watch for decreased central venous pressure with a concomitant rise in blood pressure.
• Monitor the patient for complications of pericardiocentesis, such as ventricular fibrillation, coronary artery or cardiac chamber puncture (indicated by hemorrhage with clots), and pneumothorax (indicated by sudden dyspnea and dropping blood pressure).

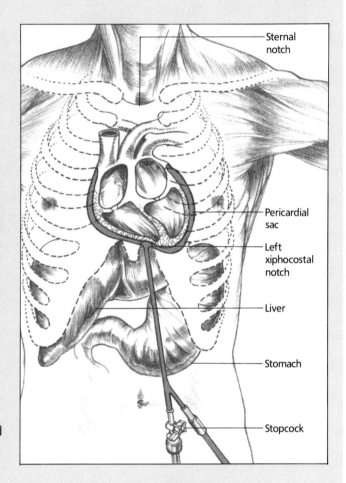

Sternal notch

Pericardial sac

Left xiphocostal notch

Liver

Stomach

Stopcock

Ongoing nursing interventions

Once the patient has been stabilized, your nursing responsibilities include assessing him to detect and prevent complications and tamponade recurrence, and teaching him about the disorder and its treatment.
• Stay alert for signs and symptoms of recurring tamponade, including dyspnea, chest or retrosternal pain, weakness, malaise, chest discomfort, anorexia, and dyspnea.
• Assess the patient for signs and symptoms of infection, including fever, chills, and drainage or redness at the insertion site. Monitor the white blood cell count for elevation.

• Teach the patient about the disorder, any procedures he will undergo, and postoperative treatments (such as chest drainage systems and oxygen). Provide instruction on pulmonary hygiene.

Dissecting aortic aneurysm

Also called aortic dissection, dissecting aortic aneurysm is a localized dilation of the aorta

EMERGENCY INTERVENTIONS

Responding to dissecting aortic aneurysm

A life-threatening emergency, dissecting aortic aneurysm may quickly progress to cardiac tamponade, aortocoronary fistula, or exsanguination. Focus emergency measures on stabilizing the patient's hemodynamic status and preparing him for surgery.

Administer oxygen as ordered. Monitor the patient's blood pressure, pulses, and respirations. Palpate all peripheral pulses for quality and amplitude. Assess skin color, capillary refill, and urine output. Monitor pulmonary artery pressure and central venous pressure.

Administering antihypertensive drugs and colloids

• Give antihypertensive drugs, as ordered, before and during aortography (if time permits this diagnostic test). Expect to give nitroprusside to reduce systolic pressure to below 120 mm Hg. This drug decreases the perioperative risk by making extension or rupture of the dissection less likely.
• Administer isotonic fluids or colloids, as ordered, to maintain pulmonary artery wedge pressure between 12 and 15 mm Hg. This pressure, slightly higher than normal, maximizes cardiac output.

Performing emergency surgery

• If the patient develops a grave complication during initial assessment and management, prepare him for immediate surgery—a median sternotomy or a thoracotomy, depending on the location and extent of the aneurysm in the thoracic aorta. The surgeon exposes the aneurysm and applies clamps above and below it. Then he excises it and replaces it with a preclotted Dacron or Teflon graft sutured in end-to-end fashion. If the aortic valve is insufficient, the surgeon replaces it.

Aneurysms are described according to shape or location. A saccular aneurysm is a vascular outpouching with a small neck that adheres to the arterial wall and involves only a portion of the vessel circumference. A fusiform aneurysm is a spindle-shaped enlargement encompassing the entire aortic circumference. Dissection is most common in the ascending aorta but also occurs in the transverse and descending aorta. (See *Classifying dissecting aortic aneurysm.*)

Dissecting aortic aneurysm most commonly affects men between ages 45 and 70—especially those with Marfan syndrome or congenital heart disease.

Causes

An aortic aneurysm can be congenital or acquired. A congenital aneurysm typically results from Marfan syndrome, Ehlers-Danlos syndrome, coarctation of the aorta, or rheumatic vasculitis.

Arteriosclerosis is the most common cause of acquired aortic aneurysm. A staphylococcal, streptococcal, or salmonella infection also may cause aneurysm; the infection usually originates at the site of arteriosclerotic plaque or a preexisting arterial lesion. Hypertension can induce a descending aortic dissection by destroying the medial vessel layer and decreasing intimal adherence, weakening the aortic wall.

Trauma also may cause an aortic dissection. A descending dissection commonly follows a traumatic injury that shears the aorta transversely, as with an acceleration-deceleration injury (such as a motor vehicle accident) or a penetrating chest injury (such as a stab wound).

Pathophysiology

Dissecting aortic aneurysm occurs when a disorder that increases hemodynamic stress on the aorta damages the media (middle layer), causing the intima (innermost layer) to separate from the media. As the vessel weakens and becomes less elastic, the media and adventitia (outermost layer) stretch outward. Blood flow pressure on the weakened wall ultimately leads to an intimal tear, with hemorrhagic separation of the aortic wall. Blood

characterized by a separation between the layers of the vascular wall, allowing blood to accumulate between the layers, forming an aneurysm. A surgical emergency, it causes death if the aneurysm ruptures. (See *Responding to dissecting aortic aneurysm.*)

Classifying dissecting aortic aneurysm

These drawings illustrate the DeBakey system of classifying dissecting aortic aneurysm (shaded areas) according to location. Dissections can also be classified by their location relative to the aortic valve. Thus, types I and II are proximal; type III is distal.

Type I
In this type of dissection, the most common and lethal, intimal tearing occurs in the ascending aorta, and the dissection extends into the descending aorta.

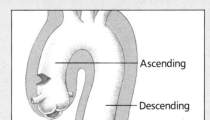

Type II
In this type of dissection, which occurs most commonly with Marfan syndrome, dissection is limited to the ascending or transverse aorta.

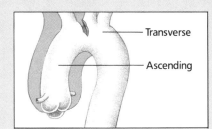

Type III
In this form of dissection, the intimal tear is located in the descending aorta and expands distally.

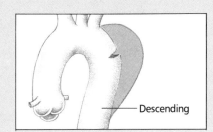

enters the media, forming an outpouching, or dilation. Stress from the resulting turbulent blood flow then dissects the layers of the media, forming a false channel between it and the intima. The heart's contractile force extends the dissection distally and proximally. The column of blood may extend varying distances along the length of the aorta.

With arteriosclerosis, the most common cause of ascending aortic dissection, atheromatous plaque forms in the intimal surface of the artery. The lesion impairs nutrition to the media, causing medial degeneration and weakening. The weakened aortic wall gradually distends the lumen.

Complications
Rupture of an aortic aneurysm into the pericardium leads to acute cardiac tamponade. Even with prompt surgical intervention, this crisis proves fatal in more than 50% of patients.

Assessment
History
An aneurysm typically doesn't cause symptoms until it begins to dissect. Then intense pain occurs (from compression of surrounding structures, from the dissection itself, or both). The pain may resemble MI-related pain and often is misdiagnosed as such.

Be particularly suspicious if the patient reports sudden onset of a severe tearing, ripping, or stabbing pain. The pain may radiate from its point of origin in the direction of the dissection.

Ask the patient where he feels the pain. Interscapular pain suggests dissection in the descending aorta; anterior chest pain signals a dissection in the ascending aorta; pain in the neck, throat, jaw, or teeth suggests an ascending or transverse dissection.

If your patient also complains of hoarseness, dyspnea, throat pain, dysphagia, or dry cough, suspect a transverse aneurysm that's compressing surrounding structures.

Physical examination
Your physical findings help confirm the diagnosis. Try to assess the patient's general appearance, blood pressure, neurologic deficits, and other factors. Keep in mind, however, that in

an emergency, you may not have time to do all of this, so assess him as well as you can.

General appearance. A patient with an aortic dissection will appear pale or cyanotic, diaphoretic, and acutely dyspneic.

Blood pressure. A descending dissection causes elevated blood pressure and a significant differential in systolic pressure between the right and left arms (from occlusion of the brachial arteries). In an ascending dissection, systolic blood pressure is equal bilaterally. If the patient is hypotensive, suspect cardiac tamponade, aneurysm rupture, or dissection of the brachiocephalic vessels, which occludes flow to the brachial artery (the site of blood pressure assessment).

Peripheral pulses. Ascending dissection may cause an abrupt loss of carotid, radial, and femoral pulses. This finding may stem from direct compression by the aneurysm or from occlusion of the arterial lumen by a flap of intima. In either case, however, the loss of pulses is transient because arterial blood pressure affects the position of the aneurysm or intimal flap. In descending dissection, you're less likely to detect peripheral pulse deficits. When they occur, they usually involve the left subclavian and femoral arteries. Carotid and radial pulses may be present and equal bilaterally.

Heart sounds. Stay alert for a diastolic murmur, reflecting aortic insufficiency in ascending dissection. The murmur, which may have a musical quality, may be more audible in the right sternal border at the second intercostal space.

Neurologic deficits. An aortic dissection may cause syncope, transient paralysis, weakness, or even an altered LOC. Although these changes typically occur in ascending dissection, lower extremity deficits may occur with either ascending or descending dissection.

Diagnostic tests
In an asymptomatic patient, aortic dissection is usually diagnosed incidentally, through postero-

anterior and oblique chest X-rays that show widening of the aorta and mediastinum.

Laboratory tests. These tests rarely help confirm dissection. However, with significant hemorrhage or blood sequestration in the aneurysm, the hemoglobin level may be reduced. LDH and bilirubin levels may be elevated from hemolysis of blood within the aneurysm.

Aortography (aortic angiography). This study is the most important diagnostic tool in confirming dissection. The aortogram identifies the tear site and determines the extent of the dissection.

12-lead ECG. This test helps rule out acute MI as the cause of chest pain. However, it's nonspecific for aortic dissection. The ECG commonly shows left ventricular hypertrophy from chronic hypertension.

Other tests. MRI and computed tomography scans help confirm and locate the dissection.

Ongoing treatment
After emergency surgery and other immediate interventions, the patient will require close observation for complications. The doctor may order isotonic solutions or colloids to maintain hemodynamic stability.

If the patient underwent emergency aneurysm repair, he'll require postoperative care as after any type of chest surgery. If sternotomy was done using cardiopulmonary bypass, he'll need close monitoring of hemodynamic parameters, vital signs, urine output, and chest tube drainage. If the aorta was clamped during surgery, the patient must be observed for signs of renal compromise.

Ongoing nursing interventions
After surgery, the patient is especially prone to atelectasis and pneumonia from cardiopulmonary bypass and incisional discomfort. Focus your care on relieving postoperative discomfort, detecting and preventing complications, and teaching the patient about his medical condition and required drug therapy.

• If your patient underwent cardiopulmonary bypass, assess him closely for signs and symptoms of shock or excessive bleeding (100 ml/hour for 3 consecutive hours). Report these findings to the doctor immediately.

• If your patient's aorta was clamped during surgery, stay alert for clinical and laboratory indicators of renal dysfunction—reduced urine output and urine creatinine levels, and increased specific gravity and BUN levels.

• To relieve pain, administer analgesics as prescribed, especially before activity. Assist with turning, coughing, deep breathing, and intermittent positive-pressure breathing as necessary.

• Monitor the patient for signs of infection—fever, incisional redness or drainage, and an elevated white blood cell count. Report these signs to the doctor.

• Before discharge, teach the patient why he must comply with antihypertensive therapy. Describe possible effects of antihypertensive medication. Teach the patient how to monitor his blood pressure. Instruct him to call the doctor immediately if he has a sharp pain in the chest or the back of the neck, which may indicate a recurrence of aortic dissection.

Cardiac arrest

The complete cessation of heart contractions, cardiac arrest severely impairs cardiac output and causes hypoperfusion of the capillary bed. Because brain damage and death occur within minutes, immediate intervention is the patient's only hope. (See *Responding to cardiac arrest,* pages 42 and 43, *Defibrillating your patient,* page 44, and *Administering ACLS drugs,* pages 45 and 46.)

Causes
Immediate precipitating causes of cardiac arrest include ventricular fibrillation, ventricular asystole, and electromechanical dissociation. However, the underlying cause is usually CAD or a complication of CAD.

Ventricular fibrillation may result from acute inferior-wall MI with damage to the sinoatrial node; toxic doses of sympathomimetic drugs (such as dobutamine and dopamine); or antiarrhythmic drugs (such as quinidine and disopyramide), which decrease the fibrillation threshold. Ventricular asystole may stem from hypertrophic cardiomyopathy, acute anterior-wall MI complicated by bundle-branch block, or toxic doses of parasympathomimetic drugs (such as neostigmine and bethanechol).

Cocaine abuse also has been linked to cardiac arrest. The mechanism is unclear, although researchers suspect the drug's potent vasoconstrictive effect increases the heart rate and blood pressure, causing an extremely increased oxygen demand.

Cardiac arrest during surgery, although uncommon, can result from asystole induced by general anesthetics with negative inotropic properties. Hypovolemia, hypoxemia, or hypercapnia during surgery also can induce cardiac arrest. Vagal stimulation associated with surgery can lead to bradycardia and, in turn, cardiac arrest. This most commonly results from ophthalmic surgery or abdominal surgery involving traction on the gallbladder.

Invasive procedures that irritate the myocardium also can induce cardiac arrest. Examples include pulmonary artery catheter insertion, cardiac catheterization, and pacemaker insertion. Vagal stimulation caused by endotracheal intubation, bronchoscopy, and colonoscopy can precipitate bradycardia and asystole, leading to cardiac arrest.

After surgery, the lethal triad of hypothermia, acidosis, and hypokalemia can induce ventricular fibrillation and, in turn, cardiac arrest. This is most common during the early postoperative phase, when the patient's body temperature is low (from vasoconstriction associated with increased afterload). As vasoconstriction reduces perfusion (especially to the lower extremities), acidosis ensues. As acidosis progresses, oxygen use declines and anaerobic metabolism occurs. If the patient also becomes hypokalemic from diuretics administered during surgery or from increased hydration caused by I.V. solutions, myocardial irritability results, triggering ventricular fibrillation.

Hyperkalemia increases the risk of cardiac arrest in many patients. When the potassium

Responding to cardiac arrest

If your patient suffers cardiac arrest, his life could depend on your ability to quickly assess his condition and initiate lifesaving measures.

Suspect cardiac arrest if the patient suddenly collapses and lacks a pulse in major vessels. Then call for help and begin cardiopulmonary resuscitation (CPR) immediately.

Initiating CPR

• Start chest compressions at a rate of approximately 60 per minute. *Important:* If the bedside monitor alarm sounds, don't assume that the monitor is accurate. Instead, check for a pulse before initiating compressions. Performing compressions on a patient with a pulse can cause further myocardial damage.
• If the patient isn't breathing, insert an oral airway into a hand-held resuscitation bag and connect the bag to 100% oxygen. Deliver manual ventilations (approximately 12 per minute) until the code team arrives.
• If the patient is sharing the hospital room, have his roommate removed, if possible.

Establishing I.V. access

• Bring an emergency equipment cart to the bed. Have a colleague insert a peripheral I.V. line and instill dextrose 5% in water at a keep-vein-open rate. This line will serve as the patient's lifeline, providing access for emergency medications.
• Keep in mind that establishing I.V. access early is crucial. As circulatory collapse progresses, inserting an I.V. line becomes increasingly difficult.
• Ensure the patency of any existing I.V. lines. If I.V. access is unavailable, the endotracheal tube offers an alternative route for epinephrine, atropine, and lidocaine delivery.
• Remove the headboard of the bed for easy access during intubation.

Establishing your role in the code team

• When the code team arrives, stay with the patient to provide pertinent information, including the patient's condition when you found him, his medical history, any allergies, and the name of the attending doctor. As appropriate, carry out your duties as a member of the code team.

• During a cardiac arrest, code team members usually assume preassigned roles. The team leader has overall responsibility for running the code, overseeing resuscitation efforts, and directing major lifesaving interventions. Basic rescuer 1 calls for another rescuer and starts one-person CPR. Basic rescuer 2 calls the code team and performs two-person CPR with basic rescuer 1. The nurse anesthetist, anesthesiologist, or respiratory therapist maintains a patent airway, intubates the patient as necessary, administers oxygen as directed, and monitors respiratory status.
• The medication nurse brings a code cart and prepares and administers all medications. (In some hospitals, a pharmacist assists with medication preparation.) The equipment nurse sets up adjunctive emergency equipment, takes the patient's vital signs, and helps with medications as needed. The go-between nurse stays flexible, helping when needed. The recorder nurse documents resuscitation efforts and writes postarrest progress notes.

Initiating ACLS

• As soon as all members of the code team arrive, advanced cardiac life support (ACLS) begins. ACLS aims to provide adequate ventilation; begin, maintain, and support a hemodynamically effective heart rhythm; and maintain and support restored circulation. Specific therapies used in ACLS include CPR, drugs, electrocardiographic monitoring, I.V. access and management, intubation and management, defibrillation or cardioversion, and postarrest stabilization.
• Defibrillation delivers an unsynchronized electrical current to the heart, causing massive simultaneous depolarization of myocardial cells. The cells then repolarize uniformly, allowing the sinoatrial node, the heart's normal pacemaker, to resume control of heart rhythm and rate. Defibrillation is less effective if the patient has acidosis, hypothermia, hypokalemia, or digitalis toxicity. Improper technique also may render it ineffective.
• If the patient has rapid ventricular and supraventricular arrhythmias associated with hypotension, he'll require synchronized cardioversion. This technique synchronizes delivery of current with the R wave of the patient's QRS complex and depolarizes

Responding to cardiac arrest *(continued)*

the myocardium to resume pacing control of the heart. Because it avoids the vulnerable period of the ventricle (the peak of the T wave), it reduces the risk of inducing a lethal arrhythmia such as ventricular fibrillation.

• The patient must continue to receive supplemental oxygen. But remember that ventilating the patient with room air is inadequate and may lead to anaerobic metabolism, interfering with drug therapy, defibrillation, or cardioversion.

The anesthetist will intubate the patient with an oropharyngeal, nasopharyngeal, or esophageal obturator, or an esophageal gastric tube airway. The fraction of inspired oxygen is determined by arterial blood gas values.

• You may be familiar with two new treatment options for cardiac arrest: abdominal compressions and the automatic external defibrillator. Research shows that administering abdominal compressions along with cardiac compressions during CPR achieves higher systolic pressures and cardiac output than using cardiac compressions alone.

The automatic external defibrillator, used extensively by paramedics, identifies specific ventricular arrhythmias and delivers an electric current only if the patient has ventricular fibrillation. Studies show that the device delivers current faster and more effectively than a manual defibrillator. Its major benefit is in nonhospital settings, where public safety personnel can use it for early intervention.

level rises, the concentration gradient for ion exchange across the cell membrane falls and myocardial excitability decreases, leading to widening ECG complexes and finally asystole.

Trauma may cause cardiac arrest by inducing severe hypoxia and profound metabolic acidosis. The risk for cardiac arrest also increases with ectopic beats, including more than six premature ventricular contractions (PVCs) per minute, three or more successive PVCs, multifocal PVCs, bigeminy, and R-on-T phenomenon. Other causes of cardiac arrest include extreme vagal stimulation (as from straining) and extreme psychological stress.

Pathophysiology

The arrhythmias most commonly identified during cardiac arrest are ventricular fibrillation, ventricular asystole, and electromechanical dissociation. (See *Common ECG arrhythmias in cardiac arrest,* page 47.)

In ventricular fibrillation, the ventricular rhythm is rapid and chaotic, indicating varying degrees of depolarization and repolarization. The patient lacks a pulse, heart sounds, and

blood pressure. This arrhythmia commonly results from ischemia, characterized by a sudden drop in the amplitude and duration of the action potential. Reduced myocardial excitability slows electrical conduction and causes electrophysiologically unstable cell membranes. Normal myocardial cells then respond with premature impulses, making the myocardium vulnerable to reentrant arrhythmias and ultimately ventricular fibrillation.

In ventricular asystole (cardiac standstill), electrical activity in the ventricles ceases. Myocardial cells aren't depolarized, and action potentials are absent.

In electromechanical dissociation, a heart rhythm appears on the ECG monitor but myocardial contraction is ineffective. The patient lacks a palpable pulse. Electromechanical dissociation may result from massive pulmonary embolism, a malfunctioning prosthetic heart valve, or cardiac tamponade.

Complications

Cardiac arrest leads to irreversible brain damage within 4 to 6 minutes and to death within

Defibrillating your patient

Step 1
Apply low-resistance conduction gel or paste to the electrode paddles (or apply pads soaked with 0.9% sodium chloride solution to the patient).

Step 2
Turn on the defibrillator, checking to make sure the machine isn't in the synchronous mode.

Step 3
Select the appropriate energy level and activate the capacitor. Then charge the defibrillator (which may take a few seconds).

Step 4
Once the capacitor reaches the appropriate energy level, make sure the patient's cardiac rhythm is unchanged (still ventricular fibrillation or ventricular tachycardia). Quickly assess his level of consciousness.

Step 5
Order the area cleared. To avoid electric shock, check to make sure no one — including yourself — is in contact with the bed, the equipment, or the patient.

Step 6
Position the paddles and apply firm pressure (25 lb).

Step 7
Reassess the patient's cardiac rhythm. Make sure he's in ventricular fibrillation or ventricular tachycardia.

Step 8
Discharge (fire) the defibrillator. On most machines, you must press both buttons on both paddles. If the shock is delivered, you should see chest muscle contraction. If you don't, recheck the machine's power supply to ensure that the synchronizer circuit is off, the machine is plugged in, and, if a battery is used, that it's sufficiently charged.

Step 9
Assess the patient's pulse and electrocardiogram immediately after defibrillation. If ventricular fibrillation or ventricular tachycardia persists, make a second attempt as quickly as the machine will allow.

Step 10
Document the procedure, including the energy level used and the response obtained. Include an ECG strip in the documentation record.

Paddle placement for defibrillation

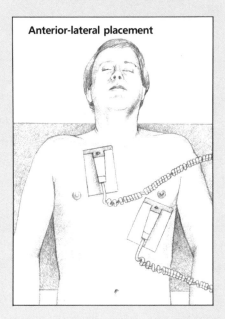

Anterior-lateral placement

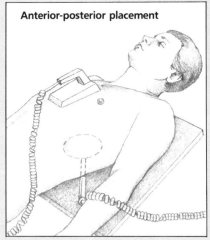

Anterior-posterior placement

10 minutes, depending on the patient's condition, the nature of the arrest, and the elapsed time between onset of symptoms and initiation of cardiopulmonary resuscitation (CPR).

The patient may develop complications after successful resuscitation. Some complications arise from improper resuscitation technique. For instance, chest compressions (precordial thumps) may cause further myocardial damage when performed on a patient with a pulse. For this reason, always establish that the patient has no pulse before performing compres-

Administering ACLS drugs

During cardiac arrest or another cardiovascular crisis, you may administer any of the advanced cardiac life support (ACLS) drugs listed here. Most act either to control the heart rhythm and rate or to improve cardiac output and blood pressure through peripheral vasoconstriction and inotropic or chronotropic cardiac effects.

DRUG AND INDICATION	DOSAGE	SPECIAL CONSIDERATIONS
Adenosine Conversion of paroxysmal supraventricular tachycardia to sinus rhythm	Give 6 mg by rapid I.V. push. If no effect within 2 minutes, give 12 mg by rapid I.V. push. Repeat 12-mg dose in 2 minutes if still no effect. Doses over 12 mg are not recommended.	• Because it lowers conduction, adenosine may produce transient heart block. • Use cautiously in patients receiving dipyridamole or carbamazepine.
Amrinone lactate Congestive heart failure	Give one 0.75-mg/kg dose I.V. over 2 to 3 minutes, followed by 5 to 10 mcg/kg/minute by I.V. infusion.	• Amrinone may exacerbate myocardial ischemia in dosages greater than 20 mcg/kg/minute.
Atropine sulfate Sinus bradycardia with hemodynamic compromise; sinus bradycardia with frequent ventricular ectopic beats; ventricular asystole	*For bradycardia:* 0.5 mg I.V. every 5 minutes to a total of 2 mg. *For asystole:* 1 mg I.V.; repeat after 5 minutes if asystole persists.	• Atropine may be given endotracheally. • Doses below 0.5 mg have parasympathomimetic effects and therefore may slow the heart rate. • Use cautiously in acute myocardial ischemia or infarction; excessive amounts may widen areas of ischemia or infarction.
Bretylium tosylate Resistant ventricular tachycardia or fibrillation	*For resistant ventricular tachycardia:* 5 to 10 mg/kg diluted to 50 ml with dextrose 5% in water (D₅W) and injected I.V. over 8 to 10 minutes. Follow loading dose with a continuous I.V. infusion at 1 to 2 mg/minute. *For resistant ventricular fibrillation:* 5 mg/kg by I.V. bolus followed by defibrillation. If indicated, increase dose to 10 mg/kg and give at 15- to 30-minute intervals to a maximum of 30 mg/kg.	• Don't use as a first-line drug. Use only if lidocaine and defibrillation fail to convert ventricular fibrillation, if lidocaine fails to prevent ventricular fibrillation from recurring, or if lidocaine and procainamide fail to control ventricular tachycardia. • Bretylium may take 2 minutes to reach the central circulation.
Dobutamine hydrochloride Heart failure	Give 2.5 to 10 mcg/kg/minute I.V.	• Dobutamine may induce reflex peripheral vasodilation. • As ordered, give with nitroprusside sodium for synergistic effect. • Monitor the heart rate closely. An increase of 10% or more may exacerbate myocardial ischemia (a common problem at dosages above 20 mcg/kg/minute). Hemodynamic monitoring is required.
Dopamine hydrochloride Shock	Give 2 to 5 mcg/kg/minute I.V. initially, and titrate according to response.	• At low dosages (1 to 2 mcg/kg/minute), dopamine dilates renal and mesenteric vessels without increasing heart rate or blood pressure. At higher dosages (2 to 10 mcg/kg/minute), it primarily stimulates beta receptors, increasing cardiac output without peripheral vasoconstriction. At dosages above 10 mcg/kg/minute, it stimulates alpha receptors, causing peripheral vasoconstriction. • Don't give dopamine in the same I.V. line as sodium bicarbonate. The alkaline solution may inactivate dopamine. • Hemodynamic monitoring is required.
Epinephrine hydrochloride Cardiac arrest	Give 1 mg (5 to 10 ml of a 1:10,000 solution) I.V. or 1 mg (10 ml of a 1:10,000 solution) endotracheally. Repeat every 5 minutes during resuscitation efforts.	• Intracardiac injection is contraindicated unless I.V. and endotracheal routes are unavailable. Intracardiac injection interrupts resuscitation efforts and may cause such complications as coronary artery laceration, cardiac tamponade, and pneumothorax. • Don't give in same I.V. line as sodium bicarbonate or any other alkaline solution.

(continued)

Administering ACLS drugs (continued)

DRUG AND INDICATION	DOSAGE	SPECIAL CONSIDERATIONS
Isoproterenol hydrochloride Hemodynamically significant bradycardia unresponsive to atropine (in a patient with a pulse)	Add 1 mg to 500 ml of D_5W. Give 2 to 10 mcg/minute by I.V. infusion. Titrate according to heart rate and rhythm response.	• Isoproterenol is not indicated in cardiac arrest. • The drug's potent inotropic and chronotropic effects increase cardiac output and work load, exacerbating ischemia and arrhythmias in patients with ischemic heart disease. • Use this drug only as a temporary measure until pacemaker therapy begins.
Lidocaine Ventricular tachycardia or fibrillation; premature ventricular contractions (PVCs) that are frequent, closely coupled, multifocal, or arranged in short bursts of two or more in succession; myocardial infarction (to prevent ventricular fibrillation)	Give 1 mg/kg by I.V. bolus, followed by 0.5-mg/kg boluses every 8 to 10 minutes, as necessary, to a total of 3 mg/kg.	• Lidocaine may be used prophylactically when myocardial infarction is suspected but not confirmed. • In ventricular fibrillation, lidocaine improves response to defibrillation. • Give only bolus doses during resuscitation efforts. After resuscitation, give a continuous infusion at 2 to 4 mg/minute. (Reduce dosage and monitor blood drug levels after 24 hours, as ordered.) • Monitor for signs of central nervous system toxicity.
Nitroglycerin Congestive heart failure; unstable angina	Give 10 mcg/minute I.V. Increase dosage in increments of 5 to 10 mcg/minute, as needed.	• Most patients respond to 200 mcg/minute or less. Mean dosage range is 50 to 500 mcg/minute. • Monitor for hypotension, an adverse reaction that exacerbates myocardial ischemia. Hemodynamic monitoring is required.
Nitroprusside sodium Heart failure; hypertensive crisis	Add 50 mg to 1,000 ml of D_5W. Initially, give 10 to 20 mcg/minute.	• Wrap drug container in opaque material; light causes drug deterioration. (However, you don't need to wrap I.V. tubing.) • Hemodynamic monitoring is required.
Norepinephrine Severe hypotension with low total peripheral resistance	Add 4 or 8 mg to 500 ml of D_5W or dextrose 5% in 0.9% sodium chloride solution. Administer the resulting concentration (8 and 16 mcg/ml, respectively) I.V., titrating according to patient response.	• Norepinephrine is contraindicated in hypovolemia. • Cardiac output may increase or decrease after norepinephrine administration, depending on vascular resistance, left ventricular function, and reflex responses. • Don't give in the same I.V. line as alkaline solutions. • Monitor blood pressure with an intra-arterial line because standard measurements may be falsely low.
Procainamide hydrochloride Ventricular arrhythmias, such as PVCs or tachycardia, when lidocaine is contraindicated or ineffective	In an emergency, give 20 mg/minute up to a total dose of 1 g. Usual dosage is 50 mg I.V. every 5 minutes until the desired response is achieved, up to a total of 1 g. Maintenance infusion rate is 1 to 4 mg/minute.	• Reduce dosage in patients with renal failure. • Guard against too-rapid infusion, which causes acute hypotension. Use particular caution in patients with acute myocardial infarction. • Monitor for widening QRS complex. If QRS complex widens more than 50%, notify doctor and discontinue infusion, as ordered.
Verapamil hydrochloride Atrial arrhythmias, especially paroxysmal supraventricular tachycardia with atrioventricular node conduction	Give 5 mg I.V. initially, followed by 10 mg in 15 to 30 minutes if the arrhythmia persists and the patient hasn't responded adversely to the initial dose.	• Monitor for hypotension, severe bradycardia, congestive heart failure, and facilitated accessory conduction in patients with Wolff-Parkinson-White syndrome.

Common ECG arrhythmias in cardiac arrest

Three arrhythmias detectable by an electrocardiogram that usually occur in cardiac arrest are *ventricular fibrillation, ventricular asystole,* and *electromechanical dissociation.* Use this chart to help you identify and define them as you monitor the patient and identify corresponding signs and symptoms.

Ventricular fibrillation

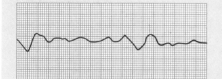

- Ventricular rhythm rapid and chaotic, indicating varying degrees of depolarization and repolarization; QRS complexes not identifiable
- Patient unconscious at onset
- Absent pulses, heart sounds, and blood pressure
- Dilated pupils; rapid development of cyanosis

Ventricular asystole

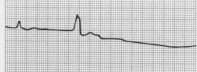

- Ventricular electrical activity absent
- Possible P waves
- Possible severe metabolic deficit or extensive myocardial damage

Electromechanical dissociation

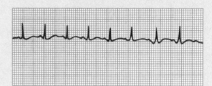

- Electrical activity but no pulse
- Organized electrical activity with no evidence of effective myocardial contraction
- Possible failure in calcium transport system (can cause electromechanical dissociation)
- Possible association with profound hypovolemia, cardiac tamponade, myocardial rupture, massive myocardial infarction, or tension pneumothorax

sions. (See *ACLS guidelines for ventricular fibrillation and pulseless ventricular tachycardia,* page 48.)

Even when performed properly, CPR can cause rib or sternum fracture, separation of the ribs from the sternum, pneumothorax, hemothorax, lung contusion, laceration of the liver and spleen, or fat emboli.

Multisystem organ failure also may occur. This complication can lead to adult respiratory distress syndrome, disseminated intravascular coagulation, shock, and neurologic deficits. (See Chapter 7, Multisystem Crises.)

Assessment
History
After initial lifesaving interventions, explore the patient's history, asking witnesses (if any) what happened. Because cardiac arrest is most commonly associated with CAD, find out if the patient has a history of CAD. Also find out if he has received sympathomimetics or parasympa-

thomimetics or if he uses cocaine. All of these drugs increase the risk of cardiac arrest.

Physical examination
The patient in cardiac arrest has an absent or extremely slow heart rate (typically less than 40 beats/minute) or a chaotic heart rhythm (ventricular fibrillation).

Expect the patient to be pulseless and unresponsive. If he's attached to an ECG monitor, check for ventricular fibrillation, ventricular asystole, or electromechanical dissociation. However, keep in mind that pulselessness *always* indicates cardiac arrest, regardless of which rhythm appears on the ECG monitor. Find out if the cardiac arrest was witnessed.

Determine if the patient is making any attempts at breathing. Assess him for signs and symptoms of reduced cardiac output, such as narrowing pulse pressure (systolic pressure usually drops more than diastolic pressure); sluggish capillary refill; mentation changes; cool,

ACLS guidelines for ventricular fibrillation and pulseless ventricular tachycardia

The following chart outlines the advanced cardiac life support (ACLS) steps you should take to treat ventricular fibrillation or pulseless ventricular tachycardia. Even if you're not ACLS certified, the chart will tell you what to expect in such an emergency.

Establish responsiveness
▼
Check pulse. If no pulse, then:
▼
Perform CPR until a defibrillator is available.
▼
Check rhythm. If ventricular fibrillation or tachycardia appears, then:
▼
Defibrillate using 200 joules
▼
Defibrillate using 200 to 300 joules
▼
Defibrillate using 360 joules.
▼
If ventricular fibrillation or tachycardia persists, then:
▼
Continue CPR
▼
Intubate as soon as possible
▼
Establish I.V. access
▼
Administer epinephrine, 1:10,000, 1 mg I.V. push every 3 to 5 minutes
▼
Defibrillate using 360 joules, 30 to 60 seconds after epinephrine
▼
Administer lidocaine 1.5 mg/kg I.V. push
▼
Defibrillate using 360 joules
▼
Administer bretylium, 5 mg/kg I.V. push
▼
Defibrillate using 360 joules
▼
Administer bretylium, 10 mg/kg I.V. push (consider sodium bicarbonate)
▼
Defibrillate using 360 joules
▼
Repeat lidocaine or bretylium
▼
Defibrillate using 360 joules.

pale, moist skin; decreased pulse amplitude; and adventitious breath sounds.

Diagnostic tests
After resuscitation, the doctor may order tests to determine the cause of cardiac arrest and to evaluate the effects of treatment.

12-lead ECG. This may pinpoint acute MI as the underlying cause of cardiac arrest.

Cardiac enzymes. Elevated levels suggest MI.

Serum potassium. An above- or below-normal serum potassium level may point to hyperkalemia or hypokalemia as the precipitating cause of cardiac arrest.

ABG analysis. ABG values may reveal extreme hypoxia or an acute acid-base disturbance as the cause of cardiac arrest.

Chest X-ray. This may identify an abnormality resulting from trauma.

Ongoing treatment
After the patient has been successfully resuscitated and is somewhat stabilized, the doctor will tailor ongoing treatment to the cause of cardiac arrest, the underlying pathophysiology, and any complications that arise.

If drug therapy fails to prevent arrhythmia recurrence, the patient may be a candidate for an implantable cardioverter defibrillator. This device is a small pulse generator implanted in the patient's abdomen. One of its three leads senses the heart rate at the right ventricle, the second lead senses rhythm and defibrillates at the right atrium, and the third lead defibrillates at the apical pericardium. The device can be programmed to suit the patient's specific needs, and it uses far less energy (25 joules on the first attempt) than an external defibrillator (360 joules). If your patient receives an implantable cardioverter defibrillator, be sure to teach him and his family about its use and provide emotional support.

Ongoing nursing interventions

Your nursing responsibilities include monitoring and ensuring an adequate cardiopulmonary status and identifying any complications that arise.

• Carefully monitor hemodynamic indicators. Assess for heart rate and rhythm changes, S_3, and jugular vein distention. Measure blood pressure, staying alert for hypotension. Check the patient's capillary refill, urine output, peripheral pulse quality, mentation, and skin color and temperature. If these indicators suggest low cardiac output, administer prescribed drugs or fluids as appropriate.

• Closely evaluate the patient's respiratory status. Auscultate for adequate breath sounds and assess the rate, depth, and quality of respirations. If the patient is on a mechanical ventilator, determine if he's assisting it. Make sure he's being ventilated according to his ABG values. If these values show persistent acidosis, administer sodium bicarbonate as ordered.

• Check for neurologic complications, such as brain anoxia, by assessing the patient's LOC using the Glasgow Coma Scale. An altered LOC may indicate cerebral edema, possibly from cerebral hypoxia during cardiac arrest.

• Assess the patient's risk of recurrence of cardiac arrest. The risk of recurrence depends on the cause of cardiac arrest. If the chance for recurrence is high, inform the patient and the family so that they can receive instruction in CPR. As appropriate, arrange for them to enroll in CPR classes.

You may want to teach the high-risk patient how to perform cough CPR. Currently under investigation, this procedure is a self-administered form of CPR using the cough reflex. When the patient recognizes symptoms of a dangerous arrhythmia, he coughs in continuous, forced spurts 1 to 3 seconds apart to help maintain consciousness for up to 30 seconds. Performing cough CPR until help arrives may convert the lethal arrhythmia to a more benign one. Coughing raises intrathoracic pressure and propels blood forward, enhancing perfusion to the myocardium and cerebrum and maintaining cardiac output.

• Teach the patient about prescribed drug therapy. If he has continuing arrhythmias, expect him to be discharged on combination antiarrhythmic therapy. Antiarrhythmics have a narrow therapeutic range, so tell the patient he'll require careful monitoring for adverse effects.

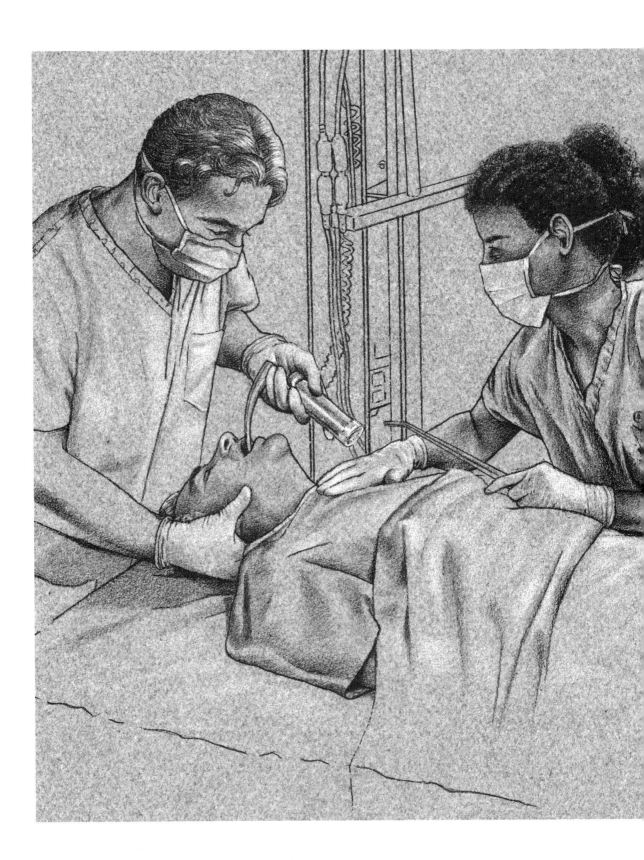

CHAPTER 2

Respiratory crises

In a respiratory crisis, you must act swiftly to avert possible death. Depending on your hospital's policy, your duties as a nurse may include performing primary assessment, carrying out life-support measures, or assisting the doctor in caring for the patient.

This chapter covers all aspects of managing respiratory crises and explains exactly what you need to know and do to safeguard your patient. Specifically, it covers pulmonary embolism, adult respiratory distress syndrome, pneumothorax, hemothorax, pulmonary edema, flail chest, and status asthmaticus. For each of these crises, you'll find a thorough discussion of its causes and pathophysiology to help you understand why you take a particular action. You'll also find coverage of complications, assessment techniques, emergency interventions, and treatment. What's more, you'll review ongoing nursing interventions, which explain your responsibilities in caring for the patient after he has received initial treatment.

Pulmonary embolism

A pulmonary embolism occurs when a mass, such as a dislodged thrombus, either partially or completely obstructs a branch of the pulmonary artery. When the embolus lodges in a vessel that's too small for it to pass through, tissue infarction occurs distal to the occlusion.

This infarction may be mild enough to not cause any symptoms. However, a massive embolism (obstruction of more than 50% of pulmonary arterial circulation) and infarction can cause rapid death. With this in mind, you should begin treating a patient with a suspected or diagnosed pulmonary embolism as soon as possible. (See *Treating pulmonary embolism.*)

Causes

An embolus may originate from a substance produced by the body: a thrombus, fat, amniotic fluid, or tumor cells. It may also be caused by something outside the body: air, clumps of bacteria, or foreign materials such as catheter fragments.

About 90% of all pulmonary embolisms result from a dislodged thrombus originating in the deep veins of the legs. Less common sources of thrombi include the pelvic, renal, and hepatic veins, the right side of the heart, and the upper extremities.

EMERGENCY INTERVENTIONS

Treating pulmonary embolism

Your first goal in treating pulmonary embolism is to maintain cardiac and pulmonary function until the obstruction resolves.

Your second goal is to prevent a recurrence of the embolism by administering heparin by continuous infusion, if necessary. Target the partial thromboplastin time to about 2 to 2½ times the control level; to achieve this, infuse approximately 25,000 units of heparin per 24 hours.

If your patient has a massive pulmonary embolism with shock or has an air embolism, he'll need additional treatment.

Massive pulmonary embolism with shock

If your patient has a massive pulmonary embolism and is in shock, he may need fibrinolytic therapy with streptokinase, urokinase, or alteplase to lyse the existing clots. At first, these thrombolytic agents will dissolve clots within 12 to 14 hours. Seven days later, these drugs lyse clots to the same degree as heparin does.

Air embolism

If your patient has had recent manipulation of a central venous catheter, you or another member of your health care team may assess the patient's problem as an air embolism.

Suspect an air embolism any time a central line has been repositioned or redressed or has had the tubing changed, which may result in air being introduced into the central line (which leads directly to the heart).

Place the patient in the left lateral decubitus position with his head down. This position should divert air in the right ventricular outflow tract to the right atrium, away from the pulmonary artery, reducing the risk of air bubbles entering the pulmonary circulation. Blood flow from the right ventricle improves, maintaining cardiac output. Because this position increases intrathoracic pressure, it helps prevent more air from being drawn into the circulation through the catheter site during inspiration.

Administer 100% oxygen through a nonrebreather face mask to relieve hypoxia and improve oxygen concentration in the blood. An air embolism is about 80% nitrogen, which easily diffuses across alveoli. Giving 100% oxygen lowers nitrogen levels in the alveoli, increasing the rate at which nitrogen is absorbed from the embolus. This reduces the size of the embolus and eliminates it through the lungs more quickly.

The thrombus forms because of vascular wall damage or abnormalities, venous stasis, or excessive coagulation. Trauma, clot dissolution, sudden muscle spasm, intravascular pressure changes, or a change in peripheral blood flow can cause the thrombus to loosen or become fragmented.

Patients at risk for developing emboli include those with preexisting lung disease, hypercapnia, and hypoxemia, which elevate the red blood cell (RBC) count (polycythemia). The polycythemia thickens the blood and creates a more sluggish flow.

In patients with congestive heart failure (CHF) and advanced pulmonary disease, clots may form in the right ventricle. Atrial fibrillation may cause the formation of mural thrombi on the endothelial walls of the right atrium, resulting in incomplete emptying of the right atrium and blood stasis. (See *Who's at risk for pulmonary embolism?*)

Pathophysiology

Normally, the lungs filter clots and other substances that are larger than the diameter of the formed elements in blood. Fibrolytic mechanisms in the lungs can dissolve small clots, but they can't dissolve a single large clot or multiple small clots without causing life-threatening symptoms.

If a thrombus breaks loose, becoming an embolus, and doesn't lodge in transit, it travels through the venous circulation to the right side of the heart and lodges in the lung in a branch of the pulmonary artery. Because of increased blood flow to the region, the embolus most commonly lodges in the right lower lobe. There the embolus may dissolve, continue to fragment, or grow. Nonthrombotic emboli, such as liquid, fat, amniotic fluid, and gaseous emboli, can change shape and pass through the pulmonary capillary bed to the left side of the heart, eventually entering the systemic circulation.

Obstruction and vasoconstriction from neurohumoral stimuli increase pulmonary artery pressure and pulmonary vascular resistance. When a branch of the pulmonary artery is occluded, a ventilation-perfusion mismatch occurs. This means that a portion of the lung is

still being ventilated, but no blood is flowing to pick up oxygen and remove carbon dioxide. To maintain adequate gas exchange, ventilation then increases in the uninvolved lung areas. The airways distal to the embolus constrict and the alveoli shrink and collapse, shifting ventilation away from the poorly perfused area. Atelectasis may follow. If the embolus enlarges, it may occlude most or all of the pulmonary vessels. Pulmonary infarction, or lung tissue death, occurs in about 10% of pulmonary embolism patients, most often those with chronic cardiac or pulmonary disease.

Complications

Complications of pulmonary embolism include hepatic congestion and necrosis, lung abscess, shock, adult respiratory distress syndrome, massive atelectasis, and venous overload.

Who's at risk for pulmonary embolism?

Early recognition and prompt diagnosis of pulmonary embolism can reduce mortality from 40% to 10%. Patients with the following conditions and disorders are at increased risk for developing pulmonary emboli and should be closely monitored:
• lung disorders, especially chronic types
• cardiac disorders
• infection
• diabetes mellitus
• history of thromboembolism, thrombophlebitis, or vascular insufficiency
• sickle cell disease
• autoimmune hemolytic anemia
• polycythemia
• osteomyelitis
• long-bone fracture
• manipulation or disconnection of central lines
• venous stasis resulting from prolonged bed rest, immobilization, or obesity
• venous injury resulting from surgery, particularly of the legs, pelvis, abdomen, or thorax; leg or pelvic fractures or injuries; I.V. drug abuse; or I.V. therapy
• increased blood coagulability caused by cancer or the use of high-estrogen oral contraceptives
• other factors, such as age over 40, burns, dehydration, eclampsia, recent childbirth (especially cesarean section), or orthopedic casts.

Assessment

History

You'll need to act quickly when you suspect pulmonary embolism, but you shouldn't skip history taking. Remember the three risk factors for pulmonary embolism: hypercoagulability of the blood, vascular wall abnormalities, and venous stasis—commonly referred to as Virchow's triad.

Determine if the patient has a history of clotting disorders, polycythemia vera, sickle cell anemia, fever, or dehydration. Ask a female patient if she's pregnant or taking oral contraceptives. Patients with vascular wall abnormalities are more susceptible to thrombus formation from local trauma, atherosclerosis, and varicose veins. Venous stasis can result from extended bed rest, obesity, and CHF with subsequent decreased myocardial contractility and atrial fibrillation.

Find out if the patient has recently had a central venous line removed, a tubing change, or new fluids infused. Air can enter the patient's circulation through the catheter or the catheter site directly into the venous circulation, causing an air embolism.

Physical examination

The most significant sign of pulmonary embolism is the sudden onset of dyspnea. During the physical examination, does the patient complain of shortness of breath for no apparent reason or pleuritic or anginal pain? The extent of lung damage, along with the size, number, and location of the emboli, determines the severity of the symptoms. Total occlusion of the pulmonary artery results in severe dyspnea. Other key signs and symptoms include hypoxia, chest pain, and coughing with hemoptysis.

A large embolus may cause cyanosis, syncope, and distended neck veins. If you observe restlessness—a sign of hypoxia—the patient may be experiencing circulatory collapse. Acute right ventricular failure may produce hepatomegaly, increased central venous pressure (CVP), and distended neck veins.

If the patient complains of chest pain, bear in mind that chest pain caused by pulmonary embolism mimics that caused by a myocardial infarction (MI). You may find that the patient has tachycardia, tachypnea, and a low-grade fever if he's experiencing impending cardiovascular or circulatory collapse. If circulatory collapse has occurred, he'll have a weak, rapid pulse rate and hypotension.

A cough that produces blood-tinged sputum may also be a sign of pulmonary embolism. You may observe chest splinting, massive hemoptysis, and leg edema as well. Also inspect the patient's neck, chest, axillae, and conjunctivae for petechiae, which may develop from fat emboli. Mental status changes include restlessness, irritability, confusion, and feelings of impending doom. Palpation may reveal a warm, tender area in the extremities, a possible area of thrombosis. Auscultation of the lungs may reveal crackles.

When you auscultate the heart, listen for a loud pulmonic closure (P_2), which may indicate pulmonary hypertension secondary to pulmonary embolism. Remember, the second heart sound (S_2) consists of the sound made by the aortic valve closing (A_2 followed by P_2). Normally, A_2 is louder than P_2. You may also note an S_3 and S_4 gallop, with increased intensity of the pulmonic component of S_2.

Don't overlook dehydration—particularly common in older people—as a risk factor for the development of pulmonary emboli. (See *Characteristic findings in pulmonary embolism.*)

Diagnostic tests

Though not always conclusive, laboratory tests may support a diagnosis of pulmonary embolism. Arterial blood gas (ABG) analysis may show a decreased partial pressure of arterial oxygen (PaO_2), indicating hypoxemia, and a decreased partial pressure of arterial carbon dioxide ($PaCO_2$), indicating tachypnea. Thoracentesis can sometimes rule out empyema, a sign of pneumonia, if the patient has a pleural effusion.

An electrocardiogram (ECG) helps distinguish pulmonary embolism from MI. If the patient has an extensive embolism, the ECG shows right axis deviation, right bundle-branch

Characteristic findings in pulmonary embolism

Pulmonary embolism produces characteristic effects that may be uncovered by physical examination, chest X-ray, electrocardiogram (ECG), and hemodynamic monitoring.

Physical examination
When assessing a patient with pulmonary embolism, look for anxiety or apprehension, headache, and fatigue; shortness of breath, cyanosis, tachypnea, pleuritic pain on inspiration (nonradiating), hemoptysis, pleural friction rub, and dry cough; and tachycardia, increased jugular vein distention, accentuated S_2, S_3, and S_4, palpitations, and pulsus paradoxus. Check for diaphoresis, pale cool skin, petechiae, fever and flu-like symptoms, symptoms of phlebitis, and recent pelvic or long-bone fracture that can lead to fat emboli.

Chest X-ray
Look for usually clear, nonspecific infiltrates initially. In later X-rays look for atelectasis with decreased ventilation, pleural effusions, prominent pulmonary arteries, and an elevated diaphragm.

ECG
Be alert for unexplained arrhythmias, an elevated ST segment, atrial flutter, and sinus tachycardia when monitoring the patient with an ECG. Also watch for transient right bundle-branch block, right axis deviation, and right ventricular hypertrophy. Observe the monitor for inverted T waves in leads V_1 and V_4 and large P waves in leads II, III, and aV_F.

Hemodynamic monitoring
Watch hemodynamic indices closely even though many may be normal. Cardiac output will be normal in most patients with pulmonary embolism, although it can be increased or decreased if the embolus affects blood flow to more than 40% of the lung field. Central venous pressure will be normal, too, although it can be elevated if the embolus affects blood flow to more than 35% of the lung field. Systemic vascular resistance and pulmonary artery wedge pressure will be normal; pulmonary artery systolic and diastolic pressures will be elevated or normal. Only pulmonary vascular resistance may be greatly elevated.

---

block, depressed ST segments, T-wave inversions (a sign of right ventricular heart strain), supraventricular tachyarrhythmias, and tall, peaked P waves. With massive pulmonary embolism, electromechanical dissociation may develop. It occurs when a patient has no pulse but the ECG shows electrical activity—usually bradycardia or second- or third-degree heart block. This patient is hemodynamically in asystole, with no discernable blood pressure and no palpable pulse, and requires immediate cardiopulmonary resuscitation. (See *Distinguishing between pulmonary embolism and MI*, page 57.)

Though inconclusive in the first 1 to 2 hours after embolism, a chest X-ray can rule out other pulmonary diseases. It may show areas of atelectasis, an elevated diaphragm, pleural effusion, and a prominent pulmonary artery. Occasionally, a chest X-ray will reveal the characteristic wedge-shaped infiltrate that suggests pulmonary infarction.

Nuclear medicine testing includes ventilation-perfusion scans, pulmonary angiography, and magnetic resonance imaging (MRI). Lung scans can be useful; however, ventilation-perfusion scans are preferred because they can show areas of normal ventilation but poor perfusion. Pulmonary angiography may reveal pulmonary vessel filling defects or a complete occlusion (an abrupt vessel ending), both of which indicate pulmonary embolism. Although pulmonary angiography is the most definitive test, it is used only if the diagnosis can't be confirmed any other way. That's because it is costly and puts the patient at risk for bleeding from the puncture site, for cardiac perforations, and for cardiac arrhythmias. MRI can more safely identify blood flow changes that point to an embolus or identify the embolus itself.

Ongoing treatment
Therapy for a patient with pulmonary embolism begins with administration of oxygen to

relieve hypoxia, followed by sedation for pain and anxiety. The sedative also helps to reduce the patient's oxygen consumption by decreasing metabolic demands. Fluids help treat hypotension and, if necessary, a vasopressor may be added.

Drug treatment
Anticoagulant therapy may consist of heparin or a combination of heparin and dihydroergotamine, which proves more effective than heparin alone. Once the patient can walk again, he'll be switched to warfarin.

Heparin is administered in a bolus dose, usually 5,000 to 10,000 units, followed by a continuous infusion of 1,000 units/hour to help prevent formation of clots. (The drug has no fibrinolytic properties, so it can't destroy clots that have already formed.) This dosage is adjusted to keep the patient's partial thromboplastin time at 2 to 2½ times the control level. A septic embolus requires antibiotic therapy, not anticoagulants, and evaluation for the infection's source, which is most likely endocarditis.

Surgery
Surgery may be necessary for patients who don't respond to conventional therapy, who experience recurrent thromboemboli, or who can't take anticoagulants. Surgery consists of vena caval ligation or plication or insertion of a vena cava umbrella that filters blood clots traveling through the systemic venous circulation to the right side of the heart. Angiographic demonstration of pulmonary embolism should take place before surgery.

Ongoing nursing interventions
• Regularly check the stools and urine of patients with either suspected or confirmed pulmonary embolism. As with any patient on anticoagulant therapy, look for occult blood in stools. Tea-colored urine may indicate hematuria and should be reported immediately.
• Watch for easy bruising, bleeding gums, epistaxis, and petechiae. Also watch for hematomas at I.V. sites after venipunctures. Don't administer I.M. injections to anyone undergoing anticoagulant therapy.

• Watch for anticoagulant treatment complications, including gastric bleeding, cerebrovascular accident, and hemorrhage.
• Assess a bedridden patient for Homans' sign: Flex the patient's knee and then firmly dorsiflex his ankle. Pain in the calf or popliteal region occurs in about 35% of patients with deep vein thrombophlebitis. Initially, thrombophlebitis may produce only localized discomfort in the leg. Eventually, it may affect a much larger area, which becomes indurated, inflamed, and extremely painful. In many cases, the inflammation follows the course of a vein.
• After the patient stabilizes, encourage him to move about and assist him with isometric and range-of-motion (ROM) exercises. Check his temperature and the color of his feet to detect venous stasis. *Never* vigorously massage his legs, which could cause thrombi to dislodge. Also discourage the patient from crossing his legs, which could promote venous stasis.
• Make sure the postoperative patient walks as soon as possible after surgery to prevent venous stasis. You may need to apply rotating tourniquets to his legs to prevent venous thromboembolism.
• During venipunctures, be careful to avoid applying a shearing force on the catheter. To prevent air emboli, clamp multiple-lumen catheters — especially those in central vessels — before changing the tubing. If the patient has a pulmonary artery catheter, be alert for signs that the balloon has ruptured: no resistance to balloon inflation and blood leakage from the balloon inflation port. Even small amounts of air in the pulmonary circulation may occlude small vessels.
• Administer analgesics for pleuritic chest pain, as ordered.
• Administer incentive spirometry to help with deep breathing, if necessary.
• Encourage the patient to drink fluids, if permitted, and assess him routinely for dehydration. After undergoing testing, some patients, particularly older patients, may feel so exhausted that they won't want to drink.
• Provide the patient with antiembolism stockings, if ordered.
• Encourage the patient to rest.

Distinguishing between pulmonary embolism and MI

Certain signs and symptoms of pulmonary embolism may mimic those of a cardiac condition. Although both disorders can be life-threatening, the interventions differ for each. When caring for a patient whose symptoms could indicate a myocardial infarction (MI) or a pulmonary embolism, you'll need to perform a quick but thorough assessment to keep your interventions on target.

To prepare yourself for this challenge, assume that you're caring for Jenny Wong, age 63, who has complications after surgical removal of an extensive neuroma from her right foot.

Assessment
You first meet Mrs. Wong 2 hours after she returns from the postanesthesia room. Her surgery was performed under general anesthesia. In reviewing Mrs. Wong's medical history, you note that she had an MI 6 years ago. Her current vital signs are as follows:
- pulse, 76 beats/minute
- blood pressure, 100/70 mm Hg
- respirations, 20 breaths/minute
- temperature, 98° F (36.7° C).

Her foot is wrapped in an elastic bandage and elevated on two pillows. Assessment of her foot reveals adequate circulation, movement, and sensation in her toes. An I.V. infusion of dextrose 5% in 0.45% sodium chloride solution is being run at 100 ml/hour.

Shortly after you leave Mrs. Wong, she calls out to the nurses' station that she's having trouble breathing. When you arrive in her room, you find her short of breath, tachypneic, apprehensive, and complaining of tightness in her chest.

Your first concern is that the pain may signal a cardiac problem. You ask Mrs. Wong if the chest tightness worsens when she takes a deep breath, knowing that the pain related to an MI is unchanged by respiration. Mrs. Wong says that the tightness is indeed worse on inspiration. You suspect that Mrs. Wong is having a pulmonary embolism.

Your continued assessment reveals that her skin is cool and moist. You obtain the following vital signs:
- pulse, 136 beats/minute and regular
- blood pressure, 90/60 mm Hg
- respirations, 38 breaths/minute and labored
- temperature, 100.2° F (37.8° C).

Auscultation reveals crackles in the right lower lobe.

Intervention
You make sure Mrs. Wong's I.V. line is patent, noting that the line hasn't been infiltrated. You also check to see if any sedatives have been ordered and call for the doctor.

When the doctor arrives, he orders a chest X-ray, an electrocardiogram (ECG), and arterial blood gas (ABG) studies. You place Mrs. Wong in semi-Fowler's position and stay with her to help reduce her anxiety. The doctor next orders oxygen at 2 liters/minute by nasal cannula to help ease Mrs. Wong's shortness of breath.

The chest X-ray results are inconclusive. Mrs. Wong's ABG study reveals a decreased $PaCO_2$ level (35 mm Hg) and a pH of 7.36, indicating an increased respiratory rate. The ECG shows tachycardia and rules out an MI. Because he is fairly confident that Mrs. Wong has a pulmonary embolism, the doctor orders a ventilation-perfusion lung scan and begins I.V. heparin therapy.

Treatment
The ventilation-perfusion scan shows pulmonary embolism. Mrs. Wong is maintained on I.V. heparin for 3 days and then converted to oral anticoagulants. Within 10 days, she is well enough to be discharged.

Because of your prompt and knowledgeable attention to Mrs. Wong's signs and symptoms, you helped detect her pulmonary embolism quickly and allowed for immediate treatment in an emergency.

Patient teaching

• Teach the patient the signs and symptoms of thrombophlebitis and pulmonary embolism; the signs of bleeding (bloody stools, blood in the urine, large bruises); and the importance of follow-up laboratory tests, such as prothrombin time, to monitor anticoagulant therapy.

• Warn the female patient that menstruation may be heavy. Instruct the male patient to use an electric razor to avoid cutting himself. Tell the patient to inform all of his health care providers, including his dentist, that he is receiving anticoagulant therapy. Instruct the patient on warfarin not to significantly vary the amount of vitamin K he takes daily because this could interfere with anticoagulation stabilization.

Adult respiratory distress syndrome

A patient with adult respiratory distress syndrome (ARDS), a life-threatening condition, experiences hypoxemia and decreased lung compliance. Diffuse alveolar infiltrates are revealed on chest X-ray and respiratory failure usually requires intubation and mechanical ventilation.

ARDS is known by various other names, including shock lung, stiff lung, wet lung, posttraumatic pulmonary insufficiency, obliterative alveolitis, noncardiogenic pulmonary edema, pump lung, hyaline lung, and Da Nang lung.

Causes

ARDS can result from direct or indirect injury to the lung. Trauma is the most common cause of ARDS, possibly because trauma-related factors (such as fat emboli, sepsis, shock, pulmonary contusions, and multiple transfusions) increase the likelihood that microemboli will develop.

Other common causes of ARDS include anaphylaxis, aspiration of gastric contents, diffuse viral pneumonia, drug overdose, idiosyncratic drug reaction, inhalation of noxious gases, hemorrhage, disseminated intravascular coagulation (DIC), eclampsia, near drowning, oxygen toxicity, and multisystem organ failure.

Less often, ARDS results from complications of coronary artery bypass grafting, hemodialysis, leukemia, acute miliary tuberculosis, pancreatitis, thrombotic thrombocytopenic purpura, uremia, and venous air emboli.

Pathophysiology

ARDS develops when the permeability of the alveolocapillary membrane increases, allowing protein and fluid to leak into the alveoli, small airways, and interstitial spaces. Alveolocapillary membrane permeability results from direct insult, such as inhalation of a lung-toxic substance, or from an indirect systemic cascade effect that results when lysosomal substances are carried to the pulmonary microcirculation. This disruption of the pulmonary capillary membrane causes injury to the type I alveolar cells and causes alveolar edema, atelectasis, and decreased lung compliance.

Leaking proteinaceous fluid leads to poor gas exchange, and flooding of the alveoli causes the type II alveolar cells to stop producing surfactant, which balances the tension between air and liquid in the lungs. Without surfactant, the alveoli collapse or become filled with fluid, making them unavailable for gas exchange. Consequently, lung compliance decreases, atelectasis develops, and the functional residual capacity—the amount of air left in the lung at the end of exhalation—decreases. The lungs become stiff and noncompliant, making it difficult for the patient to breathe. At the same time, emboli and thrombosis cause vasoconstriction and vascular occlusion in the pulmonary microcirculation, leading to hemorrhage.

As atelectasis increases, a significant right-to-left shunt takes place, with venous blood returning to the arterial circulation. As alveolar edema increases, arterial hypoxemia and intrapulmonary shunt increase rapidly. The mismatched perfusion of nonventilated and underventilated alveoli causes a severe ventilation-perfusion ratio mismatch.

A simultaneous inflammatory response occurs in the lung. It results from the increase of polymorphonuclear neutrophils (which secrete toxic mediators) within the lung. This in turn further increases capillary permeability. At the same time, complement cascade is activated, resulting in the chemotaxis of macrophages and neutrophils and in lysis of foreign antigens. Histamine, a vasoactive substance, is released from mast cells because of platelet and alveolar macrophage concentration. The patient may then develop interstitial pulmonary fibrosis from the large protein molecules in the interstitial spaces. Within 48 to 72 hours after the initial tissue injury, hyaline membranes form from the alveolar epithelial cell debris. (See *Responding to ARDS,* at right, and *Understanding ARDS,* page 60.

Complications

Severe ARDS may lead to metabolic and respiratory acidosis as well as cardiac arrest. The mechanical ventilation the patient receives, with high oxygen levels and positive end-expiratory pressure (PEEP), can lead to barotrauma and oxygen toxicity.

ARDS is fatal for one-half of the patients who develop it. One-third of ARDS patients are left with permanent reduction in pulmonary function, such as airflow obstruction and decreased vital capacity. Other patients develop bronchopulmonary dysplasia, characterized by obliteration of the bronchioles and formation of large cystic air spaces with thick fibrous walls. Bronchopulmonary dysplasia may result from using high oxygen concentrations and mechanical ventilation at high pressures.

Assessment

To establish the presence of ARDS, you'll need to question the patient about his recent and past health history. Make sure you know the causes of ARDS, and determine whether any of these are relevant in your patient's case. You'll also need to perform a physical examination and order any diagnostic tests necessary to determine the presence of ARDS.

Responding to ARDS

Untreated, adult respiratory distress syndrome (ARDS) can lead quickly to acute respiratory failure. To treat a patient with ARDS, administer oxygen with a tightly fitting mask. The oxygen mask provides continuous positive airway pressure.

You can tell if the patient's ventilatory requirements are increasing by monitoring his breathing. If his respiratory rate is greater than 35 breaths/minute and minute ventilation (respiratory rate multiplied by tidal volume) is above 10 liters/minute, he'll need to be intubated for mechanical ventilation.

Remember: The patient with ARDS usually requires oxygen therapy at greater than 50%. Paradoxically, oxygen therapy at 50% for longer than 24 hours may cause oxygen toxicity, which can contribute to the development of ARDS. Therefore, you should use the lowest possible concentration of oxygen for the shortest possible period consistent with improving your patient's oxygenation.

Using mechanical ventilation

Initially, the patient may require mechanical ventilation in the assist-control mode. Set the ventilator to deliver a tidal volume of 10 to 15 cc/kg, a respiratory rate of 12 to 16 breaths/minute, a fraction of inspired oxygen of 100%, and a positive end-expiratory pressure (PEEP) of 3 to 5 cm H_2O.

Using other devices

Other measures used with ARDS patients include pressure-support ventilation and pressure-controlled inverse ratio ventilation.

Pressure-support ventilation provides positive airway pressure during the inspiratory cycle (the most difficult part of any breath), improving the patient's oxygenation and reducing the airway resistance that occurs with traditional modes of mechanical ventilation.

Pressure-controlled inverse ratio ventilation, which provides ventilation in direct opposition to normal breathing, may be used if the patient doesn't respond to oxygen and PEEP therapy.

Understanding ARDS

The illustrations at right depict the progression of adult respiratory distress syndrome (ARDS) and what to watch for in your patient.

Response to insult
Injury reduces normal blood flow to the lungs, allowing platelets to aggregate (1). These platelets release such substances as serotonin, bradykinin and, especially, histamine (2), which inflame and damage the alveolocapillary membrane and later increase capillary permeability (3).

Development of pulmonary edema
As capillary permeability increases (4), proteins and more fluid leak out, increasing interstitial osmotic pressure and causing pulmonary edema (5).

Collapse of alveoli
Fluid in the alveoli and decreased blood flow damage surfactant in the alveoli (6). Without surfactant, alveoli collapse, impairing gas exchange.

Slowing of gas exchange
The patient breathes faster, but not enough oxygen (O_2) can cross the alveolocapillary membrane, resulting in collapsed alveoli (7). Carbon dioxide (CO_2), however, crosses more easily and is lost with every exhalation (8). Both O_2 and CO_2 levels in the blood decrease (9).

Beginning of metabolic acidosis
Pulmonary edema worsens. Meanwhile, inflammation leads to fibrosis (10), which further impedes gas exchange.

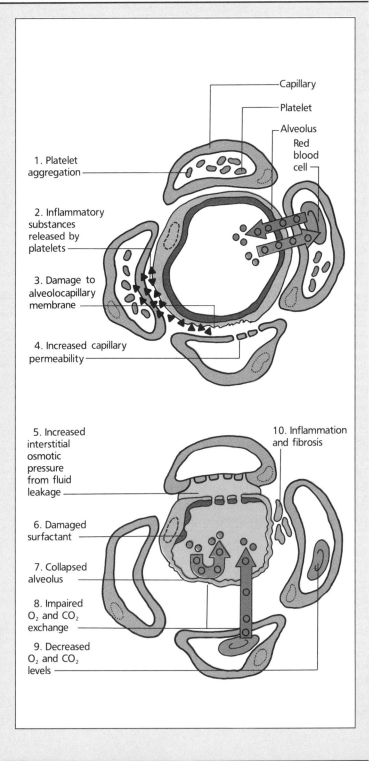

1. Platelet aggregation

2. Inflammatory substances released by platelets

3. Damage to alveolocapillary membrane

4. Increased capillary permeability

Capillary
Platelet
Alveolus
Red blood cell

5. Increased interstitial osmotic pressure from fluid leakage

6. Damaged surfactant

7. Collapsed alveolus

8. Impaired O_2 and CO_2 exchange

9. Decreased O_2 and CO_2 levels

10. Inflammation and fibrosis

History

First, find out if the patient has received a direct or indirect injury to his lung in the past 48 to 72 hours. Has the patient aspirated gastric contents, recently received multiple blood transfusions, or inhaled noxious gases? Review other likely causes of ARDS, including diffuse viral pneumonia, drug overdose, shock, and oxygen toxicity. If the patient has experienced one or more of these, he may be at high risk for ARDS.

Physical examination

Examine the patient for signs of ARDS. In the first stage, he may complain of dyspnea, especially on exertion. Respiratory and pulse rates are normal to high. You may hear diminished breath sounds when you auscultate his lungs.

As respiratory distress becomes more apparent, the patient with ARDS may have increased difficulty breathing. He'll begin using the accessory muscles of respiration. He may look pale and seem anxious and restless. He may have a dry cough or thick, frothy sputum and bloody, sticky secretions. His skin may feel cool and clammy. Tachycardia and tachypnea may accompany an elevated blood pressure. Auscultation may reveal basilar crackles.

As breathing difficulty increases, the patient may develop acute respiratory failure with severe hypoxia. Check his vital signs: The patient with ARDS has a respiratory rate above 30 breaths/minute and tachycardia, often with premature ventricular contractions and a labile blood pressure. He'll probably need intubation and mechanical ventilation. Many patients with ARDS develop refractory hypoxemia or hypoxemia that doesn't respond to conventional treatments of oxygen therapy and PEEP. Spontaneous respirations usually aren't evident, and bradycardia with arrhythmias may accompany hypotension. Metabolic and respiratory acidosis develop. Mental status can deteriorate and the patient may become comatose.

At this stage, the patient experiences a large intrapulmonary shunt—the portion of pulmonary blood flow that doesn't participate in gas exchange because it's exposed to nonfunctioning alveoli. The intrapulmonary shunt provides an index of how efficiently the lungs are exchanging gases.

You can determine the extent of an intrapulmonary shunt by calculating the arterial-alveolar (a-A) ratio. Divide the PaO_2 by the partial pressure of alveolar oxygen (PAO_2), which is derived from the alveolar air equation. The alveolar air equation is:

$$FIO_2 \times (PB - PH_2O) - \frac{PaCO_2}{0.08}$$

where FIO_2 is the fraction of inspired oxygen, PB is the barometric pressure (760 mm Hg), PH_2O is the water vapor pressure (47 mm Hg), and 0.08 is the respiratory quotient. A normal a-A ratio is greater than 0.75. An a-A ratio of less than 0.75 indicates an increased intrapulmonary shunt and ineffective gas exchange. Advanced ARDS typically shows an a-A ratio of less than 0.25.

Diagnostic tests

ABG analysis is the most common method of detecting hypoxemia, a hallmark of ARDS. With the patient breathing room air, initial ABG values usually indicate a PaO_2 of less than 60 mm Hg and a $PaCO_2$ below 35 mm Hg. The resulting blood pH usually reflects respiratory alkalosis. As ARDS worsens, ABG values show respiratory acidosis (increasing $PaCO_2$, above 45 mm Hg), metabolic acidosis (decreasing bicarbonate levels, below 22 mEq/liter), and a declining PaO_2 despite oxygen therapy.

Pulse oximetry, a noninvasive method of monitoring arterial oxygen saturation (SaO_2), doesn't take the place of ABG analysis, but it is less costly and more convenient. The pulse oximeter probe is clipped to the patient's finger or toe or the bridge of his nose. This probe connects by wire to a computer screen, where the percentages of SaO_2 and the pulse rate are displayed.

Serial chest X-rays show bilateral infiltrates in the early stages of ARDS. In later stages, X-rays show lung fields with a ground-glass appearance and eventually, with irreversible hypoxemia, whiteout of both lung fields. Another typical finding is a ventilation-perfusion mismatch, which shows the extent to which alveolocapillary units are being adequately perfused but poorly ventilated.

Differential diagnosis must rule out cardiogenic pulmonary edema, pulmonary vasculitis, and diffuse pulmonary hemorrhage. Etiologic tests may involve sputum analysis, including Gram stain and culture and sensitivity tests. Blood cultures may be used to identify infectious organisms; toxicology tests, to screen for drug ingestion. Various serum amylase tests are used to rule out pancreatitis.

Pulmonary artery wedge pressure (PAWP) may be normal or low, and the pulmonary artery systolic and diastolic pressures will be normal or increased. Other hemodynamic measurements include a normal cardiac output and cardiac index (although they can be increased or decreased), normal CVP, increased pulmonary vascular resistance, decreased oxygen consumption ($\dot{V}O_2$), decreased oxygen delivery, and normal, increased, or decreased systemic vascular resistance.

Ongoing treatment

Most patients with ARDS have a pulmonary artery catheter to monitor fluid volume status and assess mixed venous oxygen saturation ($S\bar{v}O_2$). Once the pulmonary artery catheter is inserted, obtain a wedge pressure reading. If the PAWP is above 12 mm Hg, suspect overhydration; below 6 mm Hg, underhydration.

Sedatives, narcotics, or neuromuscular blockers (such as vecuronium) may be prescribed for a patient with ARDS who's receiving mechanical ventilation. These drugs combat restlessness, decrease $\dot{V}O_2$ and carbon dioxide (CO_2) production, and facilitate ventilation.

When ARDS results from a fat embolus or a chemical injury, a short course of high-dose corticosteroids may help if given early. Treatment with sodium bicarbonate may be necessary to reverse severe metabolic acidosis. Fluids and vasopressors may be needed to maintain adequate blood pressure. Nonviral infections require treatment with antimicrobials.

Ongoing nursing interventions

• When a patient is using pressure support on a mechanical ventilator, he sets the timing of the ventilation, the inspiratory flow rate, the inspiratory rate, and the amount of tidal volume (VT). Make sure the pressure support is set to allow the patient to maintain a spontaneous VT of 10 to 15 cc/kg (250 to 350 cc/breath).

To counteract the lack of control over the minute ventilation, you or the doctor may decide to increase the rate to make sure the patient has a minimum minute ventilation. Normal minute ventilation is 5 to 10 liters/minute. (See *Understanding mechanical ventilation modes.*)

• Use pressure-controlled inverse ratio ventilation to provide direct opposition to normal breathing. During normal breathing, the expiratory phase is about twice as long as the inspiratory phase. Reversing this ratio (so that the inspiratory phase is about twice as long as the expiratory phase) will increase the functional residual capacity, increase diffusion time for air in the alveoli, and open more alveoli and small airways, thereby increasing oxygenation.

• Use PEEP and continuous positive airway pressure (CPAP) to prevent a ventilator patient's airway pressure from returning to zero. (See *Understanding PEEP and CPAP,* page 64.)

• Assess the patient's respiratory and hemodynamic status at least every 2 hours. Respiratory assessment consists of measuring the patient's respiratory rate and rhythm and evaluating ventilatory support. Is the patient triggering the ventilator? Determine the patient's spontaneous VT and the peak airway pressure needed for ventilation.

• To maintain PEEP, suction the patient only as needed. Using a closed-system suction device prevents disconnection of the ventilator circuit when suctioning, preserving the PEEP.

• Because PEEP may lower the patient's cardiac output, check for hypotension, tachycardia, and decreased urine output. As PEEP rises above 3 cm H_2O, it increases positive intrathoracic pressure, decreasing blood return to the right side of the heart and thereby decreasing stroke volume, cardiac output, and blood pressure.

• Monitor the patient for a sudden rise in peak airway pressure and triggering of the ventilator's high-pressure alarm. PEEP predisposes the patient to barotrauma: pneumothorax, pneumomediastinum, and subcutaneous emphysema. A sudden rise in peak airway pressure may indicate that the patient has tension pneumothorax, which develops when the pres-

Understanding mechanical ventilation modes

The pressure waveforms at right show the patterns of common modes of mechanical ventilation. Each graph shows the point at which inspiration starts; arrows in assist-control and synchronized intermittent mandatory ventilation (the only modes that are patient initiated) point to the beginning of patient-initiated breaths that trigger the ventilator. The graphs also show the relative duration of inspiration and expiration. The gray areas indicate inspiration; the green areas, expiration. The numbers to the left of the graphs indicate pressure in cm H_2O.

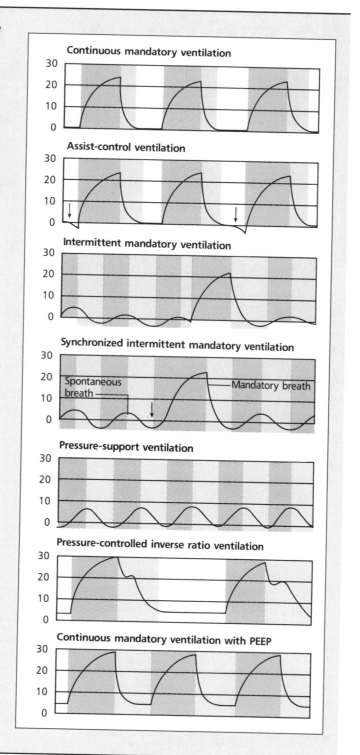

Understanding PEEP and CPAP

Certain patients may require adjunct therapy, such as positive end-expiratory pressure (PEEP) or continuous positive airway pressure (CPAP), to prevent alveolar collapse. PEEP is the application of positive pressure during expiration on a ventilator. CPAP is the application of positive pressure throughout the respiratory cycle during spontaneous breathing.

Both PEEP and CPAP prevent airway pressure from returning to zero, or atmospheric pressure. This, in turn, creates an intra-alveolar volume great enough to overcome the elastic forces of the lung, which helps reopen collapsed alveoli and prevents small-airway closure at the end of expiration. PEEP or CPAP increases functional residual capacity and substantially improves gas exchange, which decreases intrapulmonary shunting and the ventilation-perfusion mismatch. As a result, partial pressure of oxygen improves and the fraction of inspired oxygen can fall below 50% without hampering the effectiveness of therapy.

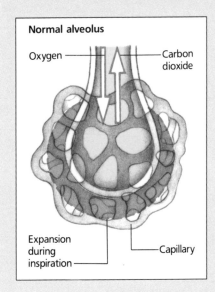

Normal alveolus

Oxygen — Carbon dioxide

Expansion during inspiration — Capillary

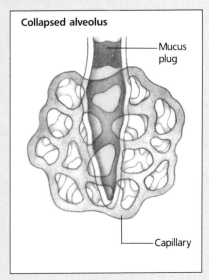

Collapsed alveolus

Mucus plug

Capillary

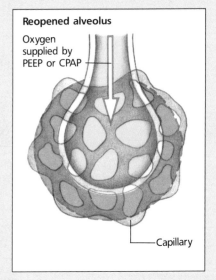

Reopened alveolus

Oxygen supplied by PEEP or CPAP

Capillary

sure in the thorax ruptures alveoli or blebs, allowing air to escape into the pleural space. Notify the doctor immediately if breath sounds become unequal or crepitus develops.
• Monitor ventilator settings often, draining condensate from the tubing promptly to ensure maximum oxygen delivery and decrease the risk of water draining into the patient's lungs. Monitor ABG levels, documenting and reporting any changes or abnormalities. (See *Responding to mechanical ventilator alarms*.)
• When the patient has a pulmonary artery catheter in place, monitor the readings frequently, watching the PAWP and checking for decreasing $S\bar{v}O_2$ levels.
• Start nutritional support early. The diaphragm and intercostal muscles require additional energy to counteract the fatigue that develops during respiratory failure. Administer tube feedings and parenteral nutrition as ordered.
• Monitor the serum albumin and phosphate levels. Hypophosphatemia is associated with weak respiratory muscles and can aggravate respiratory failure.
• Give sedatives, as ordered, to reduce restlessness and then monitor the patient's response to the medication. Because paralyzing agents are frequently used, be sure to reposition the

Responding to mechanical ventilator alarms

Mechanical ventilators have preset alarms triggered by changes in the patient's respiratory rate, which signal changes (some potentially fatal) in the patient's condition. Use this chart to determine the potential causes of these alarms and the actions you must take to resolve them.

ALARM	POSSIBLE CAUSE	ACTIONS
High pressure The pressure required to ventilate the patient exceeds the preset pressure, usually set at 10 to 15 cm H_2O above normal peak airway pressure.	• Pneumothorax, decreased lung compliance	• Assess breath sounds and chest wall expansion, percuss for hyperresonance, and verify endotracheal (ET) tube placement.
	• Excessive secretions, coughing, airway plugging	• Provide suctioning.
	• Changes in patient position	• Reposition patient.
	• Kinked ventilator tubing	• Unkink tubing; check ventilator circuit.
Low pressure The resistance to the inspiratory flow is less than the preset amount, usually set at 10 cm H_2O below peak airway pressure.	• Patient disconnected from ventilator	• Check for disconnected patient; reconnect patient.
	• Break in ventilator circuit	• Check ventilator for loose connections; notify respiratory therapist if break not obvious or can't be corrected quickly. • Use manual resuscitator to support patient if problem can't be solved quickly.
Apnea The period of apnea exceeds preset time; ventilator defaults to assist-control mode (not available on all ventilators).	• Patient fatigue • Decreased level of consciousness (LOC)	• Assess patient for changes in fatigue and LOC. • Notify doctor if patient's condition has changed. • Alert respiratory therapist to ventilator changes.
Respiratory rate The respiratory rate falls below or exceeds the preset rate.	• Patient anxiety	• Reassure patient; use relaxation techniques.
	• Hypoxia	• Evaluate for signs and symptoms of hypoxia, such as decreased LOC, confusion, cyanosis, tachycardia, and arrhythmias; assess need for arterial blood gas analysis or pulse oximetry reading.
Low exhaled volume The exhaled tidal volume falls below preset alarm volume.	• Leak in ET or tracheal tube cuff	• Assess ET or tracheal tube cuff for patency; add air if needed and if cuff pressure doesn't exceed 18 mm Hg (22 cm H_2O).
	• Airway secretions, increasing airway resistance, decreased lung compliance	• Suction airway secretions, assess peak airway pressure, and assess breath sounds and chest wall expansion.
	• Increased respiratory rate	• Assess patient respiratory rate.
	• Leak in ventilator system	• Assess ventilator circuit for leaks; notify respiratory therapist.

patient every 2 hours to prevent skin breakdown and promote aeration of all lung fields.
• Closely monitor fluid and electrolyte status. Diuretics may be ordered, depending on the underlying cause, but must be administered cautiously. Evaluate fluid status by monitoring intake and output, the patient's daily weight, and his PAWP, and by assessing for mucous membrane and axillary moisture and adventitious breath sounds. Watch for overhydration,

which can exacerbate pulmonary edema.

• Maintain joint mobility by performing passive ROM exercises. If possible, help the patient perform active exercise.

• Provide meticulous skin care. To prevent skin breakdown, reposition the endotracheal (ET) tube from one side of the mouth to the other every 24 hours. Change the tape or securing device on the ET tube when it becomes wet or soiled.

• Be alert for signs of treatment-induced complications, including arrhythmias, DIC, GI bleeding, infection, malnutrition, paralytic ileus, pneumothorax, pulmonary fibrosis, renal failure, thrombocytopenia, and tracheal stenosis.

• Provide emotional support and any necessary teaching to both the patient and his family. Answer their questions as fully as possible. Explain the disorder and the signs and symptoms that may occur. Review the treatment that may be required and provide simple demonstrations. Tell the recuperating patient that recovery will take some time and that he will feel weak for a while.

Pneumothorax

An accumulation of air or gas between the parietal and visceral pleurae is called pneumothorax. The amount of air or gas trapped in the intrapleural space determines the degree of lung collapse. The three types of pneumothorax—tension, open (traumatic), and closed (spontaneous) pneumothorax—are also classified by size. A small pneumothorax occupies 15% or less of the pleural cavity; a moderate pneumothorax, 15% to 60%; and a large pneumothorax, more than 60%. In tension pneumothorax, air in the pleural space is under higher pressure than air in adjacent lung and vascular structures. Without prompt treatment, a tension or large pneumothorax results in fatal pulmonary and circulatory impairment. (See *Responding to tension pneumothorax.*)

Causes

In tension pneumothorax, positive pleural pressure develops from a penetrating chest wound, chest tube occlusion or malfunction, lung or airway puncture by a fractured rib associated with positive pressure ventilation, mechanical ventilation (after chest injury) that forces air into the pleural space through damaged areas, or high-level PEEP that causes alveolar blebs to rupture. Tension pneumothorax commonly follows blunt trauma in which a tear in the pulmonary parenchymal tissue fails to seal. Each inspiration traps air in the pleural space, resulting in positive pleural pressure. This, in turn, causes collapse of the ipsilateral lung and significant impairment of the patient's venous return, which can severely compromise cardiac output and may cause a mediastinal shift. Decreased filling of the great vessels of the chest results in diminished cardiac output and lowered blood pressure.

Open pneumothorax occurs when air flows between the pleural space and the outside of the body. It can be caused by a penetrating chest injury (such as a gunshot or knife wound), insertion of a central venous catheter, chest surgery, transbronchial biopsy, thoracentesis, or closed pleural biopsy.

Closed pneumothorax occurs when air reaches the pleural space directly from the lung. It can be caused by blunt chest trauma, rupture of emphysematous bullae, high intrathoracic pressures that occur during mechanical ventilation, tubercular or cancerous lesions that erode into the pleural space, interstitial lung disease (such as eosinophilic granuloma), and air leakage from ruptured, congenital blebs adjacent to the visceral pleural space.

Pathophysiology

You can better understand what causes pneumothorax by briefly reviewing the physiology of the lungs and pleurae. Normally, the area between the visceral pleura (which envelops each lung, separating it from the mediastinal structures) and the parietal pleura (which lines the thoracic cavity) is air-free. It contains a thin layer of lubricating fluid that allows the two surfaces to glide smoothly over each other during inspiration and expiration. If air or blood enters this pleural space, it separates these surfaces by overcoming the negative pressure that holds them together.

As the air pressure in the pleural cavity becomes positive in open pneumothorax, the lung collapses on the affected side, resulting in substantially decreased total lung capacity, vital capacity, and lung compliance. The resulting ventilation-perfusion mismatch can lead to hypoxia.

As air continues to accumulate and intrapleural pressures rise in tension pneumothorax, the mediastinum shifts away from the affected side and decreases venous return. This forces the heart, trachea, esophagus, and great vessels to the unaffected side, compressing the heart and the contralateral lung. (See *Differentiating among types of pneumothorax*, page 68.)

Complications

A large pneumothorax or a tension pneumothorax can lead to fatal pulmonary and circulatory impairment.

Assessment

History

Find out if ordinary chest movement, breathing, and coughing have made the patient's chest pain worse. Has he been experiencing shortness of breath. If so, for how long?

Physical examination

When you inspect the patient, you'll probably find asymmetrical chest wall movement with overexpansion and rigidity on the affected side. He may show signs of cyanosis.

Upon palpation, you may detect crackling beneath the skin, indicating subcutaneous emphysema and decreased vocal fremitus. Palpation may also reveal tympany on the affected side with unequal, diminished, or absent breath sounds. Mediastinal shift and tracheal deviation are late signs.

Percussion may demonstrate hyperresonance on the affected side, and auscultation may disclose decreased or absent breath sounds over the collapsed lung. Closed pneumothorax, which releases only a small amount

EMERGENCY INTERVENTIONS

Responding to tension pneumothorax

Even if a chest X-ray hasn't yet confirmed tension pneumothorax, suspect it if the patient reports sudden, sharp chest pain and shortness of breath. Also, if the patient is on mechanical ventilation, tension pneumothorax is likely if he suddenly develops hypotension, high airway pressures, increased respiratory rate, or increased anxiety.

Closed (spontaneous) pneumothorax, which releases only a small amount of air into the pleural space, may cause no signs and symptoms. Tension pneumothorax, which usually causes dyspnea, rapid breathing, and extreme anxiety, must be treated immediately.

If less than 30% of the lung collapses, treatment is conservative, consisting of bed rest and careful monitoring of the patient's blood pressure, pulse rate, and respiratory rate. If more than 30% of the lung collapses, chest tube drainage is necessary. If symptoms are moderate, needle aspiration (thoracentesis) is performed.

After the chest tube and drainage system are in place, encourage the patient to breathe deeply and exhale fully to drain the pleural space and promote lung reexpansion. Remind him to do this at least once an hour.

A flutter valve may be used in addition to or instead of a water seal to maintain one-way flow of drainage.

Provide analgesics for pain. Monitor vital signs for indications of shock, respiratory distress, and mediastinal shift.

If the patient is on mechanical ventilation, remove him from the ventilator and provide manual ventilation with a manual resuscitation bag. Notify the doctor immediately and prepare for insertion of a chest tube or a large (16G) needle.

of air into the pleural space, may not cause signs and symptoms.

The patient with tension pneumothorax will have dyspnea, rapid respirations, and extreme anxiety. Other assessment findings include a narrowed pulse pressure and hypotension.

Differentiating among types of pneumothorax

Open (traumatic) pneumothorax
This disorder results from entry of air (as shown by the arrows) into the pleural space through a chest wall opening.

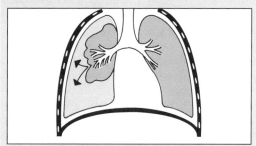

Closed (spontaneous) pneumothorax
The chest wall remains intact in this injury. Air (shown in the shaded area) enters the normally airtight pleural cavity through the lung's surface.

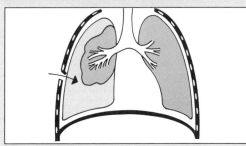

Tension pneumothorax
When an increasing amount of air becomes trapped in the pleural space, tension pneumothorax may develop. As air and tension increase, the lung and mediastinum are compressed and shifted toward the unaffected side.

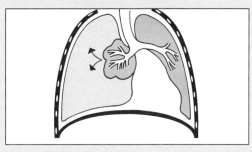

Diagnostic tests
Chest X-rays reveal air in the pleural space and, possibly, a mediastinal shift, which confirms the diagnosis. ABG studies may show hypoxemia, possibly accompanied by respiratory acidosis and hypercapnia. SaO_2 levels may fall initially but typically return to normal within 24 hours.

Ongoing treatment
Medical treatment for closed pneumothorax is fairly conservative, unless the patient shows signs of tension pneumothorax (increased pleural pressure) as well. If the patient's lung collapse is less than 30% and he has no dyspnea, treatment includes bed rest, careful monitoring (blood pressure and pulse and respiratory rates), oxygen administration and, possibly, aspiration of air with a large-bore needle attached to a syringe.

Recurring closed pneumothorax requires thoracotomy and pleurectomy. These procedures prevent recurrence by causing the lining of the lung to adhere to the parietal pleura. Analgesics may be prescribed to relieve pain.

Ongoing nursing interventions
For chest tube drainage
• Keep the patient as comfortable as possible. He'll usually prefer an upright position.
• Give analgesics as needed.
• Assess the patient regularly, noting the rate, depth, and ease of his breathing. Monitor vital signs every hour for indications of shock, increasing respiratory distress, and mediastinal shift. Palpate the tissue around the insertion site for any subcutaneous air and auscultate for changes in his breath sounds that indicate improving or worsening respiration.
• Watch for pallor, gasping respiration, and sudden chest pain. Watch for signs of tension pneumothorax (falling blood pressure and rising pulse and respiratory rates), which could· be fatal if not treated promptly.
• Change the dressing around the chest tube insertion site at least every 24 hours. Keep the site clean and watch for signs of drainage and infection.

Managing chest drainage problems

PROBLEM	INTERVENTIONS
Patient positioned improperly	• Keep the collection chamber below chest level. • Place the patient in semi-Fowler's position when in bed to promote drainage. • Avoid dependent loops in the tubing; coil the tubing flat on the bed and then let it fall in a straight line to the drainage unit.
Absent tidaling (rise and fall of solution in the rod submerged in the water seal)	• Check for kinked tubing and unkink it. • Inspect the connections for clots.
Air leak	• Apply pressure to the skin around the chest tube insertion site. Observe if the bubbling stops; if so, the leak may be in the patient end of the tube and additional sutures are needed at the insertion site. • Briefly clamp the chest tube close to the patient. If the leak persists, it is in the tubing. Continue to briefly clamp the tubing at intervals to determine where the leak is. • Keep connections taped securely and the chest dressing occlusive.
Accidental disconnection of the chest tube from the chest drainage system	• If the patient doesn't have an air leak, the tube can be briefly clamped or pinched shut until the tube is reconnected to the drainage system. • Reestablish the system quickly.
Accidental removal of the chest tube	• Apply direct pressure to the chest tube site. • Cover area with a sterile dressing and call the doctor immediately.

• Don't dislodge or reposition the tube. If the chest tube becomes dislodged, immediately place a petroleum gauze dressing over the opening to prevent rapid lung collapse.

• Watch for air leakage (bubbling in the water-sealed chamber), which can result from a hole or tear in the lung. Continuing air leakage indicates the lung's failure to heal and may necessitate surgery. Be careful not to create tension pneumothorax with a dressing that's too tight. (See *Managing chest drainage problems.*)

• Watch for increasing subcutaneous emphysema by checking around the neck or at the tube's insertion site for crackling beneath the skin. For the patient receiving mechanical ventilation, watch for difficulty breathing in time with the ventilator and pressure changes on the ventilator gauges.

• Teach the patient what pneumothorax is and what causes it. Explain all diagnostic tests and procedures. If the patient is to have surgery or chest tubes inserted, explain why he needs these procedures. Reassure him that the chest tube will make him more comfortable. Encourage the patient to perform deep-breathing exercises every hour when awake. Discuss the potential for recurrent closed pneumothorax and review its signs and symptoms. Emphasize the need for immediate medical intervention if these occur.

For the patient with a thoracotomy

• Urge the patient to control coughing and gasping during the procedure.

• Monitor vital signs every hour after thoracotomy.

• For the first 24 hours, assess respiratory status by checking breath sounds hourly.

• Observe the chest tube site for leakage, and note the amount and color of drainage.

• Help the patient walk, usually on the first postoperative day, to promote deep inspiration and lung expansion.

Hemothorax

Commonly accompanied by pneumothorax, hemothorax occurs when blood enters the pleural cavity. Depending on the amount of blood and the underlying cause of bleeding, hemothorax can cause varying degrees of lung collapse.

Causes

Hemothorax usually results from either blunt or penetrating chest trauma. Less commonly, it results from thoracic surgery, pulmonary infarction, neoplasm, dissecting thoracic aneurysm, or anticoagulant therapy. Hemothorax can also result from a lacerated liver or perforated diaphragm.

Pathophysiology

Hemothorax produces shock quickly, with less ventilatory impairment than pneumothorax. Blood collects in the pleural space, partially or completely collapsing the lung. This blood may come from damaged intercostal, pleural, or mediastinal vessels or from the internal mammary artery or the lung's parenchymal vessels. As the pleural space fills with blood, the underlying lung tissue is compressed on the affected side. The compression of the lung tissue results in alveolar collapse and impaired gas exchange.

When hemothorax results from trauma, it may be self-limiting. As the blood accumulates in the chest, it creates pressure on the source of bleeding, which may result in a reduction or complete stoppage of the bleeding. This limits the amount of blood in the thorax and the amount of lung collapse.

Complications

Hemothorax may result in mediastinal shift, ventilatory compromise, lung collapse and, without successful intervention, cardiopulmonary arrest. (See *Treating hemothorax*.)

Assessment

History

A patient with hemothorax usually has a recent history of trauma. He may complain of chest pain and the sudden onset of breathing difficulty, which may be mild to severe, depending on the amount of blood in the pleural cavity.

Physical examination

When you examine the patient, you'll probably detect tachypnea, dusky skin color, diaphoresis, tachycardia, hypotension, and hemoptysis. If hemothorax progresses to respiratory failure, you may note restlessness, anxiety, cyanosis, and stupor. As the patient's chest rises and falls, you may notice that the affected side expands and stiffens; the unaffected side may rise with the patient's gasping respirations (asymmetrical lung expansion).

Percussing the patient, you may detect dullness over the affected side of the chest. Auscultation may detect decreased or absent breath sounds over the affected side.

Diagnostic tests

ABG studies may reveal a normal or low PaO_2 level and a high $PaCO_2$ level. The hemoglobin level may be decreased, depending on the amount of bleeding that has occurred. A chest X-ray may reveal pleural fluid and detect a mediastinal shift. It may also show pleural effusion.

Thoracentesis, performed for diagnosis and therapy, may yield blood or serosanguineous fluid. Fluid specimens are sent to the laboratory for analysis.

Ongoing treatment

Mild hemothorax usually clears in 10 to 14 days; after that, the patient should be observed for further bleeding for a week to 10 days.

Both chest tube drainage and suction may be used. The diameter of the chest tube must be large enough to prevent clots from blocking it. If chest drainage doesn't improve the patient's condition, a thoracotomy may be necessary to remove blood and clots and to control bleeding. Other treatment measures include oxygen therapy, I.V. therapy to restore fluid volume, and administration of analgesics.

Ongoing nursing interventions

• Make sure appropriate blood products are available.

• Monitor the patient's hemoglobin and hematocrit levels for falling trends that may indicate continuous bleeding.

• If the patient is receiving autotransfusion, monitor him for complications, including blood clotting, hemolysis, coagulopathies, thrombocytopenia, particulate and air emboli, sepsis, and citrate toxicity (from the acid citrate dextrose solution).

• Give oxygen by face mask or nasal cannula if ordered.

• Give I.V. fluids and blood transfusions, as ordered, to treat shock. Use a CVP line to monitor treatment progress.

• Monitor ABG levels often. Also check the white blood cell count and coagulation studies to determine blood replacement needs.

• Watch for complications signaled by pallor and gasping respirations.

• Monitor the patient's vital signs diligently, usually every 1 to 2 hours until he stabilizes, and then every 4 to 6 hours. Watch for increasing pulse and respiratory rates and falling blood pressure, which may indicate shock or massive bleeding. Be prepared to get the patient ready for surgery.

• Give pain medications, as ordered, and document their effectiveness.

• Assist with thoracentesis, if performed.

• During chest tube drainage, record the volume, color, and character of the drainage at least hourly. Immediately report a chest tube that's warm and full of blood or a rapidly rising bloody fluid level in the drainage collection chamber. If the patient drains more than 150 ml/hour for several hours or more than 1,500 ml daily, notify the doctor. The patient may need emergency surgery. Follow your hospital's policy for milking the chest tube. If you can see bloody drainage or clots, milking may be permitted to keep the tube patent. (See *Milking a chest tube,* page 72.)

• Keep petroleum gauze at the bedside in case the chest tube dislodges. If it does, place the gauze over the chest tube site, taking care not to cover the wound so tightly that tension pneumothorax results. Don't clamp the chest tube. Change the chest tube dressing as necessary. Watch for signs of infection at the insertion site. Avoid all tubing kinks, tape all chest tube connections, and tape the tube securely to the patient's chest.

• Explain all procedures to the patient and his family and include them in care-related decisions whenever possible. Encourage the patient to ask questions about his care. To promote gas exchange, encourage the patient to perform deep-breathing exercises every hour when he's awake.

Treating hemothorax

Emergency treatment goals for a patient with hemothorax include:
• stabilizing the patient's condition
• stopping the bleeding
• oxygenating the patient
• restoring fluid volume
• administering blood transfusions, as necessary, to treat shock
• performing thoracotomy, if necessary, to remove blood and blood clots and to control bleeding
• reexpanding the affected lung.

In severe hemothorax, thoracentesis is performed to remove blood and other fluids from the pleural cavity and a chest tube is inserted.

Autotransfusion

The hemothorax patient's own blood may be filtered and reinfused by autotransfusion if his blood loss is close to or more than 1 liter.

A large-bore chest tube connected to a closed drainage system is used to collect the patient's blood from a wound or chest cavity. The blood then passes through a filter, which catches most potential thrombi (including clumps of fibrin and damaged red blood cells), before being collected in a collection bag. The blood is reinfused immediately, directly from the bag, or it may be processed in a commercial cell washer that reduces anticoagulated whole blood to washed red blood cells for later infusion.

Milking a chest tube

Despite recent questions about the effectiveness and safety of milking, it remains the most reliable method of keeping a chest drainage tube patent and clear of clots. Milking dislodges and pushes forward any clots or fibrin in the tubing and creates a brief and surprisingly high pulse of suction as the compressed section of tubing is released and then reexpands.

The longer the section you compress, the more suction you create. The transient suction may exceed -100 cm H_2O when as little as 4" (10 cm) of tubing is milked. It averages almost -300 cm H_2O when 18" (45 cm) is milked and often exceeds -400 cm H_2O when the entire length is milked.

Although no proof exists that milking causes permanent damage to tissue, bruising and entrapment (in which lung tissue or coronary vessels are entrapped in the eyelets of the chest tube) have been reported.

Determining the appropriateness of milking

Weigh the benefits and risks of chest tube milking. Milk when the tubing is most likely to be blocked by a clot—especially when fresh bleeding develops—instead of routinely on every patient's chest tube. Blood remaining in the pleural space for a few hours rarely clots, serous drainage itself is un-likely to obstruct the tubing, and air alone can't clog it. Milking definitely isn't necessary with a heart surgery patient who has a mediastinal sump tube because a continuous flow of air through the tube's vent keeps it patent.

Performing proper technique

When milking seems appropriate, try a gentle technique first, such as squeezing hand over hand along the tube and releasing between each squeeze, or folding several sections of tubing and then squeezing them.

The usual technique is to grip and stabilize the tubing with the thumb and forefinger of one hand, sliding the thumb and forefinger of the other hand along the tubing from that point toward the collection chamber to compress a section of tubing. Then release your first hand. Regrip the tubing where you stopped, repeating the procedure along the entire length of the tubing. Use an alcohol swab or hand lotion as a lubricant to make milking easier.

Alternatively, you may use a special chest tube roller. You may also progressively squeeze sections of the tubing hand over hand, folding several sections of tubing back and forth on each other and squeezing them, or milking *toward* rather than *away* from the chest.

Pulmonary edema

A common complication of cardiac disease, pulmonary edema is an accumulation of fluid in the extravascular spaces of the lung. The disorder may occur as a chronic condition. It may also develop quickly and rapidly become fatal, as in the case of acute pulmonary edema. Pulmonary edema may also progress to respiratory and metabolic acidosis with subsequent life-threatening cardiac or respiratory arrest. (See *Responding to pulmonary edema.*)

Causes

Pulmonary edema usually results from left ventricular failure caused by arteriosclerotic, cardiomyopathic, hypertensive, or valvular heart disease. Cardiogenic pulmonary edema, the most common form of pulmonary edema, is marked by increased capillary hydrostatic pressure and usually results from MI, mitral stenosis, decreased myocardial contractility, left ventricular failure, or fluid overload.

The following factors may also predispose the patient to pulmonary edema: barbiturate or opiate poisoning, CHF, excessive or overly rapid infusion of I.V. fluids, impaired pulmonary lymphatic drainage (from Hodgkin's disease or obliterative lymphangitis after radiation), inhalation of irritating gases, left atrial myxoma (which impairs left atrial emptying), pneumonia, and pulmonary veno-occlusive disease.

Pathophysiology

Pulmonary edema involves both systemic circulation and microcirculation. Cardiogenic pulmonary edema occurs when the left ventricle can't effectively pump blood from the heart. Subsequently, the blood backs up into the lungs, impairing oxygen exchange and its delivery to the tissues. At the microcirculation level, pulmonary edema results from high capillary hydrostatic pressure forcing fluid out of capillaries into the interstitium.

Noncardiogenic pulmonary edema usually stems from increased capillary permeability caused by an imbalance between two opposing pressures, forcing fluid out of the capillaries into the interstitium. Alternatively, decreased colloid osmotic pressure can decrease the amount of fluid kept in the capillaries. (See *Understanding pulmonary edema,* page 74.)

Assessment

History

The patient's history may include predisposing factors for pulmonary edema, such as arteriosclerosis, hypertension, valvular heart disease, or cardiomyopathy. He'll typically complain of a persistent cough, especially a dry, hacking cough. He may report a cold, dyspnea on exertion, or orthopnea (increased dyspnea when lying flat). He may also experience paroxysmal nocturnal dyspnea (awakening with severe dyspnea and wheezing).

Physical examination

On inspection, you may note restlessness and anxiety. With severe pulmonary edema, the patient's breathing may be visibly labored and rapid. His cough may sound intense and produce frothy, bloody sputum. In advanced stages, the patient's level of consciousness decreases. Respirations are shallow and rapid. You may observe Cheyne-Stokes respiration, indicating an underlying acid-base imbalance.

Typical palpation findings include neck vein distention. In acute pulmonary edema, the skin feels sweaty, cold, and clammy. Fremitus may be palpated over the chest. On percussion, you may detect dullness secondary to fluid accumulation in the dependent areas of the lung.

Auscultation may reveal crackles in the de-

Responding to pulmonary edema

If you detect inspiratory crackles, dry cough, or dyspnea, suspect pulmonary edema. Don't wait for chest X-ray results.

Treatment aims to reduce extravascular fluid, improve gas exchange and myocardial function, and correct the underlying disease (if possible). High concentrations of oxygen can be administered by cannula or mask, although many patients with pulmonary edema can't tolerate a mask. If the patient's arterial oxygen levels remain too low, assisted mechanical ventilation may improve oxygen delivery to the tissues and usually improves his acid-base balance. Intubation and mechanical ventilation with positive end-expiratory pressure may be instituted to reduce intrapulmonary shunting.

Drug therapy

Morphine is the most effective medication for treating pulmonary edema. It sedates the patient and acts as a vasodilator. (Vasodilators increase cardiac output by decreasing left ventricular pressure.) A bronchodilator such as aminophylline may decrease bronchospasm and enhance myocardial contractility.

Diuretics, such as furosemide, ethacrynic acid, and bumetanide, may also be prescribed to increase urine output, which helps to mobilize extravascular fluids. Inotropic medications may be given to increase cardiac output by increasing myocardial contractility. Antiarrhythmics such as lidocaine may be administered to treat cardiac arrhythmias caused by pulmonary edema.

pendent areas of the lungs; the location of the crackles may change, based on the patient's position. In severe pulmonary edema, you may hear wheezing as the alveoli and bronchioles fill with fluid and the crackles become more diffuse. Heart sounds may reveal a diastolic (S_3) gallop, often associated with CHF, and an S_4 murmur. Additional findings include worsening tachycardia, falling blood pressure, thready

Understanding pulmonary edema

The pulmonary microcirculation consists of arterioles, capillaries, and venules. Normally, the thin capillary walls are permeable to fluid but not to blood cells and other large particles, such as proteins and glucose. Fluid constantly flows out through capillary walls into the interstitium. An equal amount of fluid flows into the capillaries and the pulmonary lymphatic network.

Normal pulmonary fluid movement
This fluid movement ordinarily depends on the equal force of two opposing pressures, *pulmonary capillary hydrostatic pressure,* which forces fluid out of capillaries and into the interstitium, and *plasma oncotic pressure,* which keeps fluid in the capillaries because of the force created by protein molecules.

Pulmonary capillary hydrostatic pressure is stronger in the arterioles, so fluid is pushed out of these vessels and into the interstitium. In venules, however, plasma oncotic pressure is stronger, pulling fluid *into* the capillaries.

How pulmonary edema develops
Normally, the extensive pulmonary lymphatic network helps maintain a balance between these two pressures by absorbing any excess fluid. A small amount of fluid also evaporates in the alveoli and is exhaled.

Acute pulmonary edema develops when this delicate balance is upset. In cardiogenic pulmonary edema, abnormally high pulmonary capillary hydrostatic pressure forces fluid out of the capillaries into the interstitium. In most noncardiogenic types, however, the problem stems from increased capillary permeability, not high hydrostatic pressure. Leaky capillaries allow protein-rich fluid to escape. Because of its high oncotic pressure, this fluid tends to pull more fluid with it.

Normally, the right ventricle propels blood to the lungs, where gas exchange takes place. In cardiogenic pulmonary edema, left ventricular failure causes backward pressure, forcing fluid out of the vessels and impairing gas exchange. High hydrostatic pressure (represented in the illustration below by the larger arrows) overcomes capillary oncotic pressure (smaller arrows), forcing fluid out of the vessels and into the interstitium and alveoli.

Normal

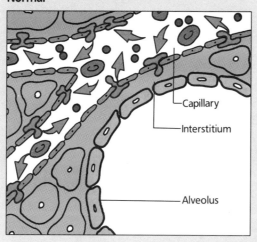

Capillary

Interstitium

Alveolus

Abnormal

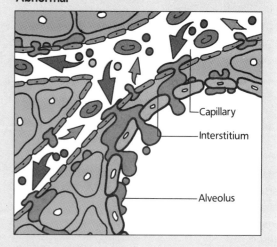

Capillary

Interstitium

Alveolus

Characteristic findings in pulmonary edema

Pulmonary edema causes characteristic effects that may be detected by physical examination, arterial blood gas (ABG) analysis, hemodynamic monitoring, or an electrocardiogram (ECG).

Physical examination
- Tachycardia
- Decreased blood pressure
- Confusion
- Increased respiratory rate and depth
- Shortness of breath
- Crackles, wheezing
- Nocturnal cough
- Increased orthopnea
- Frothy white or pink sputum
- Increased jugular vein distention
- Cyanotic extremities
- Prolonged peripheral capillary refill time
- Pulsus alternans
- S_3, S_4
- Clammy, pale skin
- Decreased urine output

ABG analysis
- Respiratory alkalosis
- Decreased arterial oxygen saturation
- Normal right-to-left shunt
- Increased arterial-alveolar gradient
- Reduced ventilation-perfusion ratio
- Normal dead space to tidal volume ratio
- Diminished mixed venous oxygen saturation
- Increased arteriovenous oxygen difference

Hemodynamic monitoring
- Reduced cardiac output and cardiac index
- Normal to slightly elevated central venous pressure
- Increased systemic vascular resistance
- Increased pulmonary artery systolic and diastolic pressures
- Elevated pulmonary artery wedge pressure
- Normal to increased pulmonary vascular resistance
- Increased left ventricular stroke work
- Increased oxygen consumption
- Decreased oxygen delivery

ECG
- Acute or previous myocardial infarction (MI), as indicated by Q waves or documented subendocardial MI
- Left ventricular hypertrophy (axis deviation)
- Elevated ST segments
- Inverted T waves
- Q waves

pulse, and decreased cardiac output. In advanced pulmonary edema, breath sounds diminish. (See *Characteristic findings in pulmonary edema*.)

Diagnostic tests
Although you can often diagnose pulmonary edema from clinical features, certain diagnostic tests provide more definitive information. ABG analysis usually shows hypoxemia with a variable $PaCO_2$ level, depending on the patient's degree of fatigue. The hypoxemia is a direct result of ventilation-perfusion mismatch. ABG results may also identify metabolic acidosis that stems from increased levels of fixed acids, such as lactic acid.

Chest X-rays show diffuse haziness of the lung fields and, usually, cardiomegaly and pleural effusion. An enlarged heart and promi-

nent pulmonary arteries and veins may be apparent on the chest X-ray. Kerley B lines (small fluid densities in the lung periphery) appear when interstitial edema is present, and alveolar infiltrates appear as the alveoli fill with fluid. The infiltrates are seen in the dependent areas of the lung. Pulse oximetry and ABG analysis may reveal decreasing SaO_2 levels.

Pulmonary artery catheterization identifies left ventricular failure, indicated by an elevated PAWP, which is usually above 18 mm Hg and frequently over 30 mm Hg. These findings help to rule out ARDS, in which PAWP usually remains normal or low.

In many patients, cardiac output and cardiac index are decreased. Pressures on the right side of the heart, as well as systemic vascular resistance, may be elevated. $\dot{V}O_2$ will be increased, and oxygen delivery decreased.

An ECG may disclose evidence of a previous or current MI. In cardiogenic pulmonary edema, you may see left ventricular hypertrophy, elevated ST segments, Q waves, and inverted T waves. ECG changes in noncardiogenic pulmonary edema usually include tachycardia without other changes.

Ongoing treatment
The primary goal in the treatment of cardiogenic pulmonary edema is improving cardiac output. Most of the therapies you'll administer aim to reduce preload and afterload. (See *When your patient has pulmonary edema.*)

Drug treatment
Treatment of myocardial dysfunction includes positive inotropic agents, such as digoxin and amrinone, to enhance contractility. Pressor agents may be given to enhance contractility and to promote vasoconstriction in peripheral vessels. Antiarrhythmics may also be given, particularly in arrhythmias related to decreased cardiac output. Occasionally, arterial vasodilators, such as nitroprusside, can decrease peripheral vascular resistance, preload, and afterload.

Morphine may reduce a patient's anxiety and dyspnea and dilate the systemic venous bed, promoting blood flow from pulmonary circulation to the periphery. Morphine reduces preload by limiting venous return.

Surgery
Performing a phlebotomy can reduce preload by limiting venous return to the heart. Phlebotomy will also remove hemoglobin, which may worsen the patient's hypoxemia.

Other treatments
Patients who don't respond to conventional therapy may be treated with an intra-aortic balloon pump. The balloon pump augments diastole in the left ventricle, thereby increasing cardiac output.

Ongoing nursing interventions
• Help the patient relax to promote oxygenation, control bronchospasm, and enhance myocardial contractility. You'll need to reassure him, because he'll be frightened by his inability to breathe normally. Provide emotional support to his family as well.
• Place the patient in high Fowler's position to enhance his lung expansion. Administer oxygen as ordered. Assess the patient's condition frequently, and document his responses to treatment.
• Reposition the patient at least every 2 hours. Because of the decreased blood flow to the skin, patients with pulmonary edema develop pressure ulcers easily. Certain hospital beds are effective in preventing pressure ulcers in high-risk patients.
• Monitor ABG and pulse oximetry values, oral and I.V. fluid intake, and urine output. The patient's fluid and sodium intake will be restricted.
• In the patient with a pulmonary artery catheter, pulmonary end-diastolic pressure and PAWP are measured at least hourly. Check the cardiac monitor frequently and document any change in the ECG rate or pattern immediately. Watch for complications, such as electrolyte depletion. Also watch for complications of oxygen therapy and mechanical ventilation, such as oxygen toxicity, pulmonary barotrauma, hypotension, decreased cardiac output, and tachycardia.
• Monitor vital signs every 15 to 30 minutes when administering nitroprusside in dextrose 5% in water by I.V. drip. During use, protect the solution from light by wrapping the bottle or bag with aluminum foil or placing it in a protective bag. Discard unused nitroprusside after 4 hours. Watch for arrhythmias in patients receiving digoxin and for marked respiratory depression in patients receiving morphine. Carefully record the time morphine is given and the amount administered.
• Review all prescribed medications with the patient and urge him to comply with his medication regimen to avoid future episodes of pulmonary edema. Explain all procedures to the patient and his family, and emphasize the importance of reporting early signs of fluid overload.

When your patient has pulmonary edema

Pulmonary edema requires prompt detection and aggressive treatment. To help guide your care, suppose that you're caring for Jacob Wyckoff, age 50, who was admitted to the intensive care unit (ICU) 5 days ago with an acute anterior wall myocardial infarction (MI). Mr. Wyckoff was transferred to your telemetry unit yesterday and has had no recurrent chest pain since admission.

Quick assessment
While making your afternoon rounds, you enter Mr. Wyckoff's room to find him struggling to breathe. A quick assessment reveals a rapid and labored respiratory rate of 32 breaths/minute. His heart rate is 136 beats/minute and irregular. The cardiac monitor shows atrial fibrillation. Mr. Wyckoff says he still feels no chest pain. His blood pressure is 150/94 mm Hg. Auscultation reveals crackles and wheezes two-thirds of the way up in both lung fields. You suspect pulmonary edema.

Rapid intervention
Knowing you need to help Mr. Wyckoff quickly, you administer 4 liters of oxygen by nasal cannula (for which Mr. Wyckoff has a p.r.n. order) and page the doctor. You elevate the head of the bed 30 degrees.

The doctor obtains arterial blood gas (ABG) results that reveal a pH of 7.47, PaO_2 of 60 mm Hg, $PaCO_2$ of 30 mm Hg, and HCO_3^- of 22 mEq/liter. He also orders a chest X-ray.

Mr. Wyckoff's condition continues to deteriorate. He starts to cough up pink, frothy sputum. His chest X-ray reveals blurred vascular outlines, butterfly markings (typical of alveolar edema), and whiteouts, confirming pulmonary edema. Electrocardiogram (ECG) changes are consistent with his previous anterior wall MI plus atrial fibrillation.

Immediate drug treatment
You give Mr. Wyckoff morphine, as ordered, to decrease his discomfort and anxiety and to promote vasodilation. Morphine also helps reduce oxygen demands and oxygen consumption. You also administer furosemide, as ordered, to reduce preload and afterload. This drug's diuretic effect relieves pulmonary congestion by lowering hydrostatic pressure.

Mr. Wyckoff's atrial fibrillation is contributing to his pulmonary edema by preventing the atrium from contracting efficiently and emptying during systole. Although digoxin isn't a first-line drug in pulmonary edema, Mr. Wyckoff needs it to improve his left ventricular contractility. You also give aminophylline, as ordered, to relieve bronchospasm.

Mr. Wyckoff is still on a continuous cardiac monitor. Be sure to watch for premature ventricular contractions, which may herald ventricular tachycardia.

To help reduce Mr. Wyckoff's anxiety, explain the procedures and answer his questions.

Lack of response
Despite prompt interventions, Mr. Wyckoff doesn't respond well. An hour after initiating treatment, you note these findings:
• heart rate, 142 beats/minute and irregular
• respiratory rate, 40 breaths/minute
• blood pressure, 114/68 mm Hg
• urine output, 40 ml/hour
• PaO_2, 52 mm Hg
• $PaCO_2$, 50 mm Hg
• HCO_3^-, 20 mEq/liter
• pH, 7.28
• atrial fibrillation apparent on the ECG. (A 12-lead ECG also reveals widespread ischemia.)

Because Mr. Wyckoff's urine output is low, the doctor doubles the furosemide dosage. Mr. Wyckoff is then intubated and transferred to the ICU, where he is placed on mechanical ventilation and prepared for insertion of a pulmonary artery catheter. You record his initial readings: pulmonary artery pressure, 40/27 mm Hg (normal range is 20 to 30 mm Hg systolic and 5 to 15 mm Hg diastolic); pulmonary artery wedge pressure, 25 mm Hg (normal is 4 to 12 mm Hg); and arterial blood pressure, 112/68 mm Hg. The doctor starts a nitroglycerin infusion, which will reduce preload and, to a lesser extent, afterload, by dilating vascular smooth muscle.

(continued)

When your patient has pulmonary edema *(continued)*

Improvement

Two hours after the nitroglycerin infusion was started, Mr. Wyckoff's respiratory rate declines to 22 breaths/minute. Crackles are audible only at the lung bases. His blood pressure has stabilized at 120/70 mm Hg, and his apical pulse is down to 100 beats/minute and regular.

Responding to the furosemide, he produced almost 2 liters of urine in an hour. But an S_3 is still audible, indicating that his ventricular failure isn't completely resolved.

Still, his most recent ABG values show how much he has improved: PaO_2, 80 mm Hg; $PaCO_2$, 38 mm Hg; HCO_3^-, 22 mEq/liter; and pH, 7.40.

After 3 days of treatment in the ICU, Mr. Wyckoff's pulmonary edema clears up and serial ECGs remain negative for a new or extended MI. He is then transferred back to your unit.

Your quick but systematic assessment of Mr. Wyckoff when he first entered your unit led to a diagnosis of pulmonary edema. Alerting the doctor allowed initiation of the physical, mechanical, and drug treatments that brought Mr. Wyckoff out of the crisis.

• If the patient takes digoxin, show him how to monitor his own pulse rate and warn him to report signs of toxicity. Encourage him to eat potassium-rich foods to lower the risk of toxicity and of cardiac arrhythmias. Explain the reasons for sodium restriction, and make sure he knows which foods are high in sodium. If he takes a vasodilator, teach him the signs of hypotension and emphasize the need to avoid alcohol. Discuss ways he might conserve his physical energy.

Flail chest

In flail chest, one of the most serious thoracic cage injuries, two or more adjacent ribs are fractured in two places (anteriorly and laterally) or the sternum may be detached, resulting in a free-floating section.

Causes

Flail chest results from blunt chest trauma, most often caused by motor vehicle accidents, sporting accidents, fights, and blast injuries. (See *Responding to a flail chest injury.*)

Pathophysiology

Multiple rib fractures cause a section of the chest wall to detach, moving inward rather than outward during inspiration. Known as paradoxical chest movement, the movement of this flail section responds to the changes in intrathoracic pressure rather than assisting in respiration. As negative intrathoracic pressure increases during inspiration, the flail section is drawn inward instead of moving outward with the rest of the thoracic cage.

During exhalation, the negative intrathoracic pressure drops and the flail section is pushed outward rather than moving inward with the rest of the thoracic cage. The lung tissue underlying the flail section can't expand and fills with air on inspiration. The result is alveolar collapse and development of atelectasis. If the flail section is large, oxygenation is compromised. (See *Flail chest: Paradoxical chest movement,* page 80.)

Complications

Pulmonary contusion, pneumothorax, and myocardial contusion can all develop from flail chest. Hypoxia, which can lead to respiratory failure if left untreated, can also develop from flail chest. Whenever there has been enough trauma to result in flail chest, suspect underlying pulmonary contusions and interstitial or alveolar bleeding.

Assessment
History
When you take the patient's history, he will almost always reveal an incident of trauma.

Physical examination
Inspection may reveal bruised skin, paradoxical chest movement, rapid and shallow respirations, shortness of breath, increased difficulty breathing, and cyanosis. Palpation may reveal tenderness of the thorax. The patient may also have tachycardia, hypotension, a falling PaO_2 level, and respiratory acidosis. If there is damage to the underlying lung tissue, the patient may have hemoptysis.

Diagnostic tests
A chest X-ray will confirm rib and sternal fractures, pneumothorax, flail chest, pulmonary contusions, lacerated or ruptured aorta, lung compression, or atelectasis with hemothorax.

Ongoing treatment
Paralyzing agents, such as pancuronium, atracurium, or vecuronium, may be used to prevent the patient from breathing on his own and to allow the ventilator to control his chest wall movement during respiration. Sedate the patient when using a neuromuscular blocker. This will help prevent the frustration and anxiety the patient would feel from not being able to move.

Patients receiving neuromuscular blockers need to be monitored closely to make sure they're receiving the correct amount. The smallest drug dosage is used to achieve a level of paralysis from 75% to 90%. Currently, no laboratory tests give an accurate indication of the level of paralysis and thereby the appropriate dosage.

The best way to monitor patients receiving neuromuscular blockers is with a peripheral nerve stimulator, which you can use at the bedside. The ulnar nerve is stimulated by a

EMERGENCY INTERVENTIONS

Responding to a flail chest injury

Suspect flail chest if you observe paradoxical chest wall movement. Stabilize the flail section immediately by placing the patient in semi-Fowler's position with the flail side down. You can also stabilize the segment by taping the area with wide tape, placing a sandbag on the area, or applying manual pressure over the flail section.

Provide emergency care
Emergency care goals, in order of priority, are to:
• maintain a patent airway
• stabilize the flail chest
• control bleeding
• maintain adequate ventilation
• establish an I.V. line for fluids and medications.

Relieve mild respiratory distress
If the patient is in mild respiratory distress, administer oxygen via nasal cannula or mask. For severe respiratory distress, hypoxemia, and hypercapnia, immediate intubation and mechanical ventilation will be required. The use of positive- pressure mechanical ventilation will provide an internal pneumatic splint for the flail section. Positive end-expiratory pressure may be ordered to maintain positive pressure in the lung and to prevent alveolar collapse. Other care measures include obtaining an arterial blood gas sample and connecting the patient to a cardiac monitor.

low-voltage stimulus from a small battery-powered device. Four pulsations are delivered to the nerve at 0.5-second intervals. Watch for twitching in the fingers. The level of paralysis is determined by the number of twitches produced by the four pulses. No twitch is considered a 100% block; one twitch is considered a 90% block. Tests are performed every 15 minutes for the first hour and every hour thereafter.

If the injury is severe or prolonged mechanical ventilation is expected, the patient may require surgery to stabilize the flail section.

Flail chest: Paradoxical chest movement

Inspiration
The chest wall normally expands during inspiration, drawing air into the lungs. But in flail chest, the flail section retracts as the patient inspires, as shown in the illustration below. Atelectasis sets in as lung tissue beneath the injury can't expand.

Expiration
As the illustration below shows, the flail section moves in a direction opposite to the rest of the chest wall, bulging out during expiration. Consequently, the patient can't expel air effectively.

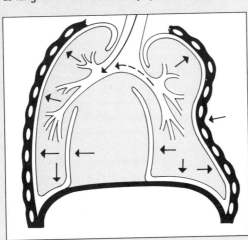

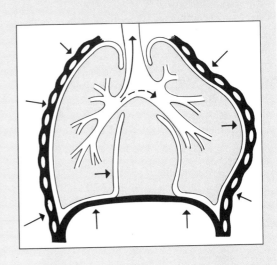

Ongoing nursing interventions
• Explain all procedures and equipment to the patient and his family. Provide emotional support to the patient, especially during times of pain and anxiety.
• Watch the patient carefully to detect paradoxical movement of the flail section.
• Monitor the patient for complications, such as hemothorax or pneumothorax.
• Monitor the patient's oxygenation via pulse oximetry or serial ABG levels, as ordered.
• Control the patient's pain as much as possible. Pain may cause voluntary and involuntary splinting, resulting in hypoventilation, hypoxemia, hypercapnia, and atelectasis. Patients may receive narcotics, such as morphine or meperidine.
• Monitor the patient closely for evidence of respiratory depression.

• If the patient isn't on a mechanical ventilator, provide nasotracheal suctioning, if ordered, to maintain a patent airway. If the patient is on a mechanical ventilator, provide suctioning every 2 hours as needed with a closed suction system to prevent oxygen desaturation. Preoxygenation with 100% FIO_2 before suctioning will also decrease the risk of desaturation. The use of chest physiotherapy may be indicated to help clear secretions.
• Keep the patient in an upright position to help improve lung expansion. At least every 2 hours, change his position by logrolling him to provide stabilization and comfort. Try to turn him to his unaffected side when possible to improve alveolar perfusion. If he has posterior rib fractures, don't position him on his back. Make sure the patient understands why he must be positioned properly.

• Have the patient cough and breathe deeply every 2 hours. Assist him by splinting the tender sites with a pillow or cough bear. If the patient isn't ventilated, encourage him to use an incentive spirometer every 1 to 2 hours.
• Maintaining fluid balance in the patient with flail chest is essential, so you should replace any lost blood with whole or packed RBCs. A contused lung handles water poorly because body fluid shifts from intravascular to extravascular spaces around damaged tissues. Consequently, the patient may need plasma or serum albumin to maintain fluid volume. These colloidal fluids keep fluid in the pulmonary capillaries, helping to maintain adequate circulation.

Status asthmaticus

A prolonged asthmatic attack that doesn't respond to conventional asthma therapy with bronchodilators, status asthmaticus can be fatal even with optimal therapy. The condition can last for days to weeks.

Causes
Status asthmaticus is a complication of asthma. An asthma attack can be caused by a variety of stimuli or precipitating factors, including dust, pollen, animal dander, food and cooking odors, perfume or cologne, cleaning products, air pollutants, mold spores, grains, exercise, and cold, dry air.

Medications, such as aspirin, nonsteroidal anti-inflammatory drugs, and beta-adrenergic agents (including eyedrops), can also trigger asthma attacks. Additionally, viral infections, overuse of bronchodilators, an autonomic nervous system imbalance, and psychological or emotional upheaval can bring on an attack in an asthmatic patient. (See *Responding to status asthmaticus*, page 82.)

Pathophysiology
Asthma is a disease of reversible airflow obstruction, characterized by bronchospasm, inflammation and edema of the airway mucosa, and increased sputum production.

When the patient inhales one of the substances to which he is hypersensitive, abnormal (IgE) antibodies stimulate mast cells in the lung interstitium to release histamine. Airway inflammation results from the release of inflammatory mediators from epithelial cells, epithelial mast cells, and macrophages. These substances cause migration and activation of eosinophils and neutrophils, which in turn cause alterations in epithelial integrity, abnormalities in autonomic neural control of the airway, changes in mucociliary function, and increased airway responsiveness.

Histamine attaches to receptor sites in the larger and smaller bronchi, where it causes swelling in smooth muscles. Mucous membranes become inflamed, irritated, and swollen. It also causes fatty acids called prostaglandins to travel via the bloodstream to the lungs, where they enhance histamine's effect. Histamine stimulates the mucous membranes to secrete excessive mucus, further narrowing the bronchial lumen. Goblet cells secrete a viscous mucus that's difficult for the patient to cough up. When the patient inhales, the narrowed bronchial lumen can still expand slightly, allowing air to reach the alveoli.

On exhalation, increased intrathoracic pressure closes the bronchial lumen completely. Air can get in but can't get out. Mucus fills the lung bases, inhibiting alveolar ventilation. Blood, shunted to alveoli in other lung parts, still can't compensate for diminished ventilation, and respiratory acidosis results. (See *How status asthmaticus progresses*, page 83.)

Complications
Respiratory alkalosis, respiratory acidosis, hypoxia, hypoxemia, and cyanosis may all develop from status asthmaticus. Ultimately, it can cause respiratory failure.

Assessment
History
Ask the patient when the attack began and what triggered it. Have the symptoms limited the patient's walking, sleeping, and talking?

Responding to status asthmaticus

Your priorities in responding to a patient with status asthmaticus are to reduce bronchoconstriction, treat hypoxemia, and, if necessary, transfer him to the intensive care unit (ICU) for possible intubation and mechanical ventilation.

Reduce bronchoconstriction

If you suspect status asthmaticus, reduce bronchoconstriction as soon as possible by administering ordered bronchodilators and assessing the patient's vital signs. Be alert for pulsus paradoxus. Provide emotional support and patient teaching to help reduce ineffective breathing, as necessary. Regularly assess the patency of the I.V. line, or establish one if needed. Also regularly monitor his respiratory rate, pattern, and depth.

Treat hypoxemia

Treat hypoxemia with oxygen therapy to keep the partial pressure of arterial oxygen (PaO_2) above 65 mm Hg or the arterial oxygen saturation (SaO_2) greater than 90%. Monitor oxygenation with periodic arterial blood gas samples and continuous pulse oximetry. Asthmatic patients don't tolerate a mask well, so use a nasal cannula at a fraction of inspired oxygen (FIO_2) of 2 to 4 liters/minute (30% to 35%).

Changes in patient position, intermittent airway plugging, and pulmonary vasodilation may result in decreasing SaO_2 levels. While monitoring the partial pressure of arterial carbon dioxide and the SaO_2, limit older patients with chronic airflow obstruction to an FIO_2 of 24% to 28%.

Provide intensive care

When a patient with increasingly severe asthma doesn't respond to drug therapy, he is usually admitted to the ICU for treatment. The patient may require intubation and mechanical ventilation. Rising carbon dioxide levels, falling pH, and increasing respiratory fatigue are signs that call for intubation and mechanical ventilation.

Review his medication history, especially since the asthma attack began. Ask the patient how often he uses his metered-dose inhaler and what type of medications he is using. These may include bronchodilators, such as albuterol, metaproterenol, or theophylline.

Find out if the patient has been to the emergency department in the past few days and how often he has needed emergency treatment in the past. Has he been taking his prescribed medications? How often has he needed intubation? Patients with a history of syncope during asthma attacks or of requiring intubation are at increased risk for a fatal attack.

Physical examination

The patient who develops status asthmaticus is usually apprehensive, pale, breathless, and exhausted from fighting for air. Also, he is usually severely dyspneic and has great difficulty walking and talking. You may also detect signs of hypoxemia: anxiety, restlessness, and confusion.

Other signs of status asthmaticus include tachypnea, tachycardia, dehydration, and wheezing. You may hear inspiratory and expiratory wheezing without placing the stethoscope on the patient's chest. Often, the patient uses the accessory muscles of respiration. His expirations will be active and prolonged, with an I:E ratio of 1:2 to 1:4. In a severe attack, you may not hear the patient's wheezing because he lacks sufficient air movement in his chest. Coughing may be almost impossible for him. His heart sounds will be distant; his pulse, rapid and thready.

Pulsus paradoxus, a drop of more than 12 mm Hg in systolic blood pressure during inspiration, indicates a severe airflow obstruction. The paradoxical pulse is linked to decreased filling of the right atrium, decreased lung compliance, and increased intrathoracic pressure.

Percussion of the chest will reveal hyperresonance. Palpation may reveal vocal fremitus. Other assessment findings include increased pulse rate, blood pressure, and respiratory rate. Diaphoresis, pallor, cyanotic nail beds, and flaring nostrils are other signs to look for.

Diagnostic tests

Tests that diagnose status asthmaticus include pulmonary function tests, ABG studies, and chest X-ray.

Pulmonary function tests reveal signs of airway obstructive disease (decreased flow rates and forced expiratory volume at 1 second [FEV_1], low-normal or decreased vital capacity and increased total lung and residual capacity, and decreased peak expiratory flow rate [PEFR]). The patient with status asthmaticus may have a difficult time performing these tests. PEFR requires only a forceful breath—rather than a full, sustained exhalation—and therefore is easier for the patient to perform. FEV_1 and PEFR are monitored over time to determine trends in lung function. Falling PEFR and FEV_1 indicate worsening airway obstruction.

Typically, the patient with asthma has decreased $PaCO_2$ and PaO_2. In status asthmaticus, however, the $PaCO_2$ may be normal or increased, indicating severe bronchial obstruction. Once the patient has stabilized, the spirometric values (FEV_1 and forced expiratory flow) remain abnormal, necessitating frequent ABG analyses or pulse oximetry measurements. Residual volume remains abnormal for the longest period—up to 3 weeks after the attack.

Laboratory tests may reveal an increased serum IgE concentration from an allergic reaction and an increased eosinophil count in the complete blood count with differential. ABG analysis can detect hypoxemia and guide treatment.

Despite hypoxemia, the patient's $PaCO_2$ level is usually normal because he compensates by hyperventilating and partially because CO_2 diffuses readily through the bloodstream. However, his $PaCO_2$ level may increase if he's exhausted and approaching respiratory failure.

As the patient tires and respiratory muscles become fatigued, CO_2 retention and accumulation of lactic acid may cause his pH to fall. If the patient is falling asleep or looks cyanotic, he may be developing acute respiratory failure. Other indicators of impending respiratory fail-

PATHOPHYSIOLOGY

How status asthmaticus progresses

Potentially fatal, status asthmaticus arises when impaired gas exchange and heightened airway resistance increase the work of breathing. This flowchart shows the stages of status asthmaticus.

> Obstructed airways hamper gas exchange and increase airway resistance, leading to labored breathing.

> Initially, the patient hyperventilates, lowering the $PaCO_2$. Respiratory alkalosis and hypoxemia may develop quickly.

> The patient tires rapidly. His respiratory rate drops to normal.

> Later, $PaCO_2$ rises to higher than baseline level. (An asthmatic patient's $PaCO_2$ is usually low.)

> The patient hypoventilates from exhaustion.

> Respiratory acidosis begins as the partial pressure of arterial oxygen drops and $PaCO_2$ continues to rise.

> Without treatment, the patient experiences acute respiratory failure.

ure include a $PaCO_2$ level above 40 mm Hg, FEV_1 or PEFR below 25% of predicted values, wide fluctuation in PEFR or FEV_1, or a less than 10% improvement in PEFR or FEV_1 over initial values after treatment.

Chest X-ray can diagnose or monitor the progress of the attack. The X-ray may show hyperinflation with areas of focal atelectasis.

Skin testing may be used to identify specific allergens. Test results are read in 1 to 2 days to detect an early reaction and then again after 4 to 5 days to reveal a late reaction. Bronchial challenge testing is used to evaluate the clinical significance of allergens identified by skin testing.

Ongoing treatment

Treatment consists of beta-agonist bronchodilators, corticosteroids, oral sympathomimetics, sympathomimetic aerosol therapy (such as metaproterenol and albuterol), epinephrine injected subcutaneously for rapid effect, terbutaline, aminophylline, and theophylline.

Bronchodilators are given via aerosol therapy at intervals dictated by the severity of the patient's symptoms. This may be as often as hourly or it may be continuous.

Systemic corticosteroids, such as methylprednisolone, are given I.V. to reduce inflammation and edema of the airway mucosa. Dosage depends on the patient's size, the severity of the attack, and his previous steroid therapy (if any).

ABG analysis and pulse oximetry are used to assess respiratory status, particularly after ventilator therapy or a change in oxygen concentration. If the patient is hypoxemic, aerosol therapy is given with oxygen rather than compressed air.

Antibiotics are indicated if the patient shows signs of infection. Fluid replacement may also be necessary.

Ongoing nursing interventions

• During the acute phase, maintain respiratory function and relieve bronchoconstriction while allowing mucus plug expulsion. Reassure the patient during an attack, and stay with him. Place him in semi-Fowler's position and encourage him to relax as much as possible.
• Administer oxygen via nasal cannula or mechanical ventilation.
• Monitor ABG levels and pulse oximetry values for trends in oxygenation.
• Administer drugs and I.V. fluids as ordered.
• Monitor the patient for dehydration, which may increase the thickness of the secretions and make them harder to remove; this, in turn, may cause airway plugging.
• Administer aminophylline I.V. as a loading dose. Follow with an I.V. drip, as ordered. Monitor the patient for aminophylline toxicity and for nausea, vomiting, tachycardia, and anxiety. Older patients with hepatic or cardiac insufficiency or those taking erythromycin are predisposed to aminophylline toxicity. Because young patients and those who smoke or take barbiturates have increased aminophylline metabolism, they require a larger dose. Monitor the aminophylline drip rate carefully, using an I.V. infusion pump.
• Don't use sedatives and narcotics because they can depress the respiratory system.
• With long-term corticosteroid therapy, watch for cushingoid signs and symptoms. Orally inhaled corticosteroids—beclomethasone, flunisolide, and triamcinolone— may be ordered for long-term use; atropine-like medications may also be ordered.
• Focus your patient teaching on preventing recurring attacks. Teach the patient and family the triggers and early warning signs (wheezing and shortness of breath) of asthma. Teach the patient how to use the metered-dose inhaler correctly. Advise him about possible adverse reactions associated with the medications he's receiving, and instruct him to notify his doctor if reactions occur.
• Urge the patient to drink plenty of fluids (at least 3 quarts daily) to maintain hydration and prevent thickening of airway secretions. Show him how to breathe deeply. Instruct him to

cough up secretions accumulated overnight and to allow time for medications to work. He can best loosen secretions by coughing correctly—inhaling fully and gently, then bending over with his arms crossed over the abdomen before coughing.

• Teach the patient and his family about diaphragmatic and pursed-lip breathing. Encourage the patient to perform relaxation exercises whenever he feels himself becoming anxious.

• Encourage the patient to maintain a well-balanced diet to prevent respiratory infection and fatigue. Help him identify foods that trigger an attack. Teach the patient and his family to avoid known allergens and irritants, such as aerosol sprays, smoke, and automobile exhausts. Refer the patient to community resources, such as the American Lung Association and the Asthma and Allergy Foundation of America.

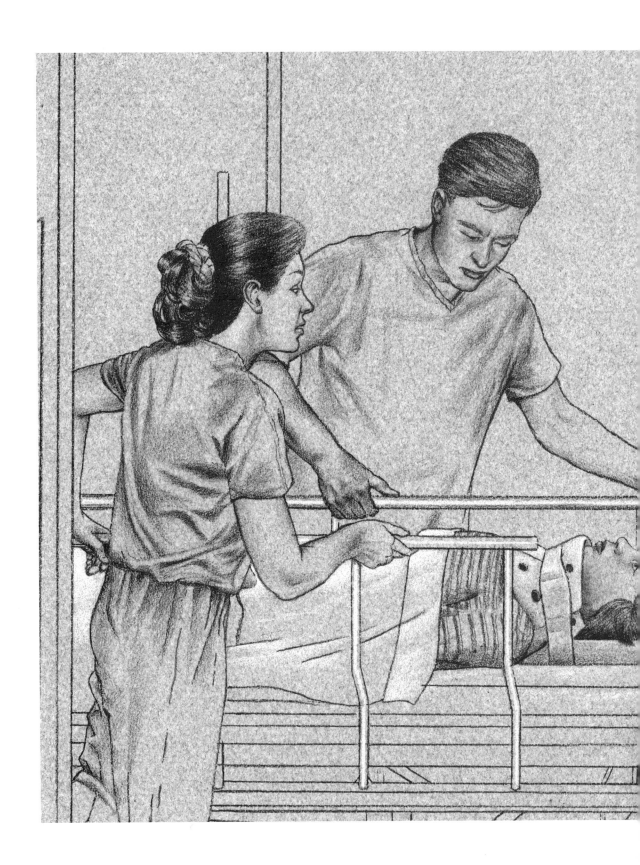

CHAPTER 3

Neurologic crises

A neurologic crisis can challenge all of your nursing assessment and intervention skills. It involves complex pathophysiologic and systemic interactions, so it compromises not just the neurologic system but other vital systems as well. Without early recognition and prompt treatment, your patient stands little chance of surviving the crisis or avoiding serious deficits.

To avert disaster, you must assess your patient's level of consciousness, perform a quick neurologic examination, and stabilize any spinal injuries. Then you need to maintain close continuing assessment. Your initial findings provide crucial baseline information. But in a neurologic crisis, the patient's condition may change rapidly. In fact, his chances for recovery may hinge on your ability to recognize when his condition is deteriorating.

In this chapter, you'll find the information you need to effectively and confidently manage patients with common neurologic crises, including closed head injury, ruptured cerebral aneurysm, arteriovenous malformation, status epilepticus, neurogenic shock, and myasthenic crisis.

Closed head injury

A closed head injury (CHI) is an injury to the head in which the skull remains intact or sustains only a linear fracture. Types of CHI include concussion, contusion, acceleration-deceleration injury, shearing injury, and diffuse axonal injury.

CHI may be primary, resulting from direct impact, or secondary, occurring as a consequence of a primary injury. To save your patient's life, you must take appropriate measures at once. (See *When your patient has a closed head injury.*)

Causes
CHI results from a head trauma that doesn't expose skull contents to air. For instance, a *concussion* results from jarring of the brain, which causes a transient loss of consciousness. Blunt head trauma usually is responsible for a *contusion,* or bruising of the brain. This injury has various forms. In a *punctate contusion,* petechial bruising occurs, usually from a shearing force. In a *coup injury,* the contusion occurs at the point of impact—for example, when the head suddenly strikes something and the brain strikes the inside of the skull. A *contrecoup injury* occurs when trauma causes the brain to rebound against the skull surface directly opposite the point of impact.

An *acceleration injury* occurs when the head strikes a moving object, such as a baseball bat; a *deceleration injury,* when the head

---

EMERGENCY INTERVENTIONS

When your patient has a closed head injury

If you suspect that a patient has a closed head injury, apply and maintain a cervical collar until the doctor rules out cervical spine injury. Then assess and ensure an open airway, breathing, and circulation.

Perform a neurologic assessment
Next, perform a brief neurologic assessment. If the patient has a Glasgow Coma Scale score below 10, prepare him for intubation to maintain airway patency and initiate hyperventilation therapy, as ordered. Hyperventilation is induced 'to constrict the vessels and control cerebral blood flow and intracranial hypertension. Aim for a partial pressure of carbon dioxide in arterial blood of 33 to 35 mm Hg.

As ordered, arrange for an immediate computed tomography scan of the head. Insert a large-bore I.V. needle and draw blood for arterial blood gas (ABG) analysis, blood chemistry studies, a complete blood count, and blood typing and cross-matching. If appropriate, prepare the patient for insertion of an arterial line to permit frequent ABG evaluation.

Administer mannitol
If the patient has dilated pupils and an altered level of consciousness, administer 50 to 100 g of mannitol I.V., as ordered, to reduce cerebral edema. Titrate the dose to the patient's weight. Elevate the head of the bed 30 to 45 degrees. Maintain mean arterial pressure above 80 mm Hg and systolic blood pressure above 100 mm Hg. Monitor cardiac output, and notify the doctor if it falls below 5 liters/minute.

Other measures
As ordered, administer 0.9% sodium chloride solution to expand volume. Insert an indwelling urinary catheter to permit accurate intake and output measurement. As appropriate, prepare the patient for emergency surgery or placement of an intracranial pressure monitoring device.

Classifying cerebral edema

Depending on the cause, cerebral edema may be vasogenic, cytotoxic, hydrostatic, or interstitial. For each form of cerebral edema, this chart describes the pathologic process, cause, and treatment.

TYPE	PATHOLOGIC PROCESS	CAUSE	TREATMENT
Vasogenic	• Altered permeability of blood-brain barrier permits proteins and water to leak into brain interstitium.	• Trauma • Tumor	• Furosemide
Cytotoxic	• Failure of sodium-potassium pump renders cells unable to maintain osmolarity gradient and allows water to flow passively into cells.	• Hypoxia • Ischemia	• Mannitol
Hydrostatic	• Rising pressures force water out of vascular compartment and into interstitium.	• Hypertension	• Antihypertensive drugs
Interstitial	• Ventricular obstruction increases hydrostatic pressure, allowing fluid to diffuse into spaces around ventricles.	• Hydrocephalus	• Intraventricular catheter or shunt

strikes a stationary object, for instance, the floor. In an *acceleration-deceleration injury* (also called a *coup-contrecoup injury*), the brain is injured directly at and opposite the point of impact.

A *shearing injury* is caused by twisting of the brain on the brain stem. A *diffuse axonal injury* occurs when the force of the impact is spread throughout the entire brain, causing axons to stretch or become disrupted, altering their ability to conduct impulses. These injuries usually result from high-velocity trauma such as a motor vehicle accident.

Pathophysiology

Enclosed by the rigid skull, the brain is further protected by three meninges, or membranes, and cushioned by cerebrospinal fluid (CSF). However, when a direct or indirect force is applied to the skull, the brain may become mobile, striking the sides of the skull and creating shearing forces through itself and through the meningeal layers. A concussion, contusion, diffuse axonal injury, shearing injury or, as a latter consequence, a hematoma may result.

CHI alters the delicate balance between brain volume and pressure, increasing the risk of secondary head injury. A secondary head injury is the brain's response to such trauma as cerebral edema, increased intracranial pressure

(ICP), hemorrhage, or hematoma. (See *Classifying cerebral edema.*) Normally, the sum of the volume components within the skull — brain volume, blood volume, and CSF volume — remains constant. If the volume of one component increases, the volume of another must decrease to maintain a constant volume-pressure relationship. After CHI, vasoconstriction occurs at the injury site to stop bleeding. This reduces perfusion to the injured area and stimulates capillary permeability, resulting in cerebral edema and increased ICP. When the brain becomes ischemic, autoregulation of cerebral blood flow fails, triggering anaerobic metabolism, which may lead to cell death.

CHI also compromises cerebral perfusion pressure (CPP). Normally, autoregulation maintains a constant cerebral blood flow regardless of pressure within the arteries. This self-regulating mechanism remains intact when CPP exceeds 50 mm Hg, but it becomes defective when CPP falls below 50 mm Hg and fails completely when CPP drops to 40 mm Hg or less. Once autoregulation is impaired, systolic pressure regulates cerebral blood flow. Other factors that alter the balance of cerebral blood flow and perfusion include the partial pressures of arterial oxygen (PaO_2) and carbon dioxide ($PaCO_2$). For instance, hypoxemia (PaO_2 below 60 mm Hg) and hypercapnia ($PaCO_2$ above

45 mm Hg) produce cerebral vasodilation, which increases cerebral blood flow.

Complications

Neurologic complications of CHI include increased ICP, cerebral edema, brain herniation, cerebral hemorrhage, hematoma, and brain infarction. (See *Supratentorial herniation syndromes*.)

Systemic problems also may arise, such as aspiration pneumonia, thrombocytopenia, seizures, arrhythmias, hypotension or hypertension, diabetes insipidus, and syndrome of inappropriate antidiuretic hormone (SIADH).

Assessment

History

If initial reports suggest CHI, assume that the patient has a spinal cord injury and take appropriate measures to immobilize the spine — or verify that rescue workers have done so.

A patient with an altered level of consciousness (LOC) or memory loss may be unable to supply information about the injury or his medical history. So you'll need to ask rescue workers or family members for a brief history. Focus on the following points:
• When and how did the injury occur?
• What was the injury mechanism? Was the patient struck with a moving or stationary object? Was he in a motor vehicle accident?
• What force or velocity was involved in the injury?
• Where was the point of impact?
• If the patient was in a motor vehicle accident, was he wearing a seat belt? Did his head strike the windshield or roof? Was he trapped in the vehicle?
• Did the patient lose consciousness? If so, for how long?
• Has the patient's condition deteriorated since the injury? If so, how?
• Has he complained of a headache or neck pain?
• Did he vomit after the injury?

Physical examination

Obtain vital signs and perform a brief examination to establish a baseline. Evaluate the patient's neurologic status, and use the Glasgow Coma Scale score to gauge his LOC. (See *Using the Glasgow Coma Scale,* page 92.) Assess his pupils for equality, reaction to light, accommodation, and the consensual light reflex.

Next, test the patient's oculomotor responses and evaluate his respirations for abnormal patterns. (See *Identifying abnormal respiratory patterns,* page 93.)

Evaluate his motor strength and assess primitive reflexes, such as Babinski's, glabellar, and sucking reflexes.

Examine the patient's scalp for abrasions and lacerations, palpate his skull for elevations or depressions, and inspect his face. If you find periorbital ecchymoses (raccoon's eyes) or posterior auricular ecchymosis (Battle's sign), suspect a basilar skull fracture. Inspect the ears and nose for drainage, which may indicate a basilar skull fracture with associated CSF leakage.

Diagnostic tests

The doctor will order an emergency computed tomography (CT) scan of the head to determine the type, location, and size of the injury; to gauge the amount of cerebral swelling; and to detect intracerebral air or fractures. (However, in a concussion, a CT scan won't detect a lesion.) A CT scan augmented by xenon inhalation helps demonstrate areas of diminished perfusion.

To evaluate the brain stem more closely or to help confirm a diffuse axonal injury, the doctor may order a magnetic resonance imaging (MRI) scan to eliminate radiologic skull distortion. A tissue biopsy must be done, however, to confirm a diffuse axonal injury.

Visual, somatosensory, and brain stem evoked response studies help evaluate brain stem and hemispheric function. These studies may provide information that helps to confirm or rule out a specific diagnosis and to establish the prognosis. Visual evoked response studies also help predict increased ICP.

Positron emission tomography scanning — a combination of radioisotope scanning and CT scanning — identifies various metabolic patterns and helps to diagnose such conditions as cerebral ischemia and determine the cause of seizures. The patient is injected with a positron-

Supratentorial herniation syndromes

In brain herniation, a potential complication of closed head injury, cerebral edema or a space-occupying lesion causes intracranial pressure to rise in the affected area. This uneven pressure causes the brain mass to shift toward areas of less pressure, depressing vital structures and causing herniation.

Herniation can occur through the tentorial notch, under the falx cerebri, or through the foramen magnum. One of three distinct herniation syndromes may result.

Cingulate herniation
Cingulate herniation occurs when the falx cerebri is laterally displaced across the midline.

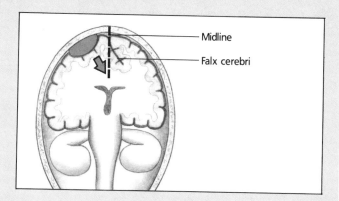

Central herniation
In central herniation, downward movement of the brain displaces the ventricles and pushes the brain stem through the foramen magnum.

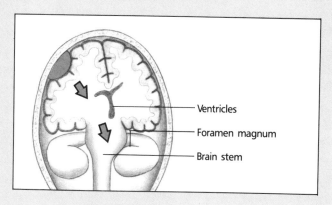

Uncal herniation
In uncal herniation, the tip of the temporal lobe (uncus) moves through the tentorial notch, compressing the midbrain and brain stem.

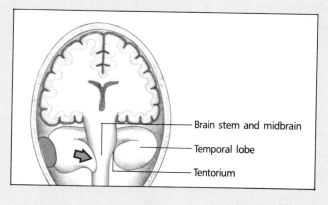

Using the Glasgow Coma Scale

For the patient with a neurologic crisis, the Glasgow Coma Scale serves as a reliable, objective tool for assessing and documenting the level of consciousness. It measures three faculties—eye opening, motor response, and verbal response to stimulation. You assign a number to each possible response within these categories. The lowest score is 3, and the highest possible score is 15. A score of 7 or less indicates coma.

If the patient is intubated, the doctor may instruct you to designate a "T" for "tube/tracheotomy" rather than assign a verbal score. The highest score this patient can receive is 11 T.

TEST	RESPONSE	SCORE
Eye opening	Spontaneous	4
	To speech	3
	To pain	2
	None	1
Best motor response	Obeys command	6
	To painful stimuli:	
	Localizes pain	5
	Withdraws	4
	Abnormal flexion	3
	Extension	2
	None	1
Best verbal response	Oriented	5
	Confused	4
	Inappropriate words	3
	Incomprehensible sounds	2
	None	1

emitting radionuclide that easily crosses the blood-brain barrier. As the compound is metabolized within the brain, a detector measures the intensity of positron emission and converts the pattern into a tomogram. Unfortunately, the high cost of this technique limits it to a few major medical centers.

Ongoing treatment

After the patient receives initial treatment and is somewhat stabilized, medical management focuses on controlling ICP and cerebral edema as ordered. Patients with hematomas or epidural, subdural, or intracerebral hemorrhages will require surgery.

To help lower ICP, the doctor may order mechanical ventilation to induce hyperventilation by blowing off carbon dioxide. (Decreasing carbon dioxide levels constrict cerebral vessels and reduce cerebral blood flow.) During hyperventilation therapy, maintain a $PaCO_2$ of 33 to 35 mm Hg, as ordered. If this range is insufficient to control ICP, you may need to maintain $PaCO_2$ at 30 mm Hg.

Drug treatment

Expect to institute hyperosmolar dehydration therapy to limit the amount of free water available in the circulation. Mannitol, an osmotic diuretic, is the initial drug of choice. It produces diuresis, stabilizes the cell membranes, enhances cardiac output and oxygen delivery, and reduces red blood cell sludging in injured areas. The usual loading dose is 1 to 1.5 g/kg, followed by 50 g every 4 to 6 hours until serum osmolality rises above 300 mOsm/ liter.

Some evidence suggests that mannitol is less effective when the blood-brain barrier is disrupted. In fact, the drug may leak into the interstitium of the brain, worsening cerebral edema. Consequently, the doctor may order concomitant furosemide to achieve the desired serum osmolality because this drug acts selectively on injured tissue.

To further lower ICP, the doctor may order a barbiturate such as thiopental. Barbiturates must be given cautiously because of their serum half-life and tendency to accumulate in adipose tissue, creating a reservoir that produces tissue concentration and prolongs drug clearance. If the patient needs high and frequent intermittent doses of thiopental to control ICP, barbiturate coma therapy may be indicated to slow the metabolic rate, decrease cerebral blood flow, and reduce ICP. During this therapy, monitor for signs and symptoms of barbiturate toxicity, such as hypotension and

Identifying abnormal respiratory patterns

To help assess the patient with a closed head injury, evaluate his respirations. The type of abnormal respiratory pattern may suggest the level of injury, as this chart shows.

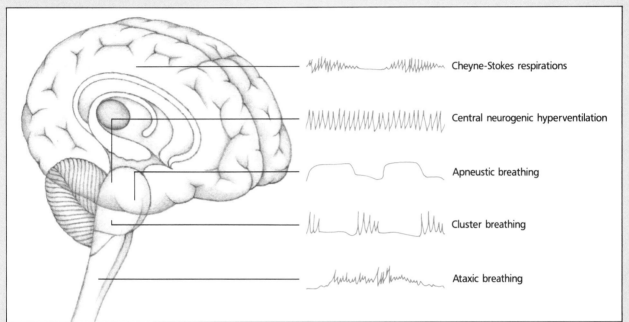

Cheyne-Stokes respirations

Central neurogenic hyperventilation

Apneustic breathing

Cluster breathing

Ataxic breathing

ABNORMAL PATTERN	LEVEL OF INJURY	POSSIBLE CAUSES	NURSING CONSIDERATIONS
Cheyne-Stokes respirations Deep, rapid respirations followed by gradually slower respirations and a period of apnea	• Cerebral hemispheres (usually bilateral); less commonly, cerebellum, midbrain, or upper pons	• Bilateral cerebral infarction, encephalopathy, metabolic disease	• Be aware that Cheyne-Stokes respirations reflect increased sensitivity to carbon dioxide (leading to abnormal increases in respiratory rate and depth) and reduced cerebral stimulation (causing apnea).
Central neurogenic hyperventilation Continual, regular, rapid respirations (at least 24 breaths/minute) with increased respiratory depth	• Lower midbrain or upper pons	• Anoxia, midbrain tumor, midbrain or pontine infarction or ischemia	• Don't assume that this pattern has a neurogenic cause unless the partial pressure of oxygen in arterial blood exceeds 70 mm Hg for 24 hours.
Apneustic breathing Prolonged inspiration with a pause at the point of maximum inspiration. Lasting for 2 to 3 seconds, this pause may alternate with an expiratory pause.	• Middle or lower pons	• Pontine infarction, severe meningitis	• Widespread brain stem damage disrupts the respiratory control center in the middle to lower third of the pons.
Cluster breathing Clustered periods of irregular breathing interspersed with periods of apnea occurring at irregular intervals	• Lower pons or upper medulla	• Tumor or infarction in medulla	• This pattern suggests serious brain damage.
Ataxic breathing Irregular, unpredictable respirations, with deep and shallow breaths and pauses occurring at random	• Medulla	• Cerebellar or pontine bleeding, compression from supratentorial tumor, severe meningitis	• This pattern reflects a disorder in the medulla, the major respiratory center, and signals a rapid deterioration in the patient's condition.

decreased cardiac function. If you're also administering vasopressors or inotropic drugs to maintain blood pressure and support barbiturate use, assess the patient for resistance to vasopressor therapy.

To calm the patient, the doctor may order a sedative—probably a short-acting, reversible one, such as fentanyl or morphine, to avoid narcosis.

If the patient's mean arterial pressure (MAP) remains low despite attempts to augment volume, the doctor may add vasoactive substances to raise his MAP and thus maintain CPP above 60 mm Hg.

Surgery
Surgery for the patient with a CHI may involve a burr hole or a craniotomy. To create a burr hole, the surgeon removes a small, circular portion of the skull. This relatively low-risk procedure allows speedy hematoma evacuation, although an unusually located clot could escape detection.

Craniotomy is gaining favor as the aggressive treatment of choice after head trauma. In this procedure, the surgeon removes a bone flap and opens the dura to expose and wash out a hematoma. He can also visualize and excise ischemic and necrotic tissue while preserving viable tissue and creating a space into which edematous tissues can swell.

Other treatments
Other medical measures aim to maintain CPP by supporting vascular volumes and arterial pressure. For example, 0.9% sodium chloride solution is preferred to restore and maintain volume. Although an alternative solution—such as dextrose 5% in 0.9% sodium chloride solution—may be used, the doctor will avoid one that contains free water because free water readily enters the brain interstitium, producing edema.

The goal of volume management is to maintain a hyperosmotic state while ensuring normal volume status. If the patient has low filling volumes, he may require boluses of a colloid, such as plasma protein fraction or albumin.

Expect the doctor to insert a central line to measure central venous pressure (CVP) and administer diuretics. If the patient remains unstable, the doctor may insert a pulmonary artery (PA) catheter to obtain more detailed hemodynamic data.

Ongoing nursing interventions
For the CHI patient, the chief goals of ongoing care are managing ICP (thus preventing secondary brain injury) and preventing systemic complications.

Be sure to monitor the patient's neurologic status hourly and to report any deterioration promptly. Maintain the patient in a travel-ready state in case he requires an emergency CT scan for further evaluation.

Managing ICP
• Implement ICP management protocols. An ICP monitoring device is usually inserted in any patient with a Glasgow Coma Scale score of 8 or less. Assess the patient for factors that may precipitate increased ICP, and determine how effectively nursing and medical interventions are controlling his ICP.
• Obtain and document ICP readings every hour. (See *Comparing ICP monitoring techniques.*)
• Obtain MAP readings; then calculate and document CPP hourly by subtracting ICP values from MAP values.
• To ensure normal CPP and maintain vascular volumes, maintain the patient at roughly two-thirds the normal volume restoration rate. Usually, this means ensuring a total I.V. fluid intake of approximately 100 ml/hour.
• Intersperse care with frequent rest periods to prevent overstimulating the patient, which could trigger a rise in ICP.
• Elevate the head of the bed 30 to 45 degrees to help reduce ICP, and ensure proper head and neck alignment to promote venous drainage. (The jugular veins are highly sensitive to occlusion related to positioning.)
• Administer prescribed sedatives and analgesics judiciously, keeping in mind the patient's neurologic status and ICP.

Comparing ICP monitoring techniques

The patient with a closed head injury may require continuous intracranial pressure (ICP) monitoring. This chart compares major ICP monitoring techniques.

TECHNIQUE	ADVANTAGES	DISADVANTAGES
Intraventricular catheter Drainage tube inserted into cerebral ventricle to drain excess cerebrospinal fluid and control spikes in ICP due to cerebral edema	• Permits drainage of cerebrospinal fluid (CSF) to reduce intracranial volume	• Carries a high risk of infection
Camino catheter (intraparenchymal monitoring) Fiber-optic catheter placed directly into brain tissue	• Senses brain tissue pressure and shifts • Is less likely to cause infection	• Can be easily broken or pulled out • May produce readings that are slightly higher than actual intraventricular pressure • May drift
Subarachnoid screw Special screw inserted into subarachnoid space to monitor CSF pressure	• Is easier to insert than a catheter	• Requires frequent troubleshooting to eliminate air and matter in screw • Dura frequently reseals, blunting readings
Epidural sensor Tiny fiber-optic sensor inserted into epidural space through a burr hole	• Senses shifts in pressure • Is less likely to cause infection	• May produce readings that are higher than actual intraventricular pressure • May drift

• Release of tissue thromboplastin from the injured brain may lead to altered coagulation and thrombocytopenia, exacerbating intracerebral bleeding. Therefore, take measures to maintain normal coagulation, such as administering fresh frozen plasma and vitamin K, as ordered. Discontinue heparin administration in all invasive lines and apply a pneumonic compression sleeve to the legs, as ordered.
• To help manage ICP, dim the lights and minimize noise in the patient's room. If appropriate, use special audiotapes, such as soothing music or familiar voices. Instruct the patient's family to speak in soft tones and use gentle touch.
• Be aware that patients have varying responses to environmental factors. If you suspect environmental stimulation is increasing your patient's ICP, try to pinpoint the cause and then minimize or eliminate it.
• Temperature and ICP are directly related: ICP increases as body temperature rises. To maintain a normal body temperature, administer acetaminophen, as ordered, and apply heating or cooling blankets.

Preventing systemic complications
• Maintain adequate oxygenation and hyperventilation therapy. As needed, monitor arterial oxygen saturation (SaO_2) by using an SaO_2 monitor, and evaluate carbon dioxide concentration in exhaled gas by using an end-tidal carbon dioxide monitor. These monitors provide information on oxygenation trends while eliminating the need for frequent venipuncture for blood samples.
• Perform chest physiotherapy (CPT) every 4 hours to prevent aspiration pneumonia—common in patients with an altered LOC—and to mobilize secretions. If ordered, maintain the patient in Trendelenburg's position to promote lung drainage and help prevent the need for increased positive end-expiratory pressure (PEEP) to treat atelectasis and infiltration. (In one study, Trendelenburg's position improved

lung clearance and oxygenation with no adverse effects when used for up to 15 minutes in patients with ICP above 25 mm Hg.) However, be aware that this position remains controversial because many neurosurgeons believe an ICP of more than 18 mm Hg is unacceptable and should be treated more aggressively.

• If the patient's secretions become foul smelling, obtain sputum cultures and initiate antibiotic therapy, as ordered and as necessary, to treat respiratory infection.

• Hyperoxygenate and hyperventilate the patient with a hand-held resuscitation bag prior to and following suctioning. Suction the patient every 2 to 4 hours. If ICP rises during suctioning due to coughing or other causes, you may need to administer lidocaine by I.V. infusion or an endotracheal tube to reduce ICP. Coughing increases intrathoracic pressure, thereby increasing ICP.

• Monitor the patient's vital signs hourly. Assess his temperature continually, and maintain a temperature under 100° F (37.8° C).

• If the patient has a central line, maintain CVP above 10 mm Hg and pulmonary artery wedge pressure (PAWP) at approximately 15 mm Hg by administering maintenance I.V. fluids and boluses of a colloid as needed.

• Draw blood for serum electrolyte and osmolarity analysis every 4 to 6 hours, and provide electrolyte replacements, as ordered and as needed. Electrolyte imbalances, such as hypokalemia, hypomagnesemia, and hypophosphatemia, can result from diuretic use or induced hyperventilation and must be treated aggressively. Administer diuretics, as ordered, to promote free water elimination.

• Monitor coagulation factors closely, and notify the doctor if clotting time is prolonged. Maintain hematocrit above 30% to ensure adequate oxygen transport and delivery.

• Watch blood urea nitrogen and serum creatinine levels closely during dehydration therapy.

• Assess urine output closely. Suspect diabetes insipidus if you note a sudden increase in urine output and serum osmolarity (not related to diuretic therapy) combined with a significant drop in urine osmolarity and specific gravity. If urine concentration increases and serum osmolarity falls, suspect SIADH.

Ruptured cerebral aneurysm

A cerebral aneurysm is a localized dilation of a cerebral vessel, usually at an arterial bifurcation. It can produce neurologic symptoms by exerting pressure on cranial nerves and other surrounding structures. If an aneurysm ruptures, devastating consequences, even death, may ensue. Make sure that you know how to deal with this emergency. (See *When your patient has a ruptured cerebral aneurysm.*)

Aneurysms are classified according to size, shape, and cause. Congenital aneurysms are the most common type. (See *Classifying cerebral aneurysms,* page 98.)

Causes
Most aneurysms arise from a congenital defect in the middle layer of the vessel wall. Other causes include atherosclerosis, a head injury that damages the vessel wall, an embolism, syphilis, and hypertension.

Pathophysiology
The pathophysiology of cerebral aneurysms varies slightly, depending on the cause. Typically, a defect or weakness in the vessel wall leads to abnormal vessel widening along with outpouching of the innermost vessel layer. (See *How a cerebral aneurysm forms,* page 99.)

Complications
Rupture of a cerebral aneurysm may cause subarachnoid hemorrhage (SAH). The released arterial blood then becomes a space-occupying lesion that rapidly increases ICP. Rupture usually occurs during physical activity, especially strenuous exertion; thus, blood escapes under above-normal pressure, rapidly creating a hemorrhage in the subarachnoid space.

Patients who survive a rupture may experience such life-threatening complications as rebleeding, cerebral vasospasm, and acute hydrocephalus—all of which require aggressive intervention. (See *What to watch for after a ruptured aneurysm,* page 100.)

Rebleeding after an aneurysm rupture (also called rerupture) is believed to result from the body's response to clot formation and lysis. The patient's neurologic status deteriorates, with a decreased LOC and intensifying headache. If an intraventricular catheter has been inserted, frank bleeding appears in the catheter.

Cerebral vasospasm may occur from narrowing of the arteries at the base of the brain secondary to SAH. Symptoms typically develop 3 to 14 days after hemorrhaging begins, with peak incidence at 7 to 10 days.

Hydrocephalus, which also develops secondary to SAH, may be obstructive or nonobstructive. Intraventricular blood may form a clot, preventing flow through the subarachnoid space; or the blood may clog the subarachnoid villi, preventing CSF reabsorption and creating a CSF overload. Early development of hydrocephalus carries a poor prognosis because ventricular dilation increases ICP, reduces CPP, and contributes to hypothalamic dysfunction and brain herniation.

Assessment
History
Most cerebral aneurysms produce no symptoms unless they rupture. Yet, before rupture, roughly half the patients experience certain warning signs and symptoms (prodrome) that suggest aneurysm expansion. Suspect an aneurysm if your patient reports localized head pain, diplopia, blurred vision, or if you detect palsy of the third, fourth, or sixth cranial nerve.

If you suspect that your patient has a ruptured aneurysm, take immediate steps to stabilize his condition. Then proceed with a brief assessment. If the patient can't respond, ask his family for details. Find out if he has a history of head injury, hypertension, or infection.

Ask if he experienced any of the classic warning signs. If your patient has regained consciousness after an aneurysm rupture, he may report an intense headache—the worst he has ever had. If he currently has a headache, ask when it started, exactly where it hurts, and what the pain feels like. Inquire if anything specific seemed to trigger the headache. He may state that he heard a snapping or popping sound. Also note any complaints of stiff neck,

EMERGENCY INTERVENTIONS

When your patient has a ruptured cerebral aneurysm

The patient with a ruptured cerebral aneurysm requires close monitoring and expert care. Assess him briefly, and expect an altered level of consciousness and a severe headache.
• Guard against subarachnoid hemorrhage by preventing or limiting the patient's ability to cough, sneeze, or strain; by banning all external stimuli, including TV, radio, and reading material; and by not giving enemas.
• Check the patient's neurologic status every 30 minutes.
• Limit the patient's fluid intake to 1,800 ml/day.
• Arrange for an immediate computed tomography scan and possibly for cerebral angiography. Based on the results, the doctor may insert an intraventricular catheter to remove intraventricular blood, drain cerebrospinal fluid, or monitor intracranial pressure (ICP).
• As ordered, give anticonvulsants to help prevent seizures, which increase the brain's oxygen needs and trigger increased ICP.
• Arrange for laboratory tests and an electrocardiogram to establish a baseline for treatment. Depending on the clinical grade of the aneurysm, the patient may require intubation to maintain a patent airway and ensure adequate oxygenation.

photophobia, and low-grade fever—signs of meningeal irritation from blood in the subarachnoid space. (See *When to suspect a ruptured cerebral aneurysm,* page 101.)

With SAH, the patient may report a severe, migrainelike headache of sudden onset, which may be generalized or localized. A patient with a minor intracerebral hemorrhage may report nonfocal signs and symptoms, such as malaise, generalized headache, nausea and vomiting, and neck and back pain.

Development of nausea and vomiting after aneurysm rupture suggests increased ICP from cerebral edema and hydrocephalus. These findings may be accompanied by papilledema, third

Classifying cerebral aneurysms

A cerebral aneurysm may be classified according to its size, shape, or underlying cause. This chart describes some aneurysm types.

TYPE	CAUSE	DESCRIPTION
Saccular (or berry)	Congenital defect	• Berry shape with bulge or dome • Accounts for about 90% of cerebral aneurysms • Arises as a defect in medial layer of vessel wall • Usually occurs at arterial bifurcation
Fusiform	Atherosclerotic disease	• Accounts for roughly 7% of cerebral aneurysms • Reflects an irregularity of vessel wall related to loss of elasticity • Rarely ruptures; usually compresses surrounding structures • Involves basilar, internal carotid, and vertebral arteries • 3 cm or more in diameter
Microscopic	Atherosclerotic disease	• Associated with hypertension • Commonly occurs in basal ganglia and brain stem
Mycotic	Inflammatory conditions	• Accounts for fewer than 1% of cerebral aneurysms • Usually results from septic emboli caused by lodging of bacterial endocarditis in distal branches, leading to acute inflammation of vessel wall • Typically involves middle cerebral artery, either in sylvian fissure or distal artery • Usually multiple occurrences
Dissecting	Traumatic injury	• Accounts for fewer than 1% of cerebral aneurysms • Associated with facial and skull fractures • Usually involves carotid system
	Atherosclerotic disease	• Intima pulled away from wall forces blood between layers

and sixth cranial nerve palsy, and altered LOC ranging from lethargy to coma.

Physical examination
Depending on the clinical grade of your patient's aneurysm, physical findings may range from slight nuchal rigidity to deep coma. (See *Grading a cerebral aneurysm*, page 102.) In the patient with SAH, expect transient to permanent loss of consciousness. The patient with hydrocephalus usually has a decreasing LOC, pupil dilation with reduced pupillary reflexes, and deviation of the eyes.

You also may detect lateralizing signs and symptoms after an aneurysm rupture. The result of cerebral vasospasms that impair blood flow to certain brain areas, these findings may be absent if bleeding is confined to the subarachnoid space.

Note any seizures or signs of pituitary dysfunction. Observe the electrocardiogram for changes.

Take the patient's vital signs, and note any temperature elevation (which may result from SAH).

Diagnostic tests
Definitive diagnosis of both ruptured and nonruptured cerebral aneurysms requires a CT scan and cerebral angiography. A CT scan can also detect such complications as rebleeding, SAH, cerebral infarction, cerebral edema, and hydrocephalus. Four-vessel angiography helps determine the type of aneurysm and may identify hematoma and multiple aneurysms. It also differentiates an aneurysm from an arteriovenous malformation.

Lumbar puncture may be performed if the patient has a grade I or II aneurysm to detect blood in CSF, which may indicate SAH. However, this study is contraindicated in patients with large bleeds — especially those involving the cisterns — because it may induce brain stem herniation by causing rapid decompression of the subarachnoid space. Laboratory indicators of a ruptured aneurysm include an increased white blood cell (WBC) count and an elevated sedimentation rate.

Ongoing treatment
After the patient has been stabilized, medical treatment focuses on maintaining cerebral perfusion and averting or minimizing complications. To prevent rebleeding, the patient may undergo surgery.

To maintain cerebral perfusion, the doctor will order measures to balance cerebral blood flow, cerebral perfusion, and ICP. Specific mea-

How a cerebral aneurysm forms

The wall of a blood vessel consists of three layers—the tunica intima (inner layer), tunica media (middle layer), and tunica adventitia (outer layer).

In an aneurysm, the vessel wall becomes weakened, which leads to separation of the layers, abnormal widening and outpouching of the innermost vessel layers, or loss of elasticity. Aneurysms are caused by congenital defects in the cerebral arteries, arteriosclerotic changes in the blood vessels, inflammatory conditions, or trauma.

Layers of vessel wall

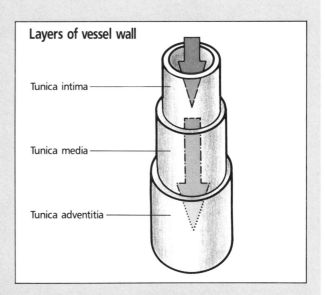

Tunica intima

Tunica media

Tunica adventitia

Dissecting aneurysm

In a dissecting aneurysm, the vessel layers separate, forcing blood between them.

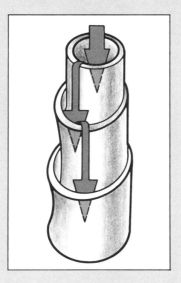

Saccular aneurysm

In a saccular aneurysm, a congenital defect of the tunica media causes widening of the vessel wall and outpouching of the tunica intima.

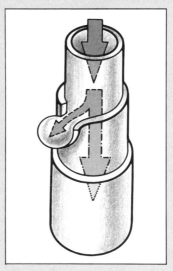

Fusiform aneurysm

In a fusiform aneurysm, loss of vessel elasticity causes vessel dilation.

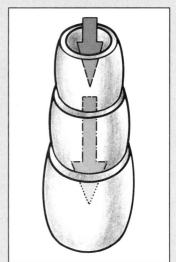

COMPLICATIONS

What to watch for after a ruptured aneurysm

If your patient has survived a ruptured cerebral aneurysm, monitor him closely for rebleeding, cerebral vasospasm, and acute hydrocephalus—potentially lethal complications. This chart lists the signs and symptoms of each complication, tells when the complication is most likely to occur, and how it should be treated.

COMPLICATION	SIGNS AND SYMPTOMS	ONSET	TREATMENT
Rebleeding	Deterioration of neurologic status, decrease in level of consciousness (LOC), intensifying headache	7 to 10 days after rupture	Sedation, bed rest, avoiding Valsalva's maneuver
Cerebral vasospasm	Decrease in LOC, motor weakness or paralysis, visual deficits, changes in vital signs (particularly respiratory patterns)	Several hours to 7 days after rupture	• Intravascular volume expanders • Induced hypertensive therapy • Calcium channel blockers
Hydrocephalus	Mental changes, disturbances in gait, general deterioration in mental and physical functions	Several hours to 7 days after rupture	Cerebrospinal fluid drainage via intraventricular catheter

sures depend on whether the patient has cerebral vasospasm or cerebral edema.

Drug treatment

The patient with cerebral vasospasm requires intravascular volume expanders (to induce hypervolemia), induced hypertensive therapy, and calcium channel blocker therapy.

The goal of intravascular volume expansion and hypertensive therapy is to increase CPP, blood flow, and oxygen delivery by maintaining MAP at 110 to 130 mm Hg. If these measures fail to increase MAP to this range, the doctor may order vasopressor therapy. Cautious administration of alpha-adrenergic drugs, such as dopamine and epinephrine, helps manage the vagal response to rising MAP by maintaining heart rate and cardiac output. During such therapy, be sure to monitor for increased urine output, keeping in mind the overall goal—to establish a positive fluid balance.

Calcium channel blockers, such as nifedipine and nimodipine (selective to blood vessels), help counter vasospasm by preventing calcium from entering vascular smooth muscle cells and causing contraction. Recent studies are focusing on the ability of calmodulin blockers and arachidonic acid inhibitors (experimental drugs that are not yet commercially available) to prevent contraction by interrupting intracellular calcium binding. Calcium channel blockers also may help reverse ischemic deficits by dilating smaller arterioles in the vascular bed.

Antifibrinolytic agents, such as aminocaproic acid, may be used to inhibit fibrinolysis—a natural process that may cause rebleeding 7 to 10 days after SAH. This therapy is most effective when started as soon as the patient is diagnosed with a ruptured aneurysm. The usual dosage is 24 to 36 g/day by continuous I.V. infusion. Be aware, however, that aminocaproic acid may cause delayed hydrocephalus as well as vasospasm, deep vein thrombosis, and pulmonary embolism.

Surgery

Surgery may be performed to prevent rebleeding of a ruptured aneurysm. Experts disagree as to the optimal timing for surgery. When performed within 48 to 72 hours of rupture in patients with a grade I or II aneurysm, surgery helps to prevent rebleeding and reduces the risk of vasospasm by removing blood before

When to suspect a ruptured cerebral aneurysm

Intense physical activity, such as labor and delivery, may cause a cerebral aneurysm to rupture. To prevent devastating consequences, you need to identify this emergency promptly.

Cynthia Martensen, age 30 and pregnant with her second child, was admitted to the hospital to give birth. She had expressed a desire for natural childbirth and because there were no contraindications, she was taken to the birthing room before labor began.

Heeding the warning signs

During delivery, Mrs. Martensen reported a sudden, extremely severe headache—a hallmark of a ruptured cerebral aneurysm. She told you that she felt nauseated and had blurred vision. You recorded the following vital signs:
- heart rate, 104 beats/minute
- respiratory rate, 28 breaths/minute
- blood pressure, 170/90 mm Hg
- temperature, 99.4° F (37.4° C).

On physical examination, you noted that Mrs. Martensen seemed irritable. You detected slight nuchal rigidity and third cranial nerve palsy—a sign of subarachnoid hemorrhage. The patient's pupils were equal, brisk, accommodating, and consensual. Mrs. Martensen moved all extremities with equal power. When you elicited positive Kernig's and Brudzinski's signs, you suspected meningeal irritation.

Averting serious consequences

You immediately reported your findings to the doctor, who suspected a grade II cerebral aneurysm. He performed an emergency cesarean delivery, and Mrs. Martensen delivered a healthy boy.

Immediately after delivery, a computed tomography scan of the head showed a small subarachnoid hemorrhage near the junction of the posterior communicating artery and the internal carotid artery. Cerebral angiography revealed a saccular aneurysm of the posterior communicating artery.

Mrs. Martensen was admitted to the intensive care unit (ICU). The doctor inserted an intraventricular catheter to remove subarachnoid blood and ordered hypervolemic and hypertensive therapy. You began to administer nimodipine, as ordered, and implemented aneurysm precautions.

Two days later, Mrs. Martensen underwent surgery to clip the aneurysm. She returned to the ICU awake and alert with no neurologic deficits.

Conclusion

Because you gave prompt attention to Mrs. Martensen's complaint of a severe headache, she may well have avoided the dire consequences of a ruptured cerebral aneurysm. Immediately reporting her vital signs to the doctor, along with the findings that indicated meningeal irritation, alerted the doctor to the need for an emergency cesarean delivery—thus preventing further exacerbation of the condition.

---

the vessel responds fully to vasospastic agents released during rupture. Early surgery also may eliminate the need for antifibrinolytic therapy and permit earlier patient mobility.

Surgery usually is delayed when the brain is edematous. However, a delay results in a more obscure anatomy and less effective autoregulation; because the surgeon must induce systemic hypotension to dissect the aneurysm safely, these problems greatly increase the risk of cerebral infarction. Roughly 65% of aneurysm patients develop cerebral vasospasm postoperatively, compared with 35% to 50%

who develop it preoperatively. However, delaying surgery markedly increases the risk of rebleeding.

Surgery may involve one of three methods—clipping, wrapping, or embolization. In *clipping*, the surgeon applies a clip to the neck of the aneurysm to eliminate its blood flow. Complications of clipping include an incomplete procedure, inadvertent clipping of a second vessel, and a slipped clip.

The surgeon may opt for *wrapping* if the aneurysm has a broad base or neck or if it involves bifurcation of a vessel that can't be

Grading a cerebral aneurysm

To gauge the severity of your patient's aneurysm, you may use the grading scale shown here. Developed by Hunt and Hess, it's based on the patient's level of consciousness and degree of neurologic dysfunction.

Grade 0
Unruptured aneurysm

Grade I
Asymptomatic, or minimal headache and slight nuchal rigidity

Grade Ia
No acute meningeal reaction but fixed neurologic deficit

Grade II
Moderate to severe headache, nuchal rigidity, third nerve palsy

Grade III
Drowsiness, confusion, mild focal deficit

Grade IV
Stupor, moderate to severe hemiparesis, possible early decerebrate rigidity

Grade V
Deep coma, decerebrate rigidity, moribund appearance

clipped. Wrapping, which involves the application of tissue adhesive or muslin around the aneurysm, may strengthen the vessel wall and prevent rupture as well as shrink the aneurysm's branching vessels. However, this method may lead to rejection because it involves the use of foreign material.

In *embolization,* the doctor places Silastic beads or coils in the brain to serve as a nidus for a thrombus, preventing blood from reaching the aneurysm. This may be done intraoperatively or by angiography. Complications include possible rejection of the foreign material and dislodgment of a bead or coil, which may then occlude an uninvolved vessel.

Other treatments
The patient with cerebral edema must undergo dehydration therapy to reduce intravascular volume and thus prevent further edema. However, great caution must be used with this therapy to avoid reducing circulating volume within the vascular compartment. A reduction in circulating volume is sensed by baroreceivers, causing vasoconstriction in an effort to maintain blood pressure and blood flow. This response alters CPP and may increase the incidence of cerebral ischemia and vasospasm and decrease vascular volume.

To manage hypervolemic therapy and prevent complications, expect the doctor to insert a PA catheter and order rapid infusion of 0.9% sodium chloride solution (300 to 700 ml) to maintain circulating volume. The goal is to increase CVP above 10 mm Hg and maintain PAWP at 18 mm Hg. Colloids may be used for cerebral edema.

Some evidence suggests that hypervolemic therapy causes hemodilution, which may precipitate further problems by reducing the blood's oxygen-carrying capacity and nutrient load. To minimize this risk, hematocrit must remain above 30%. If the patient continues to deteriorate or develops cerebral edema or cardiopulmonary complications, the doctor will switch to colloid administration to try to reduce volume and increase serum osmolarity. He may order mannitol to reduce the risk of blood sludging and enhance oxygen delivery.

To prevent acute hydrocephalus, the doctor inserts an intraventricular catheter to drain accumulated CSF and blood and reduce ICP.

Ongoing nursing interventions
Consistent nursing care helps limit the neurologic effects of a ruptured cerebral aneurysm. The goals of ongoing care include maintaining neurologic status and function, preventing rebleeding and cerebral vasospasm, and avoiding complications of surgery and immobility.

Maintaining neurologic status and function

• Assess the patient's neurologic status hourly, focusing on LOC and motor and pupil responses. Report any changes promptly.
• To ensure cerebral perfusion, maintain MAP and implement measures to reduce ICP, as ordered. Maintain accurate hourly intake and output records.
• If the patient has an intraventricular catheter, document ICP readings and take steps to prevent local infection.
• Continue to administer calcium channel blockers, intravascular volume expanders, and hypertensive agents, as ordered.
• Closely monitor the patient's vital signs.

Preventing rebleeding and cerebral vasospasm

• Implement aneurysm precautions to reduce the risk of rebleeding. These precautions include enforcing bed rest, keeping the head of the bed elevated (to promote venous drainage, decrease ICP, and prevent sudden blood pressure changes), darkening the room if the patient is photophobic, restricting visitors, maintaining sedation (usually with phenobarbital), giving ordered analgesics to relieve headache, providing a soft-foods, high-fiber diet, and having the patient avoid Valsalva's maneuver (for example, by giving him stool softeners).
• Prevent vasospasm by administering intravascular volume expanders and hypertensive agents to improve perfusion and limit ischemia, and by administering calcium channel blockers.

Preventing complications of surgery and immobility

• If the patient is recovering from surgery, maintain the aneurysm precautions discussed above during the first postoperative week.
• Monitor the patient's respiratory status to help avert hypoxia and such postoperative complications as atelectasis and pneumonia. Perform incentive spirometry every 1 to 2 hours, and monitor arterial blood gas (ABG) values. If the patient is intubated, perform CPT every 4 hours to mobilize secretions in an effort to maintain PEEP above 5 cm H_2O.

In some cases, you may use Trendelenburg's position to promote postural drainage. However, be aware that this position is controversial and should be avoided unless specifically ordered.
• Mobilize the patient early but cautiously to avoid orthostatic hypotension. Monitor routine laboratory tests, including a complete blood count (CBC) and blood chemistry analysis, which reveals the effects of hypervolemic therapy on serum electrolyte levels.

Arteriovenous malformation

An arteriovenous malformation (AVM) is a tangle of abnormal vessels with no intervening capillaries, leading to abnormal communication between the arterial and venous systems. AVMs range in size from tiny, localized tangles to huge masses involving an entire cerebral hemisphere. They also vary in location.

Affecting men and women equally, AVMs typically don't cause signs or symptoms until adulthood, especially from ages 20 to 40. Massive hemorrhage caused by AVM rupture may be lethal, so be sure to take immediate action if you suspect this crisis. (See *When your patient has an AVM,* page 104.)

Causes

Most AVMs are congenital or result from a birth injury. Because cerebral vessels develop in the pia mater at roughly 3 weeks' gestation, many AVMs are superficial, extending in a wedge shape into the parenchyma. Occasionally, they involve the lateral horn of the ventricles. The most common feeding vessel is the middle cerebral artery, although some AVMs are fed by many smaller arteries.

An AVM may form after head trauma that induces clot formation. The AVM develops as blood shunts around the clot in a compensatory effort to revascularize or recanalize blood flow.

When your patient has an AVM

Let your patient's signs and symptoms guide initial management of an arteriovenous malformation (AVM). Signs and symptoms that call for immediate intervention include hemorrhage; seizures; headache; bruits; syncope; motor, sensory, and visual deficits; and mental changes.

Ruptured AVM

If the AVM has ruptured, the doctor may insert an intraventricular catheter to drain cerebrospinal fluid or intraventricular blood and allow continuous intracranial pressure monitoring. Be sure to implement precautions to prevent rebleeding.

Bleeding and seizures

For significant bleeding or intracerebral bleeding with massive cerebral edema, prepare the patient for intubation and induced hyperventilation, and administer agents to increase serum osmolarity, as ordered. If the patient is having seizures, expect to give anticonvulsant drugs and take seizure precautions to maintain a patent airway. Analgesics may be ordered to control or alleviate the headache.

Other complications

Precautions to take against subarachnoid bleeding include cautioning the patient about coughing or sneezing and banning external stimuli, such as TV, radio, and reading. Don't give the patient enemas, and check his neurologic status every 30 minutes.

Pathophysiology

Reduced resistance in the AVM causes shunting of blood to the defect. This, in turn, increases the size and tortuousness of the involved vessels. Called the *cerebral steal* phenomenon, such shunting reduces blood flow and perfusion to surrounding tissues. These effects — increased cerebral blood flow with reduced perfusion — are an AVM's hallmarks.

Enlarging gradually, the AVM exerts pressure on surrounding structures, producing symptoms typical of a space-occupying lesion. It also may rupture directly into brain tissue or produce an SAH. Rupture typically occurs during increased activity. (See *Understanding AVMs*.)

Complications

The most common complications of an AVM are rupture with consequent hemorrhage, increased ICP, cerebral ischemia, compression of brain tissue, and hydrocephalus.

Assessment

History

Suspect an AVM if your patient complains of a vascular-type headache, has a history of seizures, or has signs and symptoms of hemorrhage, such as hemiparesis and aphasia. For many patients, seizure is the primary symptom.

If the AVM has ruptured, the patient may report an excruciating headache and other symptoms resembling those of a ruptured cerebral aneurysm. To help rule out a ruptured aneurysm, elicit answers to the following questions:
• How long has the patient had the headache?
• Exactly where does he feel the pain?
• Has he had this type of headache before?
• Has he ever had a seizure? If so, when was the first time? What was it like?
• Is he currently taking anticonvulsants?
• Has he ever had hallucinations?

If the patient has a history of seizures, unilateral headache, hallucinations, and symptoms of mild SAH, suspect an AVM rather than a ruptured cerebral aneurysm. (See *Distinguishing a bleeding AVM from a ruptured cerebral aneurysm,* page 106.)

Physical examination

Manifestations of an AVM vary with the location and size of the defect. Examine the patient for focal neurologic signs and symptoms, such as weakness, sensory loss, aphasia, and hemianopia. Observe for dementia.

Auscultate for a bruit over the eye, forehead, or neck — typical with an AVM. However, this sign may disappear once an AVM bleeds. In a pediatric patient, you may note underdevelopment of the body on the side opposite the AVM because large amounts of blood are diverted to the brain before full growth occurs.

PATHOPHYSIOLOGY

Understanding AVMs

Usually a congenital disorder, an arteriovenous malformation (AVM) is a cluster of veins and arteries that lack capillary linkage. This leads to greater blood flow from the arteries and shunting of blood to the lower pressure veins, reducing perfusion. As a result, local ischemia occurs.

With more blood flow, the AVM grows and the low-resistance, high-flow system increases. This causes even greater shunting of blood, a phenomenon called *cerebral steal*. As shunting increases, ischemic areas widen and normal arteries grow larger to maintain perfusion. This impairs blood flow autoregulation, causing an increase in cerebral blood flow and cardiac output.

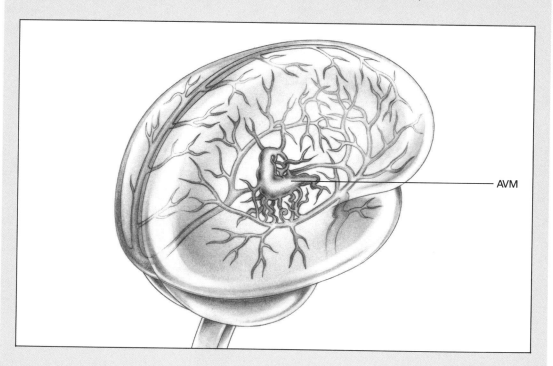

AVM

Rupture of an AVM usually involves a vein, not an artery. Therefore, hemorrhaging is less serious than with a ruptured aneurysm and typically causes hemispheric signs, such as seizures, headache, visual disturbances, and aphasia without brain stem or hypothalamic signs. Brain stem or hypothalamic signs include profound LOC depression or coma, hypertension, decerebration, decortication, and temperature increases without infection. These signs are consistent with a large bleed and tissue compression, placing pressure on vital brain centers.

Diagnostic tests

A CT scan using a contrast medium usually detects an AVM, as does an MRI scan with gadolinium enhancement. However, arteriography is the preferred test for definitive localization and serves as the basis for decisions regarding surgery. Occasionally, arteriography fails to detect an AVM after rupture—probably because vasospasm prevents shunt formation and filling of the malformation. In this case, arteriography must be repeated in 7 days to reexamine areas surrounding the hemorrhage.

Distinguishing a bleeding AVM from a ruptured cerebral aneurysm

Use this chart to help determine if your patient has a bleeding AVM or a ruptured cerebral aneurysm.

ASSESSMENT FINDING	BLEEDING A.V.M.	RUPTURED ANEURYSM
Headache	• Vascular or migraine type • Episodic	• Generalized or focal • Described as the worst headache patient has ever had • Sudden onset
Subarachnoid hemorrhage	• May be present	• May be present
Seizures	• May be present	• Usually absent
Bruits	• May be present	• Absent
Vasospasm	• Present	• Present
Precipitating activity	• Not specific	• Strenuous activity

Ongoing treatment

Once the patient is somewhat stabilized, definitive management begins. Medical treatments currently used to manage AVMs include surgery, radiation, radiosurgery, and embolization.

The decision about which medical measures to take depends on the size and accessibility of the AVM, the patient's age and condition, and whether the patient has intractable headaches, uncontrollable seizures, hemorrhage, or cerebral steal symptoms. In general, medical measures are targeted toward analgesics for control of headaches and anticonvulsants for seizure control.

Expect the doctor to order a follow-up CT scan to assess for increasing edema, rebleeding, or mass effect, which could produce permanent neurologic deficits.

Surgery

The surgeon may directly resect an AVM or clip the feeding vessels. Surgery most effectively reduces the risk of rebleeding. However, it requires prolonged and deep retraction with redistribution of blood flow, which may lead to cerebral edema. It also carries all the inherent risks of any surgical procedure.

Other treatments

Radiation. The success of this technique depends on the size and location of the malformation. It has proved most effective for AVMs of moderate size that are easily located. Proton-beam radiation may be used for a parenchymal AVM located deep within the brain or an AVM involving critical brain regions. However, this method may cause such complications as hemiparesis, hemianopia, and hemorrhage.

Radiosurgery. New radiosurgical techniques are encouraging. For instance, the gamma knife can deliver beams of ionizing radiation directly to the AVM with stereotaxic accuracy. Complications are rare, and patients recover quickly because the skull remains closed.

Embolization. Feeding arteries may be embolized directly during angiography. In this procedure, rapidly polymerizing plastics or Silastic beads are introduced into the feeding vessels to thrombose and destroy or shrink the AVM. This treatment is valuable for inoperable AVMs and may be used in conjunction with direct surgery to treat large AVMs. By occluding some vessels before surgery, this approach gives surrounding cerebral vessels time to adjust to increased blood flow, minimizing edema and possibly reducing intraoperative blood loss in highly vascular AVMs.

Embolization does carry certain risks. The patient may develop an inflammatory reaction to the foreign material and to the diverted blood flow, leading to cerebral edema and ischemia. Also, the embolizing material may become dislodged and stray into normal cerebrovascular pathways, creating a neurologic deficit, or into the systemic circulation, causing a pulmonary embolus. Sepsis may develop from instillation of foreign material or from a breach in sterile technique.

Ongoing nursing interventions

Ongoing care for the patient with an AVM resembles that for a patient with a CHI. Focus on reducing cerebral edema and ICP and monitoring for complications of treatment.

• Monitor the patient's neurologic status and vital signs closely. Promptly report any deterioration in his LOC.

• To minimize edema, administer diuretics as ordered. If necessary and ordered, initiate hyperventilation therapy to reduce ICP.

• Keep the head of the bed elevated to promote venous drainage and maintain MAP under 110 mm Hg. If pain control, sedation, calcium channel blockers, or antihypertensives fail to control blood pressure, administer nitroprusside as ordered. However, be aware that this drug has potent cerebrovasodilatory effects, particularly an increase in cerebral blood flow, which may increase cerebral edema.

• To maintain MAP and circulating volume, ensure a proper fluid balance. Keep in mind that the goal is to maintain a hyperosmolar but normovolemic state.

• If the patient has had surgery, monitor him for perfusion breakthrough phenomenon. Signs and symptoms of this syndrome include decreasing LOC, pupillary changes, and focal signs such as hemiparesis or aphasia. In this syndrome, autoregulation fails as normal cerebral blood flow and perfusion are suddenly restored to surrounding dilated vessels. Hematomas and massive cerebral edema develop as the dilated vessels fail to constrict in response to sudden hyperemia.

• Implement standard postoperative care measures, as appropriate, to ensure adequate respiratory function and oxygenation. Perform coughing and deep-breathing exercises or CPT as necessary. Monitor ABG values.

• Assess the incision site frequently for signs of infection.

• Promote early ambulation to prevent skin breakdown and allow an early return to normal functioning.

Status epilepticus

In this disorder, the patient suffers a series of rapidly repeated seizures without recovering neurologic function between attacks. Although status epilepticus may involve any type of seizure, generalized tonic-clonic seizures are the most common type; they're also the most dangerous because they increase the risk of anoxia, arrhythmias, and systemic lactic acidosis.

Most patients in neurologic critical care settings are at risk for posttraumatic seizures and metabolic disturbances stemming from their overwhelming injuries. Therefore, consider status epilepticus a potential and constant threat to your patient's well-being. Irreversible brain damage may occur if seizures aren't arrested, so make sure you know how to intervene in this medical emergency. (See *When your patient has status epilepticus,* page 108.)

Causes

In most patients, the cause of status epilepticus remains unknown. However, factors that may precipitate it include abrupt withdrawal of anticonvulsant drugs or alcohol, inadequate blood glucose levels, a brain tumor, a head injury, a high fever, central nervous system infections, and poisoning.

Pathophysiology

Epileptogenic foci are activated, leading to neurochemical changes that excite neighboring cells and create a favorable climate for generalized seizures.

Rapid, repetitive depolarization within brain cells during seizures places tremendous metabolic demands on the brain. As a result, cellular metabolic needs increase, and adenosine triphosphate and its precursors are depleted. This leads to hyperthermia and failure of the sodium-potassium pump.

Pump failure, in turn, causes cholinesterase depletion, increased cerebral blood flow, and vasodilation. Osmotic effects of the switch to anaerobic metabolism cause cellular swelling. As cells become hypoxic or anoxic, systemic metabolic acidosis occurs, and cardiovascular collapse ensues.

When your patient has status epilepticus

Ensuring a patent airway is your first priority for a patient with status epilepticus—but *don't attempt to insert an artificial airway* until his muscles have relaxed. Otherwise, his tongue may occlude the airway or his teeth may break, creating a partial occlusion.

Establish I.V. access
• Next, establish I.V. access to administer vasopressors and anticonvulsants and to allow blood withdrawal for analysis of arterial blood gases, electrolytes, and glucose. To reduce the risk of aspiration during a seizure, perform pulmonary hygiene measures every 2 to 4 hours and mobilize secretions. Keep emergency intubation equipment at hand in case the patient requires ventilatory support.
• Until the threat of aspiration passes, withhold all oral intake unless ordered otherwise. In some patients, the doctor may insert a Salem sump tube to avert gastric distention and vomiting, which may cause aspiration.

Halt seizures
• To halt seizures, expect to administer 5 to 10 mg of diazepam I.V. slowly. Repeat the dose every 15 minutes to a maximum of 30 mg. However, be aware that diazepam induces respiratory depression.

• Alternatively, the doctor may order 4 to 8 mg of lorazepam I.V., repeated in 10 minutes, or 20 mg/kg phenytoin I.V. at a rate of 50 mg/minute. During phenytoin infusion, monitor the patient's electrocardiogram (ECG) because this drug may cause hypotension, slowing the heart rate. If the ECG reveals bradyarrhythmia or heart block, withhold this drug as ordered.
• If these drugs don't halt seizure activity, the doctor may induce pharmacologic paralysis to ease intubation and ensure respiratory support. However, be aware that stopping visible seizure activity with a paralytic agent doesn't necessarily abolish the seizure. Seizure activity may continue and brain cells may die despite adequate oxygenation and blood pressure. To avoid clinical confusion about halting the seizure versus masking the motor responses, some hospitals use a short-acting, nondepolarizing muscle relaxant, such as vecuronium, in this circumstance for rapid clearance to prevent masking of the seizure activity and to eliminate fasciculations on clearance of the paralytic agent.
• As long as the seizure continues, measures should be taken to determine the underlying cause, such as analyzing blood glucose levels for hypoglycemia, and performing an echoencephalogram to detect cerebral hematoma.

Complications
Status epilepticus may cause traumatic injury from a fall as well as various life-threatening complications. For instance, aspiration may result from an altered LOC and a compromised airway. Hypoxia may stem from altered respiratory processes and airway occlusion. Anoxia may lead to brain cell death and cytotoxic cerebral edema, which in turn may cause brain herniation and metabolic disturbances. Fever, a result of hypermetabolism, increases cerebral and body metabolism. This, in turn, creates more cellular by-products. Rhabdomyolysis—muscle disintegration or dissolution resulting from increased energy consumption due to rapid, repetitive contraction—also poses a

grave risk. Death may ensue from multisystem collapse or from brain cell death.

Assessment
History
After ensuring a patent airway and adequate oxygenation, obtain a brief history by asking family members the following questions:
• Has the patient ever had a seizure before? If so, when did his most recent seizure occur?
• Does the patient take any prescription drugs? If so, which drugs does he take and when did he take the last dose?
• Has the patient been taking any street drugs or drinking alcohol?

ASSESSMENT INSIGHT

Investigating seizures

If your patient has a seizure, take appropriate emergency measures and then observe him closely. After the seizure ends, ask yourself the questions shown here. The answers may provide clues about the type of seizure, what precipitated it, and the area of the brain involved. Your observations may provide the neurologist with vital information in diagnosing and treating your patient.

NURSING QUESTIONS	IMPLICATIONS
What was the patient doing before the seizure?	May suggest precipitating factors
Where did the seizure start and how did it progress?	May suggest site of epileptogenic focus in brain
What movements occurred during the seizure? Did you detect ocular motions or automatisms (nonreflex acts performed unconsciously)?	Helps determine the type of seizure and focus of epileptic activity (Clonic movements usually mean focal seizures; automatisms usually mean temporal lobe involvement.)
How long did the seizure last?	May differentiate status epilepticus from other seizure activity; also may suggest the brain area involved and its size
How long ago did the most recent seizure occur?	May differentiate status epilepticus from other seizure activity (No recovery between events generally indicates a diagnosis of status epilepticus.)
Did the patient froth or foam at the mouth?	Helps identify the type of seizure (Frothing or foaming usually indicates tonic-clonic seizures and possibly an impaired airway.)
Did the patient's skin color change?	May signify hypoxia (if patient is cyanotic) and indicate the need for emergency intubation or tracheotomy
Did the patient lose fecal or urinary continence?	Helps determine the seizure type (For example, incontinence may occur immediately after a tonic-clonic seizure.)
What seemed to stop the seizure?	May suggest ways to treat future seizures
What happened immediately after the seizure ended (postictal phase)? For instance, did you detect changes in speech, level of consciousness, or motor ability?	Helps determine the type of seizure and brain area involved

• Has he had a recent injury, especially head trauma?
• Has he been ill recently?

Physical examination
Perform a rapid physical examination to help identify the type of seizures the patient is experiencing. Try to determine if they're partial seizures (such as focal or psychomotor seizures) or generalized seizures (for example, tonic-clonic, myoclonic, or atonic seizures). Signs and symptoms of tonic-clonic status epilepticus include nystagmus, bowel or bladder incontinence, diaphoresis, labored breathing, dyspnea, apnea, cyanosis, and mucus or saliva filling the mouth. (See *Investigating seizures.*)

Diagnostic tests
Initially, the doctor orders blood tests—CBC, electrolyte analysis, renal and liver function studies, and serum and urine toxicology studies. A CBC will reveal the WBC count and differential, which may indicate infection; electrolyte analysis, hyponatremia, hypomagnesemia, and acid-base balance; renal studies,

Subduing status epilepticus

A patient with status epilepticus faces the possibility of cardiovascular collapse and irreversible brain damage. Unremitting tonic-clonic seizures pose the greatest threat because they may induce anoxia, arrhythmias, and systemic lactic acidosis. However, expert nursing skills can ensure prompt detection and avert the ultimate complication—death.

Consider the case of Manuel Pultro, age 41, whose admitting diagnosis is head injury.

Assessing the situation

Reviewing Mr. Pultro's history, you note that his head injury results from a car accident in which he was apparently driving while intoxicated. A computed tomography (CT) scan shows a small contusion in the temporal lobe. This information helps predict the series of seizures he'll have while under your care: Both head injury and alcohol withdrawal may precipitate status epilepticus; a temporal lobe injury makes the disorder even more likely.

You perform a neurologic assessment and obtain a Glasgow Coma Scale score of 15. Then you obtain the following vital sign measurements:
• blood pressure, 110/70 mm Hg
• heart rate, 64 beats/minute
• respiratory rate, 16 breaths/minute
• temperature, 98.9° F (37.2° C).

Several hours later, you find Mr. Pultro more lethargic, although he continues to follow commands. However, his vital signs remain unchanged.

Monitoring and intervening

Suddenly, you see widespread muscle contractions followed by jerking motions (tonic-clonic contractions). Mr. Pultro doesn't respond when you call his name. He's frothing at the mouth and gurgling, and you see that he has urinated in bed. You try—but fail—to unclench his jaw. After turning him onto his side, you call for help.

The doctor orders an I.V. infusion of diazepam to halt the seizures, but this therapy fails. You obtain blood samples for immediate blood chemistry studies, toxicology studies, and a complete blood count to rule out metabolic disturbances and analyze blood alcohol and drug levels.

When Mr. Pultro becomes cyanotic and his respirations grow rapid and shallow, you give a bolus I.V. injection of phenytoin, as ordered. Knowing that he's at risk for impaired oxygenation, you attempt to secure his airway and prepare him for intubation; then you stand by to administer thiopental and vecuronium, as ordered.

Forty-five minutes later, Mr. Pultro has another seizure. Again, he fails to respond to diazepam. The doctor now diagnoses status epilepticus and orders concomitant phenobarbital I.V.

Despite the additional drug, the seizures continue. The doctor adds yet another drug—pentobarbital I.V.—to the regimen. You give an initial bolus dose of 5 mg/kg/hour for 4 hours, then infuse the drug continuously at a maintenance rate of 1 mg/kg/hour.

An end in sight

Finally, overt seizure activity stops. An EEG performed immediately will demonstrate quelling of electrical seizure activity. You continue to assess Mr. Pultro continuously and obtain these vital sign measurements:
• blood pressure, 90/50 mm Hg
• heart rate, 152 beats/minute
• respiratory rate, 20 breaths/minute
(with mechanical ventilation)
• temperature, 103.4° F (39.7° C).

As ordered, you administer additional doses of phenobarbital and phenytoin to achieve therapeutic blood drug levels in an attempt to suppress seizure activity. Five days later, you successfully wean Mr. Pultro from the barbiturate drip. Follow-up EEGs show no seizure activity.

As Mr. Pultro recovers, you continue to monitor him for complications of status epilepticus—aspiration, hypoxia, fever, and multisystem collapse.

Conclusion

Paying careful attention to Mr. Pultro's history alerted you to the likelihood of status epilepticus. By then monitoring him closely for seizures, you were able to respond quickly when he had them. The subsequent drug administrations and monitoring helped Mr. Pultro avert dangerous consequences from his seizures.

uremia; and liver function studies, metabolic disturbances. Once the patient is stabilized, he'll undergo a CT scan of the head to rule out traumatic injury or brain tumor. If needed, he'll also have an MRI scan and cerebral arteriography to evaluate for cerebral or vascular abnormalities. A lumbar puncture may be performed if the doctor suspects an infectious cause, such as meningitis, encephalitis, or a brain abscess.

An EEG supports the diagnosis, helps determine the type of seizure, and may help establish the prognosis.

Ongoing treatment
Your first priority is to maintain adequate oxygenation and an open airway. Maintain the patient on anticonvulsants or barbiturates, as ordered, to prevent seizure recurrence. In intractable cases, surgery may be indicated.

Drug treatment
If initial medical therapy doesn't halt seizures, expect the doctor to order a bolus of phenytoin accompanied by continuous monitoring of ECG and blood pressure. If status epilepticus persists, arrange to have an EEG performed immediately.

The doctor will probably order additional anticonvulsant drugs, such as phenobarbital. If these fail to stop the seizures, the patient may need a continuous barbiturate infusion. (See *Subduing status epilepticus.*)

Once seizures stop, expect to give additional drugs and to wean the patient from barbiturates. The doctor will try to identify and correct the precipitating cause of status epilepticus. In many cases, an effective therapeutic regimen comes only through trial and error — but even this doesn't guarantee complete freedom from seizures.

Surgery
A patient with intractable seizures may benefit from surgery — typically, a craniotomy with a temporal lobectomy. Usually, the surgeon excises the amygdala, anterior uncus, and hippocampus, if possible. This procedure has a success rate of approximately 70%. Roughly half of these patients require no further interventions; the other half must continue to take anticonvulsant drugs to stay seizure-free. However, in some patients, surgery causes further neurologic impairment.

Ongoing nursing interventions
Ongoing care focuses on ensuring overall patient well-being, avoiding more seizures, and preventing complications such as injury.
• Monitor ABG values during status epilepticus and for 24 hours afterward to help detect hypoxia and acid-base imbalances.
• Monitor the patient's vital signs closely to ensure adequate blood pressure and heart rate.
• Maintain I.V. access until an effective therapeutic regimen is established and maintained.
• Perform a neurologic assessment every hour. Watch for desired and adverse effects of anticonvulsant drugs, and monitor blood drug levels closely. If necessary, adjust dosages as ordered so that the patient can perform activities of daily living.
• Arrange for a nutritional consultation to counter the effects of the catabolism caused by status epilepticus. During seizures, muscles consume oxygen and nutrients create an oxygen debt, depriving other body tissues of oxygen and nutrients. Make sure you're familiar with the effects of food on the absorption rates of prescribed anticonvulsants to ensure optimal absorption and maintenance of serum levels.
• To avoid injury and minimize the risk of inducing seizures, maintain seizure precautions at all times: Enforce bed rest or supervise the patient's activities. Keep the bed side rails up and padded, and keep airway and suction equipment at the bedside. Make sure the patient wears only loose-fitting clothes.
• Teach the patient and family about seizures, and emphasize the need to get emergency care when one occurs. Instruct the patient to stay alert for prodromal (warning) signs: mood or behavioral changes and an aura, such as a metallic taste, a flash of light, or an unusual smell or sound.
• As appropriate, refer the patient to the Epilepsy Foundation of America for support.

Neurogenic shock

A state of altered blood vessel capacity, neurogenic shock is usually transitory, but it carries a high mortality. To help your patient survive this potentially fatal disorder, you must know how to identify it and intervene promptly. (See *When your patient is in neurogenic shock.*)

Causes

Any condition that interrupts vasomotor impulses may cause neurogenic shock. The most common cause is spinal cord injury above the midthoracic region, or the sixth thoracic vertebra (T6). Other causes include high spinal or deep general anesthesia, brain damage to the basal ganglia, medullary ischemia, insulin shock, and altered function of the vasomotor center in response to hypoglycemia.

Remember that any time you have to care for a postoperative patient who has undergone spinal or epidural anesthesia, you must remain alert for ascension of the anesthetic by performing frequent sensorimotor function examinations.

Pathophysiology

In neurogenic shock, a neurologic insult disrupts transmission of sympathetic impulses from the brain's vasomotor center, causing unopposed parasympathetic stimulation. This leads to loss of vasomotor tone, inducing massive vasodilation.

Blood volume then becomes inadequate to fill the enlarged vascular bed, causing relative hypovolemia, decreased venous return, and reduced cardiac output. In turn, these changes trigger compensatory mechanisms, which usually succeed in correcting relative hypovolemia and improving vasomotor tone.

EMERGENCY INTERVENTIONS

When your patient is in neurogenic shock

If you suspect that your patient is in neurogenic shock, first ensure his ABCs—airway, breathing, and circulation—and make sure that his spinal column is immobilized if he has or may have a spinal cord injury.

Evaluate oxygenation status
To help evaluate his oxygenation status, use an oxygen saturation monitor. As indicated and ordered, give supplemental oxygen and have emergency intubation equipment available.

Insert an I.V. line
Next, insert a large-bore I.V. line to administer volume expanders and vasoactive drugs. Prepare the patient for central line insertion to monitor central venous pressure. If he remains unstable, the doctor may insert a pulmonary artery catheter. Expect arterial line insertion for continuous direct blood pressure monitoring and frequent blood sampling for arterial blood gas analysis, complete blood count, and serum electrolyte and serum lactate levels.

Treat hypotension
Expect to administer dopamine to treat hypotension. As ordered, give this drug at levels above the renal dosage (3 to 5 mg/kg/minute) and titrate to pure alpha levels (up to 10 mg/kg/minute) if needed. Dopamine also will stimulate the heart rate and contractility, although you may need to give isoproterenol if the heart rate remains slow.

Insert an indwelling urinary catheter if ordered. The doctor may insert a Salem pump tube to prevent gastric distention and vomiting, which may lead to aspiration.

Next, attempt to identify and manage the condition that precipitated neurogenic shock. For a spinal cord injury, the neurosurgeon will reduce the injury—for example, by applying cervical traction. If neurogenic shock is related to hypoglycemia, administer I.V. dextrose, as ordered, to elevate serum blood glucose levels. If it's related to spinal analgesia, elevating the head of the bed 15 degrees will prevent the anesthetic from ascending the spinal cord to the medulla.

Complications

Since neurogenic shock is caused by a loss of vasomotor tone due to an interruption in sympathetic outflow, the patient will become hypotensive and bradycardic. This can produce all of the complications associated with a state of low cardiac output and low tissue perfusion — multisystem ischemia, multisystem organ failure and, ultimately, death. Additional complications unique to neurogenic shock include pulmonary overload, edema, and autonomic dysreflexia. (See *What to watch for after neurogenic shock.*)

Assessment

History

Before beginning the assessment, safeguard your patient's airway, breathing, and circulation. If you suspect or know that he has a spinal cord injury, make sure that he's properly immobilized. Then obtain his history — from family members or others if the patient can't respond himself.

With spinal cord injury, expect a recent history of trauma, such as from a fall, a motor vehicle accident, or a dive into shallow water. Find out whether the patient recently struck his head. Ask if he has neck pain or a history of neck pain; if so, determine how long ago it started. Has he noticed a change in his ability to move or feel? If so, when did it begin?

Physical examination

Examine the patient for typical signs of neurogenic shock — bradycardia, hypotension, and a low core temperature. If he has a spinal cord injury, you may detect respiratory insufficiency (depending on the injury level). Check deep tendon reflexes, auscultate for bowel sounds, and stay alert for priapism (in male patients). The patient may have an altered LOC and his skin may be warm, dry, and flushed.

With spinal cord disruption, expect sensorimotor alterations or loss of function. If possible, ask the patient to shrug his shoulders, bend his arms up, squeeze your hand, bend his knees, and wiggle his toes. (See *Evaluating levels of innervation,* page 114.) Perform a brief pinprick examination on his arms, trunk, and legs.

COMPLICATIONS

What to watch for after neurogenic shock

This chart identifies complications that may occur in a patient in neurogenic shock caused by spinal cord injury.

BODY SYSTEM	POTENTIAL COMPLICATION
Neurologic	• Loss of sensorimotor function
Respiratory	• Loss of muscle elasticity • Impaired ability to cough • Aspiration pneumonia • Atelectasis
Cardiovascular	• Hypotension • Bradycardia • Vasovagal response • Poikilothermy
Gastrointestinal	• Paralytic ileus • Loss of bowel function • Constipation, fecal impaction • Stress ulcers
Genitourinary	• Loss of voiding reflex, urine retention • Frequent urinary tract infections
Musculoskeletal	• Spasms • Heterotrophic ossification • Contractures
Skin	• Breakdown

If the patient suffered recent trauma, gently palpate the posterior neck for any pain or "step-off" (produced when one vertebra moves out of alignment, creating a protrusion in the spinal column). Inspect the affected area for swelling and ecchymosis.

Diagnostic tests

Initially, the doctor will order ABG analysis to detect respiratory alkalosis. He'll order chemistries to detect stress on the liver, heart, and kidneys and to detect hypoglycemia or insulin shock. Arrange for a lateral cervical spine X-ray, as ordered, to evaluate spinal column alignment, examine the neural foramina and disk space, identify soft-tissue injury of the re-

Evaluating levels of innervation

This chart will help you determine muscle movements to assess your patient's level of innervation. You can grade the quality of these movements on a motor strength scale. Using such a scale, 5 would be normal, 4 means range of motion (ROM) with resistance, 3 means full ROM against gravity, 2 means full ROM with gravity eliminated, and 1 means visible or palpable contractions.

LEVEL OF INNERVATION	MUSCLE INVOLVED	PATIENT INSTRUCTIONS
Third or fourth cervical vertebra	Diaphragm	• To inhale deeply
	Trapezius	• To shrug his shoulders
Fourth or fifth cervical vertebra	Deltoid	• To flap his arms • To push his shoulders forward and backward
Fifth cervical vertebra	Biceps	• To bend his arm up and make a muscle
Sixth cervical vertebra	Wrist	• To move his wrist up and down *Note:* Be sure to prevent arm supination and pronation, which the patient may substitute for the actual muscle movement.
Seventh cervical vertebra	Triceps	• To bring his arm across his chest, then straighten his arm with his thumb pointing to his chest and his supporting elbow up *Note:* The patient can substitute the deltoid and extensor biceps to perform this movement.
Eighth cervical vertebra	Hand	• To squeeze your hand • To open his hand and spread his fingers
First lumbar vertebra	Iliopsoas	• To lift his leg off the bed
	Hip rotator	• To pull his leg back
Second to fourth lumbar vertebrae	Quadriceps	• To bend his knee and straighten his leg. Tell him to support the knee with his arm if necessary.
Fifth lumbar vertebra	Ankle dorsiflexion muscles	• To pretend he's stepping on the gas pedal
First or second sacral vertebra	Ankle plantarflexion muscles	• To pull his toes toward his head

tropharyngeal space, and evaluate vertebral body integrity. For a more detailed study of areas with questionable integrity, open-mouth odontoid views and anterior and posterior views may be done.

To further evaluate the injury or help guide reduction or surgical management, the doctor will order an MRI or CT scan and myelography. An MRI scan can evaluate cord structure and injury despite an intact spinal column. A CT scan and myelography will reveal the quality of the injury reduction and vascular supply. If the patient is unconscious, a CT or MRI scan helps diagnose brain stem injury.

Other tests used to assess a spinal cord injury include somatosensory evoked response studies, which reveal how well impulses travel through the spinal cord.

Ongoing treatment

After the patient has been stabilized, ongoing medical treatment focuses on reperfusing the injured spinal cord—chiefly by maintaining nor-

mal to above-normal blood pressure—and ensuring body system functions.

Drug treatment

Hemodynamic support. Expect the doctor to
order sympathomimetic vasopressors for 3 to 5
days to raise MAP above 80 mm Hg and to
order I.V. fluids to maintain adequate circulating
volume.

Steroid therapy. Administering steroids may
speed rehabilitation, although the patient may
regain only a nerve root level. The doctor may
order high-dose steroid therapy by I.V. bolus
initially, then as a continuous infusion for up to
24 hours. (See *Administering high-dose steroids.*)

Other drug therapy. Naloxone, an opioid an-
tagonist, may reverse the effects of endogenous opioids released after spinal cord injury.
This drug also restores extracellular calcium
and may improve microcirculation.

Surgery

The patient with a spinal cord injury may undergo surgery to reduce and stabilize the injury. To prepare for surgery, he'll undergo
reduction with skeletal traction and weights.
Once he is stable or has achieved plateau, he'll
undergo surgical fixation or halo vest application. Surgery may involve anterior fusion or
posterior fusion. Both methods use bone grafts
to build a bone bridge and hardware to maintain the reduction until the bone bridge fuses.

Other treatments

The doctor may insert a PA catheter to closely
monitor intravascular volume and cardiac output. Be aware that vagal outflow commonly
continues uninterrupted despite vasopressor
therapy, causing urine output to increase. However, volume must be replaced cautiously because loss of vasomotor tone prevents an
increase in myocardial contractility and heart
rate to compensate for increased preload
brought on by volume resuscitation. This predisposes the patient to hypervolemia and pulmonary edema.

Administering high-dose steroids

When administering high-dose steroids to a patient
in neurogenic shock from a spinal cord injury, follow these guidelines to help ensure accurate dosage calculation and safe drug administration.

Initial I.V. bolus
Use this formula to calculate the total bolus dose
(in milliliters):

$$30 \text{ mg/kg} \times \frac{\text{patient weight in kg}}{\text{mg/ml (based on drip concentration)}}$$

Set the infusion pump to deliver the total bolus
over 15 minutes, and maintain the I.V. line with
0.9% sodium chloride solution for 15 minutes. As
ordered, give the initial bolus as soon as possible—
within 8 hours of the injury.

Maintenance dose
To calculate the hourly maintenance dose, use this
formula:

$$5.4 \text{ mg/kg} \times \frac{\text{patient weight in kg}}{\text{mg/ml (based on drip concentration)}}$$

Set the infusion pump to deliver an hourly maintenance dose. If the infusion is stopped inadvertently,
calculate new flow rates to make sure that the remaining dose is given within the allotted time.

Placing the patient on a kinetic treatment
table (Roto Rest bed) promotes postural drainage, offers respiratory support, and reduces
the need for mechanical ventilation. If the patient will require prolonged mechanical ventilation, the doctor may perform a tracheotomy
to provide a suction port, decrease the work
of breathing, and permit eating and speech
during ventilation.

If neurogenic shock is precipitated by insulin shock, the doctor will order the delivery of
one ampule of dextrose 50% to replenish
blood glucose levels. Serial blood glucose measurements will be performed and the patient

reestablished on his diet and daily insulin routine.

Ongoing nursing interventions

The goal of ongoing care is to maintain stability of all body systems and, if the patient has a spinal cord injury, to achieve maximal rehabilitation potential. Monitor vital signs closely, especially heart rate, blood pressure, and temperature.

Maintaining hemodynamic support

• As ordered, administer volume expanders and vasoactive drugs to maintain spinal cord perfusion. Once the patient's compensatory mechanisms are activated or sympathetic innervation resumes, wean the patient gradually from sympathomimetic therapy, as ordered, so that his body can adjust to a lower blood pressure and slower heart rate. Aim for a systolic pressure above 90 mm Hg and a heart rate of 50 to 60 beats/minute. If you have trouble weaning the patient from blood pressure support, the doctor may order ephedrine elixir to increase heart rate and blood pressure.

• Be sure to avoid Valsalva's maneuver — for example, during suctioning — to avoid slowing the heart rate further. Keep atropine at the bedside at all times in case of a vasovagal event.

• Allow only slow, progressive position changes. Orthostatic hypotension — a potential problem for any patient on prolonged bed rest — is especially likely to occur in patients lacking sympathetic innervation. Apply elastic bandages to the legs and an abdominal binder to maintain blood pressure when the patient sits upright.

Safeguarding circulation

• Deep vein thrombosis is a danger to the immobilized patient. As ordered, withhold anticoagulants for roughly 1 week to reduce the risk of increasing hemorrhage in the injured spinal cord and to prepare the patient for surgery.

• Apply pneumonic compression stockings, as ordered.

Maintaining body temperature

• Temperature regulation poses a challenge when caring for the patient in neurogenic shock. Lacking vasomotor tone, he can't shiver to retain heat or sweat to release heat below the injury level. Thus, his body temperature depends on environmental temperature, a condition called *poikilothermy*.

To maintain proper body temperature, use a heating or cooling blanket or other measures. If you apply a blanket, keep in mind that the patient can't sense heat or cold and thus risks a thermal burn. An effective way to warm a patient is across the lungs using warmed, humidified oxygen via the vent or a face mask.

Avoiding respiratory complications

• Be alert for respiratory compromise in patients with neurogenic shock. At least half of respiration takes place passively via the diaphragm, which arises from the cervical plexus at C3 to C5, whereas most defender mechanisms (intercostal and abdominal muscles for coughing) arise from thoracic vertebrae. If spinal cord injury or spinal anesthesia occurs at these levels, the patient will experience respiratory compromise secondary to reduced vital capacity and loss of forceful exhalation.

• Monitor the respiratory rate closely, and watch for signs of increased work of breathing. Perform incentive spirometry at least every 4 hours.

• If the patient can breathe spontaneously, help him perform incentive spirometry every 2 to 4 hours, and note any decrease in generated volumes. If he can't generate a flow of 1,000 ml/second, suspect impending respiratory failure.

• Ensure meticulous pulmonary hygiene. To help clear secretions, help the patient to cough, and perform abdominal thrusts and rib springing.

• If the patient is on a mechanical ventilator, perform aggressive CPT every 4 hours and hyperoxygenate him adequately before suctioning to minimize vasovagal stimulation.

• For the patient with a high-level spinal cord injury, weaning from the ventilator can prove arduous and requires the coordinated efforts of the entire health care team. Typically, weaning is attempted once the patient achieves pulmonary stability.

Obtain weaning parameters to assess whether the patient is ready to be weaned. Interventions may include a straight pressure-support mode after reducing synchronized intermittent mandatory ventilation (SIMV). This augmented mode lets him initiate his own breaths and allows alteration of the pressure support to achieve desired support volumes. Pressure support ventilation then can be reduced gradually, for example, by one or two sessions daily.

Another weaning strategy involves removing the patient from the ventilator and putting a trach collar on him twice a day, increasing his trach collar time by 15 to 30 minutes daily. Between trials, he receives pressure support ventilation and is fully ventilated at night for a rest phase. The goal is to alternate work periods with rest periods.

If the patient is being weaned by continuous positive airway pressure (CPAP), be aware that CPAP lasting more than 2 hours may cause fatigue and make him feel as if he's not really off of the ventilator.

During weaning, ensure meticulous pulmonary hygiene. If infiltrations and atelectasis occur during trach collar weaning, the patient must first be weaned to 0 cm H_2O PEEP and then advanced to trach collar weaning. PEEP will ensure that end-expiratory pressure doesn't fall below preset ventilator values.

Ensuring nutritional status and GI function
• Initially, your patient will probably have a gastric tube inserted to monitor gastric pH and gastric decompression. As ordered, insert a duodenal tube to permit early enteral feeding.
• Once feedings (enteral or oral) are successfully implemented, initiate a bowel elimination regimen that includes stool softeners and suppositories. These measures promote elimination and reduce the risk of constipation, which could precipitate autonomic dysreflexia, a disorder characterized by exaggerated responses to stimuli.
• Monitor the patient's bowel movements, which should occur at least every other day. Also, perform daily digital checks for retained stool or fecal impaction.
• Provide stress ulcer prophylaxis, as ordered, until the patient can accept gastric feedings — especially if he's receiving high-dose steroids.
• Observe the patient carefully for paralytic

ileus, common in patients in neurogenic shock. Peristalsis is mediated by the parasympathetic nervous system — specifically the vagus nerve. Because the vagus nerve exits above the first cervical vertebra, its pathway remains intact. Some experts believe this represents merely a response to the loss of homeostasis caused by the initial trauma.

Preventing autonomic dysreflexia
• Stay alert for signs of autonomic dysreflexia, including hypertension, an increased heart rate, a throbbing headache, an extremely elevated temperature, and skin flushing. If blood pressure isn't controlled, cerebrovascular hemorrhage may occur. If possible, avoid precipitating causes of autonomic dysreflexia, such as urine retention, constipation, infection, pain, pressure ulcers, and room temperature changes. Removing the offending stimulus usually eliminates this complication.

Be aware that the onset of autonomic dysreflexia usually coincides with a return of bladder tone, priapism, and muscle spasms (which typically occur as neurogenic shock resolves).

Preventing genitourinary complications
• Assess the patient's genitourinary status frequently. Observe his urine for color, clarity, and blood, and monitor urine pH and odor. Stay alert for signs of urinary tract infection — a particular risk if he has an indwelling urinary catheter.
• Once the patient's condition stabilizes and he achieves a balanced intake and output, restrict fluid intake to 2,000 to 2,400 ml/daily and perform straight catheterization every 4 hours, as ordered, progressing to every 6 hours if residual urine remains below 500 ml.

Ensuring musculoskeletal integrity
• Perform range-of-motion exercises on all muscles and joints to maintain mobility and prevent contractures and para-articular heterotrophic ossification. Turn and reposition the patient frequently to prevent pressure ulcers.
• Once neurogenic shock resolves and the spinal cord injury is stabilized, encourage the patient to exercise lightly to prevent complications related to prolonged immobility. If he de-

velops widespread muscle spasms, assess him for pain and interference with therapy. If necessary, notify the doctor and administer muscle relaxants such as baclofen as ordered.

Providing patient teaching

• Teach the patient and his family about his condition, its management and care, rehabilitation programs, and the psychological, emotional, and social implications of his condition. As appropriate, arrange for referral to a neuropsychologist trained to help patients and their families cope with a spinal cord injury.

Myasthenic crisis

This disorder is an acute exacerbation of myasthenia gravis, a chronic autoimmune and immunopathologically mediated disease characterized by abnormal muscle weakness

EMERGENCY INTERVENTIONS

When your patient has myasthenic crisis

Myasthenic crisis can progress rapidly, causing respiratory failure in less than an hour. You must take immediate steps to protect the patient's airway and help maintain adequate respiratory status.
• Every 15 to 30 minutes, assess the patient for an adequate gag reflex and ptosis, and check his speech, respirations, and amount of saliva. Perform a quick neurologic check to evaluate his motor strength.
• Monitor arterial blood gas values and administer supplemental oxygen, as ordered. Insert a large-bore I.V. line to provide access for volume expanders and other emergency drugs. To help prevent aspiration, place the patient on a soft diet. If he's extremely weak, withhold all oral intake.
• To avert respiratory failure, expect the doctor to order intubation and supportive mechanical ventilation. To avert cholinergic crisis, give atropine I.V., as ordered, as an antidote for anticholinesterase medications such as neostigmine or pyridostigmine.

and fatigability. Respiratory muscles become weak, possibly leading to respiratory paralysis and failure. The patient needs immediate intervention to ensure adequate ventilation. (See *When your patient has myasthenic crisis.*)

Causes

Conditions that may precipitate myasthenic crisis include excessive or insufficient anticholinesterase medication, fatigue, illness, emotional stress, surgery, trauma, infection, and use of such drugs as neuromuscular blocking agents, drugs with local anesthetic properties (such as quinidine, propranolol, and lidocaine), antibiotics (especially neomycin, kanamycin, and gentamicin), barbiturates (such as pentobarbital and secobarbital), and narcotics (such as morphine). In women, myasthenic crisis has been linked to pregnancy and the initiation of menstruation. Also, myasthenic crisis is more likely to occur in a hospitalized patient with newly diagnosed myasthenia gravis.

Pathophysiology

In myasthenia gravis, an autoimmune response presumably reduces the number of acetylcholine receptor sites on motor end plates. This leads to reduced amplitude of end plate potentials, which impairs muscle contraction by interfering with impulse transmission and muscle action potentials. Impaired muscle contraction, in turn, produces characteristic muscle weakness.

In myasthenic crisis, extreme muscle weakness may progress to respiratory failure. (See *What happens in myasthenic crisis.*)

Complications

Myasthenic crisis may progress to a life-threatening state within an hour. Difficulty swallowing may precipitate aspiration, and respiratory muscle failure may lead to rapid respiratory failure and death. The patient also may develop cholinergic crisis from overmedication with cholinergic drugs used to treat the crisis.

Assessment

History

After ensuring your patient's ventilation, take a brief history by asking him these questions:

PATHOPHYSIOLOGY

What happens in myasthenic crisis

These illustrations compare the normal physiology at the neuromuscular junction with the alterations that occur during myasthenic crisis.

Normal motor cell and synapse

Vesicles release acetylcholine (ACh) at special release sites. ACh then crosses the synaptic space, reaching ACh receptors. Acetylcholinesterase in the clefts rapidly hydrolyzes ACh.

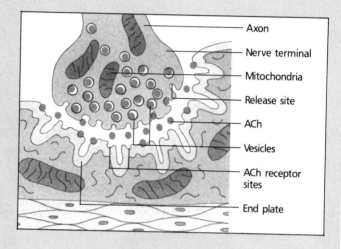

- Axon
- Nerve terminal
- Mitochondria
- Release site
- ACh
- Vesicles
- ACh receptor sites
- End plate

During myasthenic crisis

Antibodies attack and destroy ACh receptor sites, limiting the number of available receptor sites. This decreases motor end-plate action potentials, leading to extreme muscle weakness.

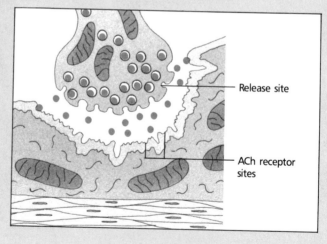

- Release site
- ACh receptor sites

• Have you ever been diagnosed with myasthenia gravis?
• When did you first notice that your symptoms were getting worse?
• Have you ever had a crisis before? If so, do you know what caused it?
• Are you taking any prescribed medications? If so, which ones and in what dosages? When did you take the last dose? Has the doctor recently adjusted the dosage? Has he recently taken you off any medications or prescribed any new ones?
• Do you take your medication consistently and exactly as prescribed?
• Have you had a recent illness or been under unusual stress?

ASSESSMENT INSIGHT

Differentiating myasthenic crisis from cholinergic crisis

Myasthenic crisis is sometimes difficult to differentiate from cholinergic crisis. Use this chart to quickly determine if your patient is experiencing myasthenic crisis or cholinergic crisis. Withdrawal of anticholinesterase drugs for 24 to 72 hours will worsen the signs and symptoms of myasthenic crisis but improve those of cholinergic crisis; however, you're unlikely to have 3 days to make a diagnosis.

FEATURE	MYASTHENIC CRISIS	CHOLINERGIC CRISIS
Heart rate	• Above normal	• Below normal
Blood pressure	• Increased	• Decreased
Demeanor	• Restless	• Restless
Secretions	• Increased	• Increased
Respiratory pattern	• Dyspnea	• Dyspnea
Muscle strength	• Weakened	• Weakened, with fasciculations
Swallowing	• Impaired	• Impaired
Speech	• Nasal	• Slurred
Bowel sounds	• Hypoactive	• Hyperactive
Vision	• Blurred	• Blurred
Ptosis	• Present	• Present
Results of Tensilon test	• Improved strength	• No change or increased weakness

Physical examination
Expect signs and symptoms of acute respiratory distress. Examine the patient for exaggerated manifestations of myasthenia gravis — muscle weakness, fatigue, ptosis, dysphagia, increased salivation, a decreased gag reflex, slurred or nasal speech, and absent facial expression. You may also detect tachycardia and hypertension. Typically, the patient seems irritable, extremely restless, and anxious. He may also report having diplopia.

Assess the strength of muscles in the head, neck, trunk, and extremities. Closely evaluate the patient's respiratory function, especially his vital capacity.

Diagnostic tests
The doctor may perform the Tensilon test (using edrophonium chloride) to distinguish myasthenic crisis from cholinergic crisis. In this test, he injects 1 mg edrophonium I.V. and then assesses the patient's motor responses by having him perform a series of muscle group movements. If signs and symptoms improve quickly after injection, the crisis is myasthenic; if they worsen, the crisis is cholinergic. (See *Differentiating myasthenic crisis from cholinergic crisis.*)

Be aware that the Tensilon test is performed only on a patient with previously diagnosed myasthenia gravis to confirm myasthenic crisis. In other patients, the diagnosis of myasthenic crisis rests largely on history and physical findings. The doctor may order anti-acetylcholinesterase receptor antibody titers, serum triiodothyronine and thyroxine levels, a thymus scan, and electromyography to confirm the diagnosis and determine which muscle groups are involved.

Ongoing treatment
After the patient has received initial treatment and is somewhat stable, the doctor will order measures to maintain ventilatory support and prevent complications. In some cases, thymectomy (thymus removal) is indicated.

If initial interventions fail to halt progression of the crisis and the patient is nearing respiratory failure, he'll be intubated for mechanical ventilation and possible tracheostomy. Ventilatory augmentation, such as assist-control ventilation or SIMV with pressure support, may be required to promote full ventilation despite weakened respiratory muscles.

Drug treatment
The doctor may discontinue anticholinesterase drugs such as neostigmine or pyridostigmine during mechanical ventilation to prevent in-

creased airway pressure resulting from drug therapy. Alternatively, he may order ipratropium, an anticholinergic that doesn't increase airway pressure, to dilate the patient's bronchioles and facilitate ventilation.

Some patients also require steroids, cytotoxic agents (such as azathioprine or cyclophosphamide), or plasmapheresis. These therapies target the immune response by attacking anticholinesterase receptor antibodies.

Surgery

Because up to 90% of patients with myasthenia gravis have thymic disease, thymectomy may be indicated to induce immunosuppression and thereby decrease the number of circulating anticholinesterase antibodies.

Ongoing nursing interventions

Focus nursing care on ensuring your patient's respiratory function, maintaining drug therapy, and preventing complications.

• Evaluate the patient's neurologic status every hour and check his muscle strength, ocular motion, speech quality, and swallowing ability. Check for diplopia and ptosis. Repeat this assessment 1 hour after medication administration, and document any changes.

• Every hour, assess the patient's respiratory rate and pattern, accessory muscle use, breath sounds, skin color, tidal volume, and vital capacity. Report any abnormalities or findings outside these desirable ranges: respiratory rate, 35 breaths/minute or less; negative inspiratory force, -20 cm H_2O or more; tidal volume between 400 and 700 ml, depending on the patient's age, sex, height, and weight; and vital capacity, 1.65 to 4.85 liters in a female and 2.79 to 6.65 liters in a male.

• Administer anticholinesterase doses exactly on schedule to maintain therapeutic blood levels of the drug. The normal guideline of 30 minutes' flexibility in scheduled administration time doesn't apply to these medications. Be aware that anticholinesterase drugs may increase bronchial secretions and precipitate bronchospasm when given in excessive amounts.

• Administer supplemental oxygen, as ordered, and use an SaO_2 monitor or a pulse oximeter to obtain continuous oxygenation data. Evaluate monitor readings in conjunction with periodic ABG values.

• Until the myasthenic crisis passes, withhold all oral intake to prevent aspiration. Perform postural drainage, turning, and suctioning every 2 to 4 hours to avoid pooling of secretions.

• Maintain nutritional support to ensure a smooth recovery after the crisis. Provide a soft diet to reduce the effort of eating. If the patient can't tolerate oral intake, provide feedings through a duodenal tube, as ordered. Many myasthenic patients can't tolerate enteral feedings and require total parenteral nutrition.

• Monitor laboratory studies, such as serum albumin and serum transferrin levels, to help determine the patient's nutritional needs.

• Develop a schedule of alternating rest and activity periods. Schedule activities requiring the greatest muscle strength early in the day, after drug administration.

• Perform range-of-motion exercises and schedule short, assisted exercise periods to reduce muscle atrophy and prevent deep vein thrombosis. To further minimize risk of thrombosis, apply pneumonic compression sleeves and give subcutaneous heparin, as ordered.

• Teach the patient and his family about myasthenia gravis and factors that may precipitate a crisis. Make sure they know how to identify signs and symptoms of myasthenic crisis. Verify that the patient understands his prescribed medication regimen and the importance of compliance, and teach him about potential adverse drug effects.

• To help the patient resume his normal roles and responsibilities, urge him to establish a daily routine that includes frequent rest periods. Refer him to the Myasthenia Gravis Foundation for information and emotional support.

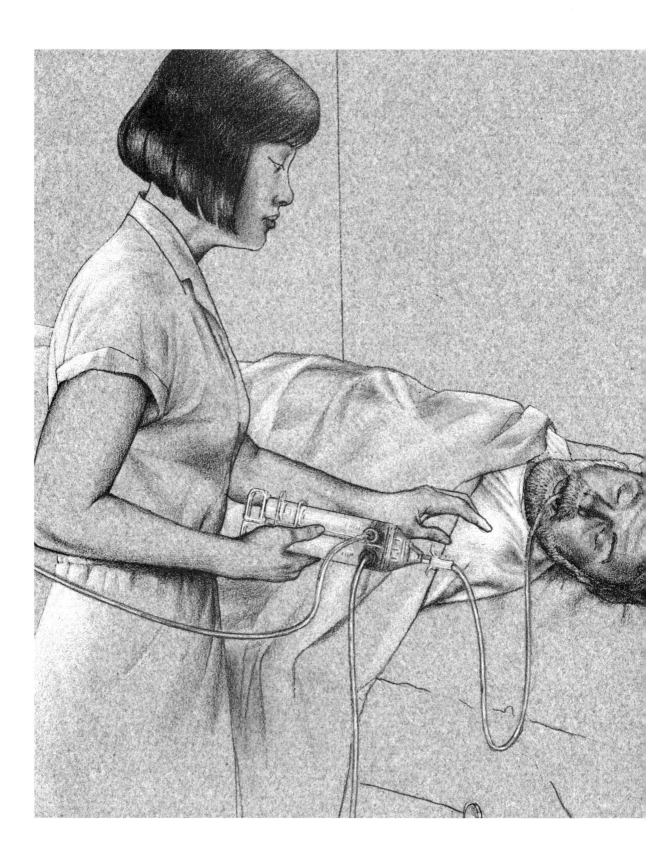

CHAPTER 4

Gastrointestinal crises

The gastrointestinal (GI) system serves two major functions. The first is digestion: the breaking down of food and fluids into simple chemicals that can be absorbed into the bloodstream and transported throughout the body, providing cells with energy. The second major function is eliminating waste products from the body.

Any serious disruption of the GI system can have far-reaching metabolic effects and may lead to a life-threatening GI crisis—a condition that can occur as a primary disorder, as a consequence of chronic disorders or injuries, or as a complication of medications or diagnostic tests.

This chapter will explain how to manage patients with certain GI crises, including ruptured esophageal varices, perforated GI ulcer, GI hemorrhage, and hepatic failure. You'll become familiar with the causes, pathophysiology, and complications of these emergencies, and you'll learn how to assess your patient rapidly

EMERGENCY INTERVENTIONS

When your patient has ruptured esophageal varices

A patient with ruptured esophageal varices is at risk for shock and requires aggressive medical care and expert nursing care.

Ensure ABCs
Focus on ensuring and stabilizing the patient's ABCs—airway, breathing, and circulation. As ordered, administer supplemental oxygen if the patient is hypoxic or in respiratory distress. If he can't breathe independently, he may require mechanical ventilation.

Monitor vital signs
Monitor the patient's blood pressure, heart rate, and respiratory rate. Initiate cardiac monitoring to check the heart rate and detect arrhythmias. Obtain noninvasive blood pressure equipment to allow blood pressure readings every 5 minutes. Insert a large-bore I.V. line to administer dextrose 5% in water, 0.9% sodium chloride solution, or both. Infuse the fluid at a rate of 250 to 500 ml/hour, as ordered, to replace volume lost through hematemesis or melena and to maintain normal vital signs.

Obtain blood samples
Collect blood samples for type and crossmatch tests, complete blood count with differential, serum electrolyte levels, coagulation studies, liver function tests, and blood urea nitrogen levels. Draw an arterial sample to assess the patient's oxygenation.

To treat hematemesis, the doctor will immediately insert a nasogastric (NG) tube and connect it to suction. He'll also use the NG tube for gastric lavage with 0.9% sodium chloride solution or water (iced or at room temperature). Accurately record the amount of fluid used for irrigation; then subtract it from the total amount of NG aspirate to assess the true amount of bleeding. Even if the patient doesn't have active bleeding, an NG tube may be inserted to prevent further hematemesis and allow accurate measurement of blood in vomitus.

and intervene to avert possible death. Finally, you'll learn about continuing treatments and interventions, including the nursing care your patient will need after surviving an acute GI crisis.

Ruptured esophageal varices

Esophageal varices are dilated, tortuous veins in the submucosa of the lower esophagus. When they rupture, they cause massive, life-threatening hematemesis. The patient with ruptured esophageal varices needs emergency treatment to control hemorrhage and prevent the progression to shock. (See *When your patient has ruptured esophageal varices.*)

Causes
Esophageal varices nearly always result from portal hypertension—increased pressure in the portal vein caused by obstruction in the portal circulation. Usually, the underlying cause of portal hypertension is a disorder of the liver or biliary system, such as alcoholic cirrhosis, hepatitis, biliary infection, liver or biliary tumors, cholelithiasis, or trauma or surgery involving the portal vein.

Pathophysiology
Normally, venous blood from the digestive tract—including the esophagus—flows through the portal vein into the liver. Portal hypertension disrupts normal circulation, causing blood to bypass the liver through collateral channels instead of flowing through it via the portal vein. A common collateral channel lies between the left and short gastric veins and the esophageal veins that open into the azygos vein. As demands on this collateral system increase, pressure within the portal vein rises. The excessive pressure causes the thin-walled esophageal veins to become varicosed.

Because the delicate varices are vulnerable to increased portal vein pressure, they rupture easily. Normal portal pressure ranges from 8 to 12 mm Hg; in portal hypertension, the pressure may rise above 30 mm Hg. Conditions

PATHOPHYSIOLOGY

What happens when esophageal varices rupture

Esophageal varices rupture when pressure in the portal vein increases, as from liver disease.

Normally, blood from the GI tract flows through the portal vein into the liver and then drains through the hepatic veins into the inferior vena cava, as shown here.

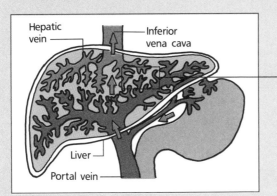

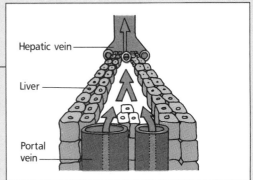

Hepatic cells are destroyed in such conditions as cirrhosis, hepatitis, liver tumors, biliary stones, infection, and biliary trauma or surgery. Damaged portions of the liver obstruct portal vein circulation and increase pressure, causing portal hypertension.

Because of portal hypertension, blood from the portal vein backs up into the thin-walled veins of the esophagus. If these veins rupture from excessive pressure, the patient will experience massive hemorrhage.

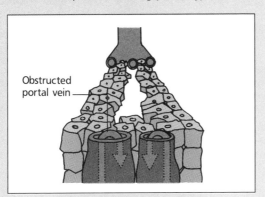

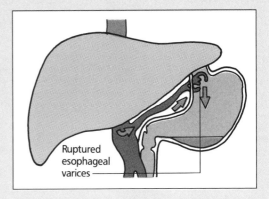

causing increased intra-abdominal pressure (such as lifting, straining, and vomiting) also may lead to variceal rupture. Ruptured varices cause massive hemorrhage in the upper GI tract and disrupt blood supply to vital organs.

(See *What happens when esophageal varices rupture.*)

Complications
Ruptured esophageal varices may lead to hypovolemic shock, exsanguination, and death.

Ruptured esophageal varices caused by alcohol abuse

Alcohol abuse is a major cause of liver disorders. And liver disorders often bring on the portal hypertension that leads to esophageal varices, which may rupture with devastating consequences.

If your patient has ruptured esophageal varices, you can't waste precious moments trying to uncover a drinking problem. But once he's stable, you'll need to take a thorough history—and not shy away from investigating any personal habits that seem relevant.

Consider the case of Jeremy Stewart, age 45, who comes to the hospital after vomiting a large amount of bright red blood.

Emergency treatment
Nurse Dana Landes quickly inspects Mr. Stewart, noting peripheral edema and an enlarged abdomen. The health care team starts emergency measures, inserting a large-bore I.V. line and nasogastric (NG) tube and performing gastric lavage to prepare Mr. Stewart for endoscopy. They draw blood for type and crossmatching, complete blood count, serum electrolyte levels, coagulation tests, and arterial blood gas analysis. Then they administer oxygen at 4 liters/minute by nasal cannula.

Stabilization and diagnosis
In the intensive care unit, the doctor performs an endoscopic examination, which reveals ruptured esophageal varices. To sclerose the varices and halt bleeding, he injects a sclerosing agent through the endoscope.

When Dana reviews Mr. Stewart's medical record, she sees the following note from the emergency department nurse: "Wife reports patient started complaining of increasing weakness, swollen ankles, and an enlarged abdomen about 6 months ago. He told her he had two black bowel movements within the last 3 hours. She says he's had no serious health problems."

As ordered, Dana administers a bolus of vasopressin, 20 units in 100 ml dextrose 5% in water over 15 minutes. Then she starts a vasopressin drip at 0.2 unit/minute. She assists with insertion of pulmonary artery and arterial catheters to closely monitor the patient's hemodynamic and pulmonary status. Every 15 minutes to 1 hour, she watches the cardiac monitor to assess for adverse effects of vasopressin and measures the patient's blood pressure, pulmonary artery pressure, and heart rate.

Once Mr. Stewart's condition seems stable, Dana tries to find out what might have caused his esophageal varices. When she asks him how much alcohol he drinks, he replies he has an occasional beer. Mrs. Stewart reports that her husband usually drinks four to six cans of beer daily—and has been doing so for at least 20 years. Dana documents this on Mr. Stewart's flow sheet.

Recovery
Within 6 hours, Dana detects no further blood in the NG tube. She discontinues vasopressin, as ordered, and continues to check for occult blood in stools.

Also, the airway may become obstructed from aspiration of vomited blood or its accumulation in the oropharynx. Mortality from ruptured esophageal varices may be as high as 60% during the first episode. In patients who survive this episode, rebleeding is likely within 1 year and carries an even higher mortality.

Assessment
History
If time allows, take a brief history from your patient or his family to determine the presence of underlying chronic liver disease or chronic alcohol abuse. Expect a report of hematemesis with blood welling up in the back of the throat. Ask about the frequency of vomiting and the amount of vomitus. Find out if the patient has pain—ruptured esophageal varices usually are painless. Also ask if he's noticed melena (tarry, black stools). (See *Ruptured esophageal varices caused by alcohol abuse.*)

Determine if the patient had a previous disorder or surgery of the biliary tract (such as gallstones, gallbladder surgery, abdominal trauma, or infection) or has a family history of GI tract disorders. Take a medication history, staying alert for drugs that may contribute to bleeding, such as aspirin, nonsteroidal anti-inflammatory drugs (NSAIDs), and anticoagulants.

Physical examination
Sudden, profuse, painless vomiting of bright red blood is the hallmark of ruptured esophageal varices. Assess vomitus for clots. Check stools for melena and occult blood. Observe for signs and symptoms of hypovolemic shock—restlessness, hypotension, tachycardia, diaphoresis, pallor, decreased urine output, and reduced central venous pressure (CVP) and pulmonary artery pressure (PAP).

Other signs and symptoms depend partly on how much blood the patient has lost. (See *Determining blood loss from clinical findings.*)

Inspection. Assess the patient for an altered level of consciousness or lethargy, jaundice, ascites, lower extremity edema, and muscle wasting. These signs reflect liver disease, a typical cause of portal hypertension and ruptured esophageal varices. You also may note dilated abdominal veins and abdominal distention.

Auscultation. Listen to bowel sounds to assess their quality and quantity. Blood in the GI tract typically causes hyperactive bowel sounds, so you should hear more than 20 sounds per minute instead of the normal 10 to 20.

Palpation. Assess for abdominal tenderness or pain, and note the location of these symptoms. Palpate for masses and liver or spleen enlargement.

Percussion. Percuss the abdomen for shifting dullness, a sign of ascites.

Diagnostic tests
With ruptured esophageal varices, a complete blood count (CBC) may reveal anemia from upper GI tract bleeding and decreased hematocrit, hemoglobin level, and platelet count. (However, hemoglobin and hematocrit don't fall until several hours after blood loss occurs.) Expect elevated liver enzyme levels (lactate de-

Determining blood loss from clinical findings

If your patient has ruptured esophageal varices, try to determine the severity of blood loss by identifying his signs and symptoms.

Findings in initial bleeding
During the initial bleeding stage, when less than 500 ml of blood is lost, you may detect only weakness, restlessness, and diaphoresis. Body temperature may rise to between 101° and 102° F (38.4° and 39° C). Bowel sounds are hyperactive from sensitivity of the bowel to blood. Blood in the bowel acts as a cathartic, causing increased bowel sounds and diarrhea.

Findings after loss of 500 to 1,000 ml
After a blood loss of up to 1,000 ml, intravascular volume diminishes further. A sympathetic nervous system response causes release of the catecholamines epinephrine and norepinephrine. This, in turn, causes the heart rate to rise in an attempt to maintain adequate blood pressure (more than 100 mm Hg systolic).

Findings after loss of 1,000 ml or more
After a loss of 1,000 ml of blood, expect classic signs and symptoms of shock. To boost blood flow to the brain and heart, catecholamine release now triggers vasoconstriction in the skin, lungs, intestines, liver, and kidneys. As blood flow to the skin diminishes, the patient's skin cools. With less blood flowing to his lungs, he hyperventilates to maintain adequate gas exchange. Expect blood pressure to drop—a sign of advanced shock indicating that the body's protective mechanisms have been overwhelmed. As intravascular volume diminishes, urine output decreases from renal reabsorption of water in response to the release of antidiuretic hormone.

hydrogenase; alkaline phosphatase; aspartate aminotransferase [AST], formerly SGOT; and alanine aminotransferase [ALT], formerly SGPT).

Prothrombin time (PT) and partial thromboplastin time (PTT) may be prolonged from liver disease or other contributing factors, such as anticoagulant use. The blood urea nitrogen

(BUN) level rises from GI bleeding.

After the patient has been stabilized, the doctor may perform esophagogastroduodenoscopy (EGD) to visualize and identify the source of bleeding, confirm the diagnosis of ruptured esophageal varices, and help determine the appropriate therapy to stop bleeding. Other diagnostic studies that may help identify the source of bleeding include ultrasonography, a computed tomography (CT) scan, and angiography.

Ongoing treatment

To halt bleeding and stabilize the patient, the doctor may use a combination of sclerotherapy, fluids and volume expanders, blood transfusions, balloon tamponade, drug therapy, and surgery.

Endoscopic sclerotherapy. During EGD, the doctor will inject a sclerosing agent through the endoscope while visualizing the bleeding varices. The sclerosing agent promotes thrombosis and sclerosis of varices, which helps to control bleeding. Gastric lavage with a nasogastric (NG) tube, begun as an emergency treatment, should continue up to and immediately prior to endoscopy to aid visualization of the upper GI tract.

Fluids and volume expanders. The patient will need I.V. fluids and volume expanders to reverse hypovolemia and prevent electrolyte imbalance. A central venous (CV) catheter or pulmonary artery (PA) catheter will be inserted to monitor his fluid status, determine fluid requirements, and evaluate the effects of therapy.

Blood transfusions. The patient with massive GI hemorrhage will need blood transfusions — preferably with fully crossmatched blood. The doctor may order whole blood or packed red blood cells (RBCs). Depending on the patient's laboratory values, he also may order administration of clotting factors, platelets, and calcium.

Balloon tamponade. To control persistent hemorrhage, the doctor may perform balloon tamponade by inserting an esophageal tube, which applies pressure on the bleeding site. The Sengstaken-Blakemore tube has two balloons (esophageal and gastric) and three lumens (one used to inflate the esophageal balloon, one to inflate the gastric balloon, and a gastric aspiration port to allow drainage and instillation of fluid and drugs). The Minnesota tube has two balloons and four lumens; the fourth lumen allows for esophageal suctioning. The doctor will choose an esophageal tube according to his preference, the patient's specific needs, or hospital policy. Assist with tube insertion as needed.

Balloon tamponade stops acute variceal hemorrhage in roughly 85% to 90% of cases — but usually just temporarily. Even after successful tamponade, approximately 20% to 60% of patients experience rebleeding with balloon deflation. Balloon tamponade also may cause such complications as aspiration of oral secretions, airway obstruction from balloon displacement, and esophageal rupture.

Drug treatment

To stop bleeding, the doctor may infuse vasopressin I.V. or intra-arterially into the superior mesenteric artery. This agent has a powerful vasoconstrictive effect that reduces portal hypertension and mesenteric blood flow by constricting arterioles. The I.V. dosage is 200 units in 500 ml of dextrose 5% in water (D_5W), given at a rate of 0.5 to 1 ml/minute by infusion device (to deliver 0.2 to 0.4 unit/minute). The doctor may order an initial bolus of 20 units in 100 to 200 ml of D_5W over 10 to 20 minutes.

Vasopressin must be used cautiously because it may cause abdominal cramps, involuntary bowel evacuation (usually diarrhea), and bowel infarction. It also may induce coronary vasoconstriction, leading to cardiac ischemia, and has an antidiuretic effect. (See *Using vasopressin to treat ruptured esophageal varices.*)

The doctor may prescribe propranolol, which reduces portal pressure through its beta-adrenergic blocking action and reduces the risk of bleeding. He may order nitroprusside or nitroglycerin to decrease peripheral vasoconstriction. Nitroglycerin can be given I.V., transdermally, or sublingually. Vitamin K may be given to promote prothrombin synthesis and increase blood clotting. The typical dosage is 10 mg given by slow I.V. infusion, I.M., or S.C.

Surgery

If vasopressin and balloon tamponade can't control bleeding, your patient may require surgery. Surgery doesn't always succeed, but it may be the only method that reduces portal pressure and directly controls bleeding. Surgical procedures used to control bleeding from esophageal varices include shunts, direct ligation of varices, and esophageal transection.

Shunting procedures aim to control bleeding from varices by diverting blood from the portal vein to collateral vessels. However, shunts carry significant risks, such as hepatic failure, hepatic encephalopathy, and hemorrhage. When performed as emergency measures, decompression shunts have a mortality of 25% to 50%. (See *Understanding decompression shunts,* page 130.)

Another surgical procedure, transesophageal ligation, helps control esophageal hemorrhage by directly cutting or ligating varices. Completed through a left thoracotomy, this procedure carries the risk of rebleeding, esophageal leakage, and death during surgery.

With esophageal transection, the surgeon makes a small gastrostomy incision to the lower end of the esophagus and then uses a circular mechanical stapling device to obliterate submucosal varices by transecting and stapling the distal esophagus. Risks associated with this procedure include rebleeding.

Ongoing nursing interventions

You'll need to monitor your patient closely. Other measures depend on his status and the procedures he undergoes.
• During EGD, provide emotional support to alleviate stress from this uncomfortable procedure.
• Monitor and document the patient's blood pressure, heart rate, respiratory rate, and urine output at least every hour.
• Closely monitor laboratory indicators of fluid and electrolyte status.
• During vasopressin therapy, maintain especially close monitoring. Assess vital signs every

---

Using vasopressin to treat ruptured esophageal varices

A patient with upper GI bleeding from ruptured varices requires immediate medical attention. If lavage doesn't control the hemorrhage, the doctor may insert a balloon tube (such as a Minnesota or Sengstaken-Blakemore tube) and apply pressure to the bleeding site. But in recent years, medical treatment with vasopressin has become increasingly popular for ruptured esophageal varices.

A posterior pituitary hormone, vasopressin is a potent vasoconstrictor that works by dramatically reducing mesenteric blood flow. It controls hemorrhaging by decreasing portal vein blood flow and pressure.

Administering vasopressin

Vasopressin can be administered by the intra-arterial or I.V. route. In studies, I.V. administration has been just as effective as intra-arterial administration, with fewer complications. Typically, I.V. vasopressin is initiated at 0.2 to 0.4 unit/minute and titrated to patient response.

Despite vasopressin's effectiveness, some studies have shown that it doesn't improve survival rates—which leads researchers to wonder if dosages used in practice are high enough. But increasing the dose would be risky. Even in standard amounts, vasopressin can cause adverse hemodynamic reactions, including hypertension, bradycardia, electrocardiographic changes, and reduced cardiac output.

Administering vasopressin with nitroglycerin or nitroprusside

Some doctors combine vasopressin with nitroglycerin or nitroprusside. These two drugs augment vasopressin's beneficial effect on portal pressure. They also help counteract vasopressin's adverse effects, including reduced cardiac output. Nitroglycerin and nitroprusside increase cardiac output by causing vasodilation, which lowers blood pressure and improves stroke volume, and by causing an increase in heart rate. Combination therapy hasn't been extensively studied, but it seems to reduce complications and improve hemorrhage control.

---

15 minutes, observe the cardiac monitor for arrhythmias, and measure urine output.
• Obtain hemodynamic readings, such as CVP, PAP, and arterial pressure, every hour or as ordered.
• Maintain a patent airway, and ensure adequate oxygenation and ventilation. If ordered, maintain mechanical ventilation or administer oxygen by nasal cannula. Carefully monitor oxygen delivery and assess the patient's respiratory status regularly through pulse oximetry

Understanding decompression shunts

Shunting controls bleeding from varices by diverting blood from the portal vein to collateral vessels. Surgical decompression shunts relieve portal hypertension associated with esophageal varices and liver disease, reducing blood flow to the varices.

Portacaval shunt

The most common procedure, *a portacaval shunt* diverts blood from the portal venous system by dissecting the portal vein away from the liver and inserting it into the inferior vena cava. Although this procedure decreases portal vein pressure, it carries significant risks. Infusion of blood into the inferior vena cava may cause acute postoperative pulmonary edema and ventricular overload. Also, it prohibits conversion of ammonia to urea (which normally occurs when portal blood flow enters the liver), predisposing the patient to chronic hepatic encephalopathy. The end-to-side anastomosis reduces portal pressure more effectively than side-to-side anastomosis.

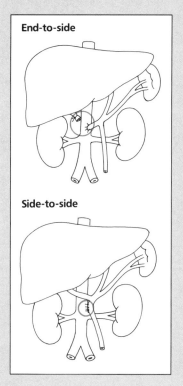

Splenorenal shunt

Recommended in portal vein obstruction and when hypersplenism accompanies portal hypertension, a *splenorenal shunt* joins the splenic vein and the left renal vein. The end-to-side anastomosis involves splenectomy, unlike the side-to-side anastomosis, which may be performed in the absence of hypersplenism.

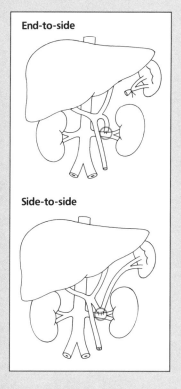

Mesocaval shunt

Indicated in portal vein thrombosis, previous splenectomy, or uncontrollable ascites, a *mesocaval shunt* joins the superior mesenteric vein to the inferior vena cava. However, neither the side-to-side nor the Dacron graft anastomosis is as effective as other shunts, and both carry the risk of thrombosis.

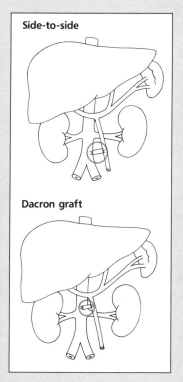

and arterial blood gas (ABG) values. Assess and document heart and breath sounds every 4 hours and as indicated.

• As ordered, administer drugs—vitamin K if the patient has prolonged bleeding times, nitroglycerin or nitroprusside if he has peripheral vasoconstriction, and vasopressin to decrease blood flow to the portal system. Be sure to follow hospital policy and procedure regarding these drugs. Assess for therapeutic and adverse drug effects.

• To maintain fluid and electrolyte balance, continue to administer fluids and blood products as needed and ordered. Monitor serial laboratory tests frequently and report suspicious values.

• If your patient has an NG tube, assess his bowel sounds before instilling drugs through the tube. Check tube placement every 4 hours. Ensure tube patency by irrigating with 0.9% sodium chloride solution or water, as ordered, after the initial lavage.

• If your patient has an esophageal tube for balloon tamponade, carefully monitor for asphyxiation caused by tube displacement. Keep scissors at the bedside so you can quickly cut and remove the tube in case asphyxiation occurs. Maintain the prescribed pressure inflation and deflation schedule to prevent tissue necrosis resulting from excessive pressure.

• Irrigate the gastric aspiration port every 4 hours to ensure its patency and accuracy in measuring instilled fluids and drainage. Keep the esophageal suction source on intermittent suction or as ordered.

• Continually monitor the patient for increased bleeding from the NG or esophageal tube as well as for hematemesis or melena. Once bleeding stops, stay alert for rebleeding from any of these sites.

• While the GI tube is in place, withhold all oral intake and administer parenteral nutrition, as needed, to support the patient's metabolic needs.

• Continue to test all vomitus, stools, and drainage for occult blood even after all obvious bleeding stops.

• Carefully measure and record intake and output. Be sure to include all I.V. fluids and medications as intake. Record all fluids instilled through the NG tube as intake and all drainage from the tube as output.

• As ordered, insert an indwelling urinary catheter as soon as possible to accurately monitor urine output. Measure and record urine output, and report output below 30 ml/hour.

• Perform frequent mouth care and provide comfort measures.

• Always wear gloves and wash hands thoroughly to avoid contamination from blood and body fluids.

• Provide emotional support and reassurance to the patient to help ease his anxiety.

• Maintain a calm, quiet environment, and encourage all personnel to approach the patient calmly.

Perforated GI ulcer

In this disorder, a peptic ulcer perforates, or erodes through, the wall of the stomach or duodenum. Approximately 10% of ulcers perforate, with the incidence of perforation rising with the patient's age. Although peptic ulcers include both duodenal and gastric ulcers, most perforations involve duodenal ulcers. (See *When your patient has a perforated peptic ulcer,* page 132.)

Treat perforation of a peptic ulcer as an abdominal emergency. Concurrent hemorrhage occurs in roughly 10% of patients. To halt the progression to hypovolemic shock, you must take quick action.

Causes
NSAIDs (such as aspirin and phenylbutazone), steroids, reserpine, and chemotherapeutic agents increase the risk of peptic ulcers and perforation by inhibiting prostaglandin synthesis. Prostaglandins help the gastric mucosa resist damage by pepsin and other acidic gastric juices.

Other causes of mucosal damage include intestinal reflux (from regurgitation of bile salts and pancreatic secretions) and gastritis, a condition characterized by hypersecretion of hydrochloric acid.

When your patient has a perforated peptic ulcer

Stabilizing cardiovascular and pulmonary status is the top priority for the patient with a perforated peptic ulcer.

Insert an I.V. line
As ordered, insert a large-bore I.V. line to provide high-volume parenteral therapy, including fluids and electrolytes, to replace lost volume and prevent shock. Expect to infuse lactated Ringer's solution and assist in placing a central venous pressure line. Monitor the patient's vital signs, and watch for signs and symptoms of hypovolemic shock. Insert an indwelling urinary catheter to measure urine output.

Prepare the patient for surgery
Prepare the patient for immediate surgery to treat peritonitis, which may develop within a few hours of perforation. The surgeon may close the perforation via laparotomy, although a patient with chronic ulcer disease will need more definitive surgery such as gastric resection.

Before surgery, keep the patient in low Fowler's position and provide emotional support to relieve his anxiety. Before the procedure is performed, insert a nasogastric tube to empty stomach contents and prevent further peritoneal contamination as ordered. The doctor may also order large doses of antibiotics to prevent sepsis.

Pathophysiology
In peptic ulcer, mucosal damage permits further erosion of abdominal wall layers, possibly causing perforation, bleeding, or both. Histamine release further stimulates acid secretion and increases capillary permeability to proteins, leading to mucosal edema. (See *How a peptic ulcer develops.*)

Continued erosion damages mucosal capillaries and submucosal blood vessels. Perforation occurs when erosion progresses through the serous membrane.

Complications
As GI contents spill into the abdominal cavity, chemical peritonitis occurs from contact with GI contents. Bacterial peritonitis follows within 12 hours and may lead to shock.

Assessment
History
A perforated peptic ulcer typically causes sudden onset of intense, constant, generalized abdominal pain. If the phrenic nerve in the diaphragm is irritated, pain may be referred to the shoulders. In severe cases, pain is accompanied by vomiting and collapse.

Check for a history of previous cyclic pain occurring on an empty stomach. The patient may report that deep breathing worsens the pain. Note a history of melena or hematemesis.

Physical examination
Observe the patient's position; usually, he's bent over or assumes a fetal position to prevent pulling on the abdominal wall. He's reluctant to move and holds his body tensely.

Expect a rigid abdomen, with rebound tenderness. Check for signs and symptoms of shock, including confusion, diaphoresis, rapid pulse, shallow respirations, and blood pressure changes. (See *Comparing peptic ulcers,* page 134.)

Diagnostic tests
An upright abdominal X-ray reveals free air under the diaphragm. As ordered, draw blood samples for type and crossmatching and for measurement of PT, PTT, CBC, electrolytes, BUN, AST, serum amylase, total bilirubin, and ABGs.

Ongoing treatment
Medical management of a patient with a perforated GI ulcer consists primarily of drug therapy, rest, dietary changes, and stress reduction. Intravenous histamine receptor antagonists will help decrease gastric acid production. Insert a large-bore NG tube, as ordered, to aid in lavage, suction, and drug administration.

PATHOPHYSIOLOGY

How a peptic ulcer develops

Peptic ulcers (gastric and duodenal ulcers) can be located in any part of the stomach exposed to pepsin, which is highly acidic. Normally, a mucosal barrier protects the GI lining from pepsin, hydrochloric acid (HCl), and other gastric juices secreted by the gastric gland. The mucus absorbs pepsin and protects underlying tissue from autodigestion by HCl.

Normal stomach and gastric gland

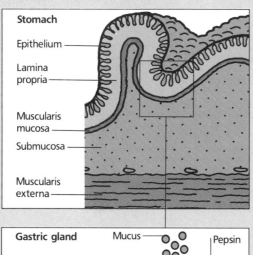

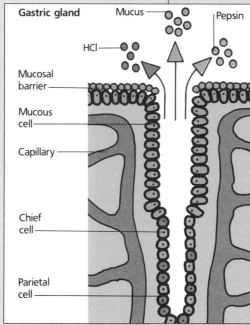

Damage to the mucosal barrier

Anything that alters or damages the barrier allows diffusion of HCl, which then damages underlying tissues and blood vessels.

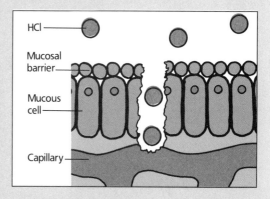

Inflammatory response

This damage triggers the inflammatory response, setting a destructive process in motion. Histamine is released, stimulating the GI tract to secrete more pepsin and HCl. Histamine also increases capillary permeability, so proteins and fluids leak out. As a result, the mucosa becomes edematous and mucosal capillaries start to bleed.

On endoscopic examination, benign ulcers look round or oval, with a punched-out area and a smooth base. Inflammation may be visible around an ulcerated area. Malignant ulcers may be larger, with an irregular, necrotic base.

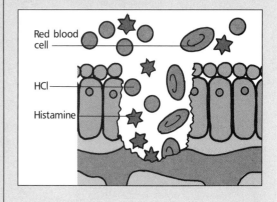

Comparing peptic ulcers

A peptic ulcer may be gastric or duodenal. Use this chart to help determine which type your patient has.

CHARACTERISTIC	GASTRIC ULCER	DUODENAL ULCER
Location	• Usually in antrum of stomach	• Usually in first ³⁄₈″ to ⁷⁄₈″ (1 to 2 cm) of duodenum
Incidence	• Typically occurs between ages 45 and 70 • Common in elderly women • Higher mortality than duodenal ulcer	• Typically occurs between ages 40 and 60 • Three times more common in men than women • Four times more common than gastric ulcer
Risk factors	• Stress, ulcerogenic drugs, alcohol abuse, smoking, gastritis	• Chronic obstructive pulmonary disease, cirrhosis, chronic pancreatitis, alcohol abuse, smoking, chronic renal failure, stress
Pain	• Occurs 1 to 2 hours after meals • Felt high in epigastrium • May be described as heartburn or indigestion • Sometimes relieved by food or liquids	• Occurs 2 to 4 hours after meals and at night • Felt in midepigastric region beneath xiphoid process • May be described as back pain, heartburn, or rhythmic pain • Relieved by food, milk, or antacids
Clinical course	• May cause weight loss • High recurrence rate • Fewer remissions than with duodenal ulcer • More likely to be malignant than duodenal ulcer • More likely to hemorrhage than duodenal ulcer	• May cause weight gain • Recurs seasonally (usually spring and fall) • Remissions and exacerbations may continue for up to 25 years after onset • Rarely malignant • More likely to cause perforation than gastric ulcer

Ongoing nursing interventions

Nursing care focuses on relief of symptoms by administering antacids every hour, providing emotional support, measuring and recording all urine output, testing all drainage for blood, and monitoring for complications.

• Postoperatively, monitor the patient's vital signs, watching for evidence of continuing peritonitis or abscess formation (such as fever, respiratory distress, and abdominal pain).

• Monitor for paralytic ileus, abdominal distention, hemorrhage, and other postoperative complications.

• Teach the patient about dietary changes, including the need to restrict or avoid intake of gastric mucosal irritants, such as alcohol and caffeine. If appropriate, arrange for a consultation with a dietitian.

• Teach the patient relaxation techniques. Increase his awareness of the causes of stress and anxiety, and urge him to eliminate or reduce these. Tell him to stop smoking if he smokes. Explain that stress and smoking stimulate gastric secretions that erode the mucosa.

• Urge him to comply with the prescribed medication regimen, designed to maintain gastric pH at a desirable level, and to avoid aspirin, corticosteroids, and anti-inflammatory drugs. These medications may inhibit mucus secretions and leave the GI tract vulnerable to injury from gastric acid.

GI hemorrhage

Hemorrhage can occur at any place along the GI tract. Acute bleeding occurs in most emergency cases of upper GI tract bleeding. To avoid hypovolemic shock from massive fluid loss, the patient needs immediate treatment. (See *When your patient has a GI hemorrhage.*)

Causes

Hemorrhage of the lower GI tract may result from such GI traumas as ulcerative colitis, diverticulosis, fistulas, cecal ulcers, tumors, angiodysplasia, and bowel infarction.

Upper GI tract hemorrhage may result from esophageal varices, peptic ulcer, and prolapsed gastric mucosa. A stress ulcer may cause massive GI bleeding several days after the initial injury. Typically arising in the esophagus, stomach, or duodenum, stress ulcers result from increased gastric acid secretion—usually in the

proximal portion of the stomach. They tend to be deep and of full thickness and thus are more likely to perforate. Stress ulcers may occur in patients with central nervous system trauma or in those who chronically ingest drugs toxic to the gastric mucosa. Such drugs fall into three categories:
• those that alter the mucosal barrier, such as NSAIDs and alcohol
• those that decrease gastric mucosal regeneration, such as corticosteroids and phenylbutazone
• those that stimulate acid secretion, such as caffeine, reserpine, and nicotine.

Pathophysiology
Because GI hemorrhage results from other disorders, its pathophysiology reflects the underlying cause (such as peptic ulcer).

Complications
GI hemorrhage may progress to hypovolemic shock and death.

Assessment
History
Tailor your assessment to the patient's condition, postponing a detailed history until he's been stabilized. Because of the patient's pain, anxiety, or confusion, he may be unable to provide you with accurate information.

If the patient reports nausea or vomiting, ask what seems to bring on or relieve the symptom. Find out if he has noticed blood in his vomitus.

Note any complaints of abdominal pain, tenderness, or pressure. With GI hemorrhage, pain may be severe. Ask if the pain is localized and if it radiates. Have the patient describe its quality, duration, and intensity. Which factors aggravate it? Which relieve it?

Find out when the patient had his last meal. Has he recently had changes in taste, swallowing problems, pain after eating, or weight loss? Has he noticed a recent change in bowel habits (such as frequency of bowel movements) or in the color or consistency of stools?

History findings may suggest the source of bleeding. Upper GI hemorrhage may cause

When your patient has a GI hemorrhage

Emergency care for the patient with a GI hemorrhage focuses on preventing or halting shock and determining the source of the bleeding.
• To improve tissue perfusion and oxygenation, insert a large-bore peripheral venous catheter to replace lost fluids and infuse blood products.
• Prepare the patient for GI endoscopy or a GI X-ray to determine the source of the bleeding.
• Monitor arterial blood gas values, perform gastric lavage to arrest active bleeding, and administer drugs to inhibit gastric secretions, as ordered.
• Hemorrhage may induce arrhythmias, so be sure to monitor the patient closely for bradycardia, heart block, ventricular tachycardia, and ventricular fibrillation.
• As ordered, insert an indwelling urinary catheter to accurately measure urine output, which reflects fluid volume.
• Once the patient is stabilized and the bleeding site identified, you may need to prepare the patient for surgery.
• Insert a rectal tube to relieve bleeding from the lower GI tract, if necessary.

bright red or coffee-ground vomitus. Depending on the underlying cause, the patient also may have intense pain. Check for a history of previous bleeding or predisposing conditions, such as peptic ulcers, tumors, and cirrhosis. Find out if the patient has had any surgery that might have contributed to GI hemorrhage.

With lower GI hemorrhage, the patient may report lower abdominal pain and cramps or cramping pain with bowel movements.

Physical examination
Physical findings vary with the underlying cause of hemorrhage and the amount of blood lost. (See *Four stages of hemorrhage,* page 136.)

Assess your patient for signs and symptoms of shock — weakness, pallor, tachycardia, hypotension, and increased respiratory rate. Obtain

Four stages of hemorrhage

STAGE	BODILY RESPONSE	EFFECT ON PATIENT
Stage I (up to 15% blood loss)	• Compensatory mechanisms (essentially sympathetic nervous system [SNS] responses, such as vasoconstriction) maintain homeostasis.	• Patient remains alert. • Blood pressure stays within normal limits. • Pulse rate stays within normal limits or increases slightly; pulse quality remains strong. • Respiratory rate and depth, skin color and temperature, and urine output all remain normal. • Capillary refill remains normal.
Stage II (up to 30% blood loss)	• Baroreceptors detect decreased venous return and cardiac output, triggering stronger sympathetic responses. • Vasoconstriction continues to maintain adequate blood pressure, but with some difficulty. • Blood flow shunts to vital organs, with decreased flow to intestines, kidneys, and skin.	• Patient may become confused and restless. • Skin turns pale, cool, and dry from shunting of blood to vital organs. Urine output decreases for the same reason. (Because other signs and symptoms are vague at this stage, decreased urine output may be the first sign of hypovolemia.) • Systolic pressure starts to fall. • Diastolic pressure may rise or fall. It's more likely to rise (from vasoconstriction) or stay the same in otherwise healthy patients with no underlying cardiovascular problems. • Pulse pressure (difference between systolic and diastolic pressures) narrows. • SNS responses also cause tachycardia. Pulse quality weakens. • Respiratory rate increases from SNS stimulation. • Capillary refill remains normal.
Stage III (up to 40% blood loss)	• Compensatory mechanisms become overtaxed. For example, vasoconstriction can no longer sustain diastolic pressure, which now begins to fall. • Cardiac output and tissue perfusion continue to decrease, becoming potentially life-threatening. (Even at this stage, however, the patient can still recover with prompt treatment.)	• Patient becomes more confused, restless, and anxious. • Classic signs of hypovolemic shock appear—tachycardia, decreased blood pressure, tachypnea, and cool, clammy extremities. • Capillary refill is delayed. • Urine output continues to decrease.
Stage IV (more than 40% blood loss)	• Compensatory vasoconstriction now becomes a complicating factor in itself, further impairing tissue perfusion and cellular oxygenation.	• Patient becomes lethargic, drowsy, or stuporous. • Signs of shock become more pronounced. Blood pressure continues to fall and pulse pressure narrows further (although if diastolic pressure "drops out," pulse pressure may widen). • Arterial blood gas analysis reveals metabolic acidosis and respiratory alkalosis. • Capillary refill is very delayed (longer than 3 seconds). • Patient may become severely anuric (output below 20 ml/hour). • Lack of blood flow to the brain and other vital organs ultimately leads to organ failure and death.

vital signs, noting fever, rapid pulse rate, hypotension, or increased respiratory rate.

Observe his body position, and determine if position changes or ambulation affects his symptoms. These may indicate the source of his pain. If he's vomiting, note the frequency of vomiting, and assess the vomitus for color, content, and odor. Inspect his abdomen. Do you notice any guarded areas, distention, or rebound?

Diagnostic tests

To determine the source of bleeding, the doctor will order GI X-rays with a radiopaque contrast medium. He also may perform GI endoscopy, such as gastroscopy, to directly visualize the gastric mucosa.

As ordered, obtain blood samples to assess hematocrit, hemoglobin level, BUN level, platelet count, mean corpuscular volume, PT, and PTT. Some of the values may be abnormal, reflecting the underlying disorder—or may result

A closer look at blood products, colloids, and crystalloids

SUBSTANCE	DESCRIPTION	NURSING CONSIDERATIONS
Whole blood	*Blood product:* Contains normal components of whole blood; one unit equals 500 ml.	• Administer over 2 to 4 hours. • Takes 12 to 24 hours for hemoglobin and hematocrit to equilibrate. • Watch for transfusion reaction and fluid overload.
Packed red blood cells (RBCs)	*Blood product:* Contains RBCs and 20% plasma (but no clotting factors and less sodium and potassium than whole blood); one unit equals 250 to 300 ml.	• Administer at a slower rate than whole blood. • Watch for transfusion reaction.
Fresh frozen plasma	*Blood product:* Contains liquid portion of whole blood separated from cells, then frozen; one unit equals 200 to 250 ml.	• Laboratory should allow 20 minutes to thaw. Use within 2 hours after thawing. • Administer one unit over 1 hour.
Plasmanate	*Blood product or colloid:* Contains 5% plasma protein fraction solution but no clotting factors; one unit may range from 50 to 500 ml.	• Infuse no faster than 10 ml/minute. (Hypotension may occur if infused too rapidly.) • Watch for hypersensitivity reaction and fluid overload. • Hyperventilation and headache may occur.
Serum albumin	*Blood product or colloid:* Contains albumin from plasma (main proteins found in blood); available in 5% and 25% solutions.	• Infuse slowly. Start infusion with 25 g and repeat after 15 to 30 minutes as needed (without exceeding 250 g in 48 hours). • Watch for fluid overload, hypersensitivity reaction, and bleeding.
Lactated Ringer's solution	*Crystalloid:* Contains sodium, chloride, potassium, calcium, and lactate, closely approximating normal electrolyte contents.	• Tailor dosage to patient's specific needs, depending on volume loss. • Can infuse rapidly (and while patient's blood is being typed and crossmatched). • Carries no risk of hypersensitivity reaction. • Watch for fluid overload.
Normal saline solution	*Crystalloid:* Contains 0.9% sodium chloride.	• Tailor dosage to patient's specific needs, depending on volume loss. • Can infuse rapidly (and while patient's blood is being typed and crossmatched). • Carries no risk of hypersensitivity reaction. • Watch for fluid overload. • Watch for electrolyte disturbances and potassium loss.

directly from the bleeding. Abnormal BUN values, for example, may indicate an increase in upper GI bleeding. And a decreased platelet count may contribute to GI bleeding.

Ongoing treatment
The source of the hemorrhage must be identified, and fluids and oxygen must be administered to maintain adequate perfusion and oxygenation. The doctor may order infusion of blood products to restore lost volume. (See *A closer look at blood products, colloids, and crystalloids.*)

The patient will need gastric lavage to arrest active bleeding and vasopressin to inhibit gastric secretion (as well as nitroglycerin or nitroprusside to counteract the adverse effects of vasopressin, if needed). Lavage may be ongoing until bleeding stops or slows. Once the patient has been stabilized and the bleeding site has been identified, he may undergo surgery to remove the cause of bleeding. A rectal tube may be inserted to relieve pressure and bleeding from the lower GI tract.

Ongoing nursing interventions

Continuing nursing interventions for the patient with a GI hemorrhage vary with the patient's needs and anticipated procedures.

• Obtain the patient's vital signs frequently.
• Continue to administer medications, as ordered.
• Monitor fluid status and record CVP (if available) and urine output hourly.
• Monitor serial laboratory values.
• If the patient will undergo surgery, administer antibiotics beforehand, as ordered, to suppress the growth of intestinal bacteria and reduce the risk of peritonitis. After surgery, monitor the patient for bleeding, hypovolemia, and other postoperative complications.
• If your patient doesn't require surgery, focus your care on permitting the bowel to rest and heal (if he had lower GI bleeding). Withhold all oral intake and keep the patient on complete bed rest to reduce intestinal motility.
• Provide measures to promote comfort and relieve pain.
• Help reduce the patient's anxiety by providing emotional support, supplying clear explanations of his condition, and informing him in advance about the procedures and treatments he'll receive.

Hepatic failure

An end-stage of liver disease, hepatic failure usually arises as a complication of conditions that cause liver dysfunction, although it can be idiopathic. It's sometimes called hepatic coma because the patient's neurologic status gradually deteriorates.

Hepatic failure may be acute and self-limiting or chronic and progressive. In advanced stages, the prognosis is poor despite vigorous treatment. A life-threatening crisis may occur if the serum ammonia level rises, causing cerebral ammonia intoxication. (See *When your patient has hepatic failure.*)

Causes

Hepatic failure typically results from cirrhosis, hepatitis, drug- or toxin-induced damage, fatty liver, portal hypertension, or surgically created portal-systemic shunts that bypass the liver and allow toxins into the blood. In patients with existing liver disease, excessive protein intake may cause cerebral ammonia intoxication by increasing the serum ammonia level.

Pathophysiology

Liver disease alters liver structure and compromises essential functions. This leads to impaired protein, fat, and carbohydrate metabolism; fluid and electrolyte imbalance; poor lymphatic drainage; reduced coagulation; and impaired detoxification of ammonia and other metabolites.

Ammonia accumulation and intoxication is the primary pathogenesis of hepatic failure and the ensuing encephalopathy. Ammonia accumulates because damaged liver cells can't detoxify and convert to urea the ammonia that is in constant supply in GI tract blood. Remaining liver functions become impaired and may be difficult to treat or control. Hepatic failure may progress insidiously to a comatose state from which patients rarely recover.

Complications

Hepatic encephalopathy, a neurologic syndrome, is a serious complication of hepatic failure and stems from an increased serum ammonia level leading to cerebral ammonia intoxication. Toxic to brain cells, ammonia inhibits neurotransmission and cerebral metabolism.

Assessment
History

If the patient has a neurologic impairment, he may be unable to provide a history or answer questions. Whenever possible, find a family member to provide or validate the history.

The patient may report fatigue and changes in mental status. Because hepatic failure is the terminal stage of liver disease, expect the history to reveal liver dysfunction. Also inquire about a history of viral hepatitis or biliary disease. Ask about exposure to hepatotoxic substances, and obtain a medication history.

Find out if the patient drinks alcohol; if so, determine the frequency and amount. Explore the family history for liver or biliary tract disease and for alcoholism. Obtain a dietary history and ask about recent appetite changes, indigestion, anorexia, and weight loss. Also inquire about recent changes in bowel habits, nausea, vomiting, or abdominal pain. If the patient has edema or ascites, find out when the problem first appeared.

If the patient is coherent at the time of admission, have him sign his name for a baseline handwriting sample. This will prove useful for later comparison because handwriting typically deteriorates as hepatic encephalopathy advances.

Physical examination
Note the patient's general appearance. Liver disease usually causes jaundice, which produces icteric skin, sclerae, and oral mucosa. Weakness and muscle atrophy may indicate malnutrition. Check for peripheral edema and ascites.

Obtain the patient's vital signs. Note rapid respirations, which may result from pulmonary compression caused by liver enlargement or ascites. Hypotension and tachycardia may reflect decreased circulating blood volume from fluid shifts related to ascites.

Auscultate for abnormal bowel sounds associated with diarrhea or constipation, which commonly accompany liver disease. Palpate for right upper quadrant tenderness, hepatomegaly, and splenomegaly. Test for a fluid wave, indicating ascites. Percuss the abdomen for shifting dullness, which also occurs in ascites.

To evaluate for hepatic encephalopathy, assess the patient's neurologic status. Hepatic encephalopathy has four stages characterized by a progressively deteriorating level of consciousness. (See *What to watch for in hepatic encephalopathy,* page 140.)

Diagnostic tests
Various test results help confirm liver dysfunction. With hepatocellular or biliary tissue necrosis, liver enzyme levels rise. Elevated alkaline phosphatase levels may indicate hepatobiliary

When your patient has hepatic failure

Immediate treatment for a patient with hepatic failure focuses on halting the progression of hepatic encephalopathy by reducing the serum ammonia level. As ordered, administer antibiotics such as neomycin to sterilize the lower GI tract. These drugs suppress the bacterial flora that break down amino acids and produce ammonia. The doctor also may order sorbitol to induce catharsis and produce osmotic diarrhea. Administer lactulose rectally or through a nasogastric tube to reduce the serum ammonia level. Continually aspirate blood from the stomach, since blood, a protein, may serve as a source of amino acids contributing to the high serum ammonia level.

Hemodialysis and exchange transfusions may be used as emergency treatments to reduce the serum ammonia level. However, hemodialysis only clears toxic blood temporarily. Exchange transfusions have drawbacks, too—they involve massive amounts of blood and produce only temporary improvement.

Monitor the patient's vital signs frequently (every 15 minutes to 1 hour), as indicated by his condition. Also monitor his electrocardiogram.

obstruction and inability to excrete bile. AST and ALT levels increase, with the degree of elevation varying with the underlying cause of liver dysfunction.

The serum glucose level may drop from malnutrition (common in alcohol-related liver disease). An increased serum ammonia level, indicating impaired hepatic synthesis of urea, is typical in advanced liver disease and hepatic failure.

A complete blood count may reveal decreases in RBC, hematocrit, and hemoglobin levels, reflecting the diseased liver's inability to store hematopoietic factors (iron, folic acid, and vitamin B_{12}). White blood cell and thrombocyte levels may drop if the patient has splenomegaly from cirrhosis.

What to watch for in hepatic encephalopathy

If your patient has hepatic failure, assess him for hepatic encephalopathy, which progresses in four stages with characteristic findings in each.

Stage 1
In this prodromal stage, expect slight personality and mood changes, disorientation, forgetfulness, slurred speech, slight tremor, periods of lethargy and euphoria, mild confusion, inability to concentrate, and hyperactive reflexes. Sleep-wake patterns typically reverse and mild asterixis (flapping tremor) may appear. Handwriting ability starts to decline.

Stage 2
The patient grows more disoriented and drowsy. He may display inappropriate behavior, mood swings, agitation, and apraxia. His handwriting becomes illegible, and asterixis may become pronounced. To elicit asterixis, ask him to extend his arms in front of him with hands flexed upward. Look for rapid irregular extensions and flexions of the wrists and fingers.

Stage 3
The patient becomes severely confused and may be combative, incoherent, and hard to arouse. He sleeps most of the time. You may detect hyperactive deep tendon reflexes and rigid extremities.

Stage 4
The patient is comatose and doesn't react to stimuli. His pupils are dilated, and he lacks corneal and deep tendon reflexes. His extremities are flaccid, and he may assume flexion or extension posturing. The EEG is markedly abnormal.

The doctor may order abdominal X-rays, a liver-spleen scan, a CT scan, or magnetic resonance imaging to identify cirrhosis or liver tumors. Superior mesenteric arteriography visualizes the hepatic vasculature to evaluate cirrhosis and portal hypertension. A liver biopsy may reveal tissue changes characteristic of cirrhosis or cancer. An EEG typically shows slow brain waves as hepatic encephalopathy worsens.

Ongoing treatment
Continuing medical treatment for the patient in hepatic failure involves further attempts to reduce his serum ammonia level. If he can tolerate oral intake, his dietary protein must be reduced and monitored. (Decreasing protein intake reduces amino acids, whose bacterial degradation in the gut is a primary source of ammonia.) If he can receive nothing by mouth, the doctor may order parenteral nutrition with controlled levels of amino acids.

Blood is a protein and may serve as a source of amino acids, contributing to a higher serum ammonia level. Therefore, any blood in the GI tract must be continually aspirated from the stomach. Lactulose is administered through an NG or rectal tube to help reduce the ammonia level and create a bacteria-free environment.

To maintain a stable blood pressure, the doctor will order fluid administration — usually D_5W. He'll avoid 0.9% sodium chloride solution if the patient has ascites. Depending on laboratory studies and the patient's condition, he may also order blood products. To monitor fluid volume and hemodynamic status, he may insert a CV catheter or PA catheter.

Before ordering analgesics and sedatives, the doctor will carefully consider use of these drugs because liver disease impairs metabolism. He'll avoid morphine because it's conjugated by the liver and may precipitate or worsen encephalopathy. Meperidine can be given because it's not metabolized by the liver.

Surgery
If the patient has ascites, a peritoneovenous shunt such as the LeVeen shunt may be used to drain ascitic fluid into the superior vena cava. Inserted with the patient under sedation and local anesthesia, the shunt consists of a peritoneal tube, venous tube, and one-way valve that controls fluid flow. The valve opens when intraperitoneal pressure exceeds superior

vena caval pressure by at least 3 cm H$_2$O. Preventing backflow of blood into the tubing, the valve eliminates the risk of clotting and shunt occlusion. To enhance fluid drainage, the patient may wear an abdominal binder and inhale against resistance via a blow bottle.

Ongoing nursing interventions

Nursing care focuses on preserving the patient's neurologic status, controlling the serum ammonia level, and maintaining stable vital signs.

• Monitor the patient's vital signs and neurologic status at least every hour. Assess his level of consciousness; orientation to person, place, and time; handwriting, if possible; and ability to follow simple and complex commands. Also check for asterixis. Notify the doctor of any neurologic deterioration.

• Monitor the electrocardiogram frequently, depending on the stage of encephalopathy and the patient's condition.

• To control the serum ammonia level, continue to administer antibiotics (such as neomycin) and cathartics (such as lactulose or sorbitol), as ordered. Restrict dietary protein. If GI bleeding is present, perform vigorous gastric lavage as ordered and suction to decrease intestinal proteins from the blood in the GI tract.

• Monitor the serum ammonia level and other ordered blood studies (such as electrolytes and CBC) at least every 8 hours. Report abnormalities to the doctor.

• Regularly record CVP or PAP, if available, to monitor the patient's fluid and hemodynamic status.

• Administer drugs to relieve pain and enhance rest as ordered.

• You may need to apply restraints — especially during stage 3 of hepatic encephalopathy, when the patient may become combative.

• Promote rest, comfort, and quiet. Provide emotional support to the patient and family, especially during the terminal stage of hepatic failure.

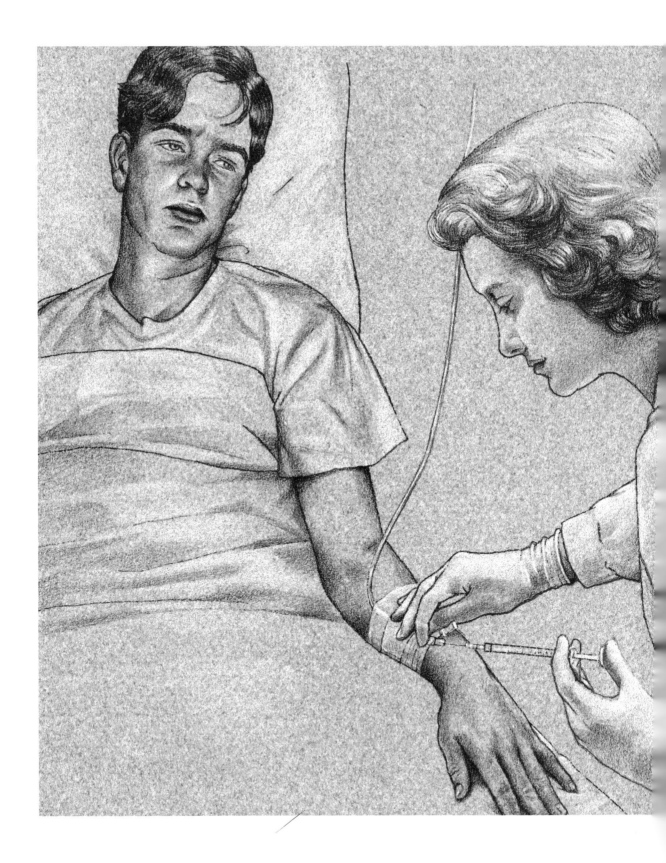

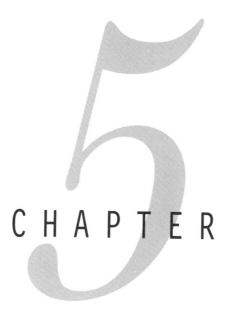

CHAPTER 5

Metabolic and endocrine crises

Metabolic and endocrine crises can be difficult to identify. After all, some are relatively uncommon, and most health care professionals have had little experience dealing with them. Others, particularly diabetic ketoacidosis (DKA) and hyperosmolar nonketotic syndrome (HNKS), are fairly common but resemble each other so closely that telling them apart during an emergency is extremely difficult.

To add to the confusion, many patients with a metabolic or endocrine crisis exhibit a decreased level of consciousness or bizarre behavioral disturbances. And, if excessive alcohol intake is an underlying problem, signs of intoxication may further cloud the clinical picture or lead to misdiagnosis.

But these potential problems don't alter the importance of promptly recognizing the signs of an endocrine or metabolic crisis — or for intervening appropriately. This chapter will help you meet the challenge. It presents the pertinent information you need to care for the patient with DKA, HNKS, thyroid storm, syndrome of inappropriate antidiuretic hormone (SIADH), adrenal crisis, metabolic acidosis, or metabolic alkalosis.

Diabetic ketoacidosis

Also called diabetic coma, DKA is an acute complication of diabetes mellitus marked by pronounced hyperglycemia and ketonemia. Reflecting an insulin deficiency, it usually occurs in patients with Type I (insulin-dependent) diabetes mellitus. For instance, it may arise if the patient has an illness that increases his insulin needs or if he omits or reduces his regular insulin dose. In some patients, DKA is the first manifestation of Type I diabetes.

DKA carries a mortality of 5% to 10%. Any delay in recognizing and treating the patient may jeopardize his life. (See *When your patient has DKA*.)

Causes
DKA results from an absolute lack or a relative deficiency of effective insulin. Causes of absolute insulin deficiency include undiagnosed Type I diabetes and, in a patient with Type I diabetes, failure to take prescribed insulin.

Common causes of relative insulin deficiency include surgery, stress resulting from infection, urosepsis, upper respiratory infection, pneumonia, trauma, myocardial infarction (MI), perirectal abscess, and periodontal abscess. Less commonly, relative insulin deficiency stems from Cushing's syndrome, thyrotoxicosis, acromegaly, or pheochromocytoma.

Pathophysiology
In DKA, the body has inadequate insulin and excessive counterregulatory hormones. These hormones — epinephrine, cortisol, glucagon, growth hormones, and thyroid hormones — are secreted in response to physical or emotional stress and counter the effects of insulin.

Insulin is responsible for normal protein, fat, and carbohydrate metabolism and inhibits glu-

cose production by the liver. When insulin levels are low, hepatic glucose production goes unchecked, causing hyperglycemia and glycosuria. Hyperglycemia, in turn, pulls water out of the intracellular spaces and into extracellular circulation. As water moves from the intracellular to the extracellular spaces, osmotic diuresis occurs. This leads to loss of water and electrolytes, promoting dehydration and intravascular volume depletion.

Insulin normally controls the release of free fatty acids (FFAs) from fat cells. Without adequate insulin, fat catabolism begins to compensate for deficient carbohydrate fuels. However, fat catabolism is incomplete; FFAs are released and carried to the liver. The liver then begins to break down stored glycogen to glucose (glycogenolysis) and to synthesize new glucose from amino and lactic acids, and fats (gluconeogenesis). Both processes worsen hyperglycemia.

In response to hyperglycemia and excessive counterregulatory hormones, the liver releases additional fuels and also uses FFAs as fuel. This release results in excessive ketone bodies — a condition called ketonemia. Although some tissues can use ketone bodies for fuel, most of these ketone bodies cannot be metabolized. Metabolic acidosis rapidly sets in, and ketone bodies are excreted into the urine (ketonuria) as the kidneys try to compensate for acidosis.

Lack of insulin also affects protein metabolism. Transport of amino acids into body cells decreases, and protein catabolism occurs. Muscle tissues then release amino acids for use as fuel, and the liver metabolizes them. Muscle tissue loses nitrogen in this reaction, causing loss of lean body mass and elevations in blood urea nitrogen (BUN) and serum creatinine levels. (See *How insulin deficiency affects protein, carbohydrate, and fat metabolism*, page 146.)

Complications
DKA leads to severe dehydration (volume depletion), hyperosmolality, metabolic acidosis, and electrolyte disturbances (such as potassium deficiency). Life-threatening arrhythmias may develop from potassium depletion. Lactic aci-

EMERGENCY INTERVENTIONS

When your patient has DKA

The patient with diabetic ketoacidosis (DKA) has a life-threatening volume depletion — a fluid volume deficit of up to 10 liters — so be prepared to replace fluids and electrolytes rapidly. You'll also need to administer insulin.

Fluid resuscitation
Initial volume expansion lowers the serum glucose level on its own, even without insulin administration. Reestablishing intravascular volume also decreases the production of the counterregulatory hormones that contribute to the rise in the serum glucose level.

Usually, you'll give 0.9% sodium chloride solution or 0.45% sodium chloride solution at 1 liter/hour until the patient's blood pressure stabilizes and his urine output measures 60 ml/hour. Typically, this takes 1 to 2 hours.

Electrolyte replacement
In DKA, osmotic diuresis causes total body potassium depletion; as dehydration resolves, potassium returns to the intracellular spaces. Insulin administration also reduces the serum potassium level by stimulating potassium uptake by adipose, muscle, and liver tissue. Therefore, potassium replacements must be administered simultaneously with fluid resuscitation, except in patients with anuria or life-threatening hyperkalemia.

The goal of potassium replacement is to maintain a normal serum potassium level, as monitored by laboratory studies and the T waves in electrocardiography.

Note: Bicarbonate administration is reserved for patients with severe acidosis (a pH below 7.1).

Insulin administration
Expect the doctor to order administration of I.V. regular insulin to reverse the two major metabolic problems in DKA — hyperglycemia and acidosis. The goal of I.V. insulin infusion is to halt hyperglycemia and acidosis without causing hypoglycemia. (Although insulin also can be administered I.M. or S.C., its absorption via these routes may be erratic.)

Typically, the doctor orders a continuous insulin infusion — usually 100 units of regular insulin in 500 ml of 0.9% sodium chloride solution, in a concentration of 0.2 units/ml. Before initiating the infusion, allow 50 to 100 ml of the mixture to run through the tubing, and then discard this amount. This allows the tubing to absorb the insulin, limiting absorption during infusion.

Use an infusion pump and administer insulin at an initial rate of 0.1 unit/kg/hour. Keep in mind that the goal is to lower the serum glucose level by 80 to 100 mg/dl/hour. (When administered I.V., insulin quickly reaches a steady state in the bloodstream, eliminating the need for an initial bolus dose.)

Adjust the infusion rate according to your patient's hourly blood glucose levels, as determined by the laboratory or a portable blood glucose meter. However, if you're using a portable meter, check the manufacturer's guidelines to verify whether it can be used in patients with severe volume depletion, dehydration, hypovolemic shock, and extremes in hematocrit.

Additional measures
During initial treatment, closely monitor your patient's level of consciousness, vital signs, and hourly blood glucose levels. Also monitor I.V. fluid administration to maintain the prescribed flow rate and to correct dehydration.

---

dosis may occur if the patient has severe metabolic acidosis without severe ketonemia or renal failure. Volume depletion may cause vascular thrombosis.

Other complications may arise from treatment of DKA. For example, reducing the patient's blood glucose level too rapidly or too much may cause hypoglycemia. A rapid blood glucose drop brought on by insulin and fluid administration may cause fluid shifts within the brain, triggering cerebral edema.

How insulin deficiency affects protein, carbohydrate, and fat metabolism

Insulin is required to maintain normal metabolism of proteins, carbohydrates, and fats. Without effective insulin, catabolism occurs, eventually leading to hypovolemia and electrolyte disturbances. A lack of effective insulin can trigger the reactions in the chart below.

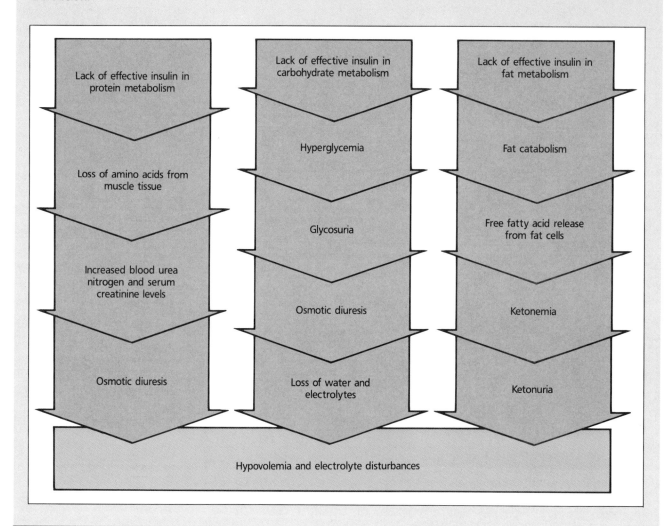

Assessment

History

Because the patient's mental status may be impaired, you may need to obtain the history from a family member or the person who accompanied the patient to the hospital. To help determine the cause of his condition, ask how he was found and in what circumstances. Find out whether he has had similar symptoms before and, if so, what the outcome was. To help establish the severity of dehydration, ask about recent food or fluid intake.

Expect a history of increased fatigue, lethargy, dry mouth, and increased thirst and urination over the last few hours or days. The patient also may have had flulike symptoms,

ASSESSMENT INSIGHT

Distinguishing DKA from insulin shock

In a diabetic patient, a coma may result from excessive blood glucose (diabetic ketoacidosis [DKA]) or from too much insulin (insulin shock). Use this chart to help determine if your patient has DKA or insulin shock.

CHARACTERISTIC	D.K.A.	INSULIN SHOCK
Onset	Gradual (over several days)	Sudden (within 24 to 48 hours)
Insulin	Insufficient insulin	Excessive insulin
Recent food intake	Normal or excessive	Usually insufficient
General appearance	Extremely ill	Very weak
Skin	Flushed, dry	Pale, moist
Respirations	Increased, air hunger (Kussmaul's)	Normal
Blood pressure	Abnormally low	Normal
Pulse	Weak, rapid	Full, bounding
Fever	Usually present	Absent
Breath odor	Acetone	Normal
Mouth	Dry	Drooling
Thirst	Intense	Absent
Hunger	Absent	Occasionally present
Vomiting	Common	Absent
Abdominal pain	Usually present	Rare
Infection	Usually present	Absent
Vision	Dim	Diplopia
Tremor	Absent	Usually present
Seizures	Absent	Present in late stages
Urine glucose level	Above normal	Absent in a second specimen
Ketone bodies	Above normal	Absent in a second specimen
Blood glucose level	Above normal	Below 60 mg/dl

such as abdominal discomfort, nausea or vomiting, and generalized myalgia. As his condition worsened, he may have exhibited deep, rapid, sighing respirations (Kussmaul's respirations).

Find out if the patient had a recent illness or infection, such as a cold, upper respiratory infection, urinary tract infection, sore throat, or GI disturbance. If he previously was diagnosed with diabetes, ask about his current insulin dosage and administration schedule and find out if he recently made changes in either of these. (See *Distinguishing DKA from insulin shock.*)

Comparing types of insulin preparations

TYPE	PREPARATION	ONSET	PEAK	DURATION	COMMENTS
Rapid acting	• Regular insulin • Prompt insulin zinc suspension (Semi-lente)	½ to 1 hour	1 to 3 hours	4 to 8 hours	Human insulins may peak earlier and may not last the full duration.
Intermediate acting	• Isophane insulin suspension (NPH) • Insulin zinc suspension (Lente)	1 to 2 hours	4 to 12 hours	18 to 24 hours	Ranges for onset, peak, and duration reflect the differences between animal and human source insulins.
Long acting	• Extended insulin zinc suspension (Ultralente)	3 to 6 hours	6 to 16 hours	16 to 28 hours	Do not use Ultralente for emergencies requiring rapid drug action.

Physical examination

The patient with DKA will seem acutely ill and severely dehydrated. Perform a complete neurologic assessment, evaluate reflexes, and check for muscle weakness, fatigue, and headache. Expect an altered level of consciousness (LOC), ranging from confusion to coma.

Assess for signs of dehydration, including dry mucous membranes; warm, dry, flushed skin; and poor skin turgor. Measure the patient's blood pressure, and suspect intravascular volume depletion if his systolic pressure drops 20 mm Hg or more when he moves from a supine to a sitting or standing position. Also assess neck vein filling, which will probably be reduced from dehydration.

Check for classic signs of DKA—acetone (fruity) breath odor and Kussmaul's respirations. These signs help rule out insulin shock.

Assess the patient's abdomen, listening closely for diminished or absent bowel sounds. Note abdominal tenderness, guarding, or rebound tenderness on palpation. These signs and symptoms probably stem from ketosis and usually resolve as the patient's biochemical status improves.

Diagnostic tests

In DKA, the serum glucose level is elevated to 250 mg/dl or more, reflecting marked hyperglycemia. Arterial blood gas (ABG) measurements show a below-normal pH (usually less than 7.3) and a serum carbon dioxide (CO_2) level of less than 18 mm Hg, indicating metabolic acidosis.

To measure serum levels of ketone bodies, serum is diluted with tap water using various dilutions. A significant number of ketone bodies in a 1:2 dilution indicates ketonemia. A urine dipstick test will show +4 glycosuria and moderate to extensive ketonuria.

Initial serum electrolyte levels may depend on the severity of dehydration. An elevated blood glucose level may cause dilutional hyponatremia. In such a case, the serum sodium level may be normal or below normal.

Total body potassium levels may decrease, yet the patient may have a high, low, or normal serum potassium value. A low value represents a total body potassium deficit and requires aggressive therapy. (Acidosis causes potassium to shift from cells to the extracellular spaces.)

The serum phosphate level may be normal on admission but later may drop as phosphate moves from cells into the extracellular space. Total body phosphate decreases as a result of osmotic diuresis.

BUN levels rise secondarily to volume depletion. The serum creatinine level may be falsely elevated because of production of acetone (a ketone body). Leukocytosis may reflect severe dehydration, although the health care team should evaluate the patient for a possible underlying infection.

Ongoing treatment

I.V. fluid replacement, started during emergency treatment, continues with 0.45% sodium chloride solution. When the blood glucose level falls to approximately 250 mg/dl, dextrose is added to the solution to allow for continuous insulin administration. Insulin is needed to correct acidosis, as it allows for the return of electrolytes to the intracellular spaces.

If the patient's temperature is above 100.5° F (38.1° C), draw a blood sample for culture to determine if he has an underlying infection. If the culture results are positive, the doctor will initiate appropriate antibiotic therapy.

Surgery

Surgery may be warranted if certain pathologic conditions contributed to DKA. For instance, an infected gallbladder or acute appendicitis may cause additional stress on the body, warranting surgery to prevent future episodes of DKA. During surgery, the patient requires close monitoring as well as I.V. administration of fluids and insulin.

Ongoing nursing interventions

Ongoing care focuses on careful monitoring and patient teaching to prevent DKA from recurring.

• Continually assess the patient's neurologic status. If his LOC remains decreased 8 to 10 hours after treatment begins, suspect increased intracranial pressure (ICP) from fluid shifts within the brain. As ordered, administer high doses of dexamethasone to help reduce ICP.

• Begin to reestablish the patient's preillness subcutaneous insulin regimen once he can tolerate oral food intake. (See *Comparing types of insulin preparations.*) As ordered, discontinue the insulin infusion 30 minutes after administering the first dose of subcutaneous insulin.

Diabetes sick-day guidelines

If your patient has diabetes, stress the importance of adhering to sick-day guidelines to prevent diabetic ketoacidosis and other crises. Instruct the patient to follow these directions.

• *Never* omit your insulin. Call your health care professional during illness because he may need to adjust the dosage. For instance, he may instruct you to take extra insulin to counter the stress of illness and the effects of the counterregulatory hormones that increase your blood glucose level.

• Test your blood glucose level at least four times a day because it may rise rapidly during illness.

• Drink plenty of fluids to prevent severe dehydration. You may want to take frequent, small sips.

• Do a urine dipstick test for ketone bodies, and notify your health care professional if the results are moderate or high.

• Contact your health care professional if your illness interferes with your food intake or if you have a fever above 101° F (38.3° C). You should also seek medical advice if you suffer persistent vomiting or diarrhea (longer than 24 hours) or if your illness lasts more than 24 hours.

• Have a family member or another person check on you frequently when you're ill because coma may develop rapidly.

• Gradually progress the patient's diet from clear liquids to the diet the patient was following prior to hospitalization, unless his diet exacerbated or provoked his condition.

• Teach the patient and family about his condition, including how to avoid future episodes of DKA. Make sure he knows how to manage diabetes during illness. (See *Diabetes sick-day guidelines.*)

• Assess the patient's ability to perform self-care activities, and give him instructions in diabetes self-care skills, such as administering insulin, monitoring blood glucose levels, planning meals, testing for urine ketone bodies, and recognizing, treating, and preventing hypoglycemia and hyperglycemia.

• Arrange for follow-up teaching and care at an outpatient diabetes clinic or with a home health nurse.

Hyperosmolar nonketotic syndrome

HNKS is a severe hyperglycemic state characterized by profound intravascular volume depletion, marked dehydration (serum osmolality above 350 mOsm), and central nervous system (CNS) depression. This syndrome may involve coma, prerenal azotemia, and electrolyte depletion. The patient's blood glucose level typically rises above 800 mg/dl. HNKS is potentially fatal, and you must act fast to save the patient's life. (See *When your patient has HNKS.*)

HNKS is most common in older adults with mild or undiagnosed Type II (non-insulin-dependent) diabetes mellitus. (See *A classic case of HNKS,* page 152.) It also may occur in patients who have a decreased thirst perception or who lack access to sufficient water.

Causes
HNKS may occur when insulin tolerance is stressed — for example, in infection, congestive heart failure, MI, cerebrovascular accident (CVA), burns, pancreatitis, pancreatic cancer, thyrotoxicosis, subdural hematoma, Cushing's syndrome, or uremia.

Other causes include use of certain medications (including thiazide diuretics, diazoxide, diphenylhydantoin, furosemide, propranolol, and glucocorticoids), medical procedures (such as peritoneal dialysis, total parenteral nutrition, and parenteral and enteral feedings), and insufficient insulin or oral antidiabetic administration.

Older persons with a coexisting condition like diabetes mellitus are predisposed to HNKS because that condition increases their risk of infection, such as a pulmonary infection, a GI virus, diabetic autonomic neuropathy (such as neurogenic bladder), or foot infections caused by peripheral vascular disease.

Pathophysiology
Hyperglycemia and hyperosmolality are the cardinal events in HNKS. Hyperglycemia normally causes osmotic diuresis, leading to water and electrolyte loss. In response to hyperglycemia and such stressors as infection and dehydration, hepatic glucose production increases. Physiologic stressors also promote production of counterregulatory hormones, which contribute to the increased blood glucose level and heightened hepatic glucose production.

When the blood glucose level exceeds the renal threshold, glycosuria results, causing osmotic diuresis, dehydration, and loss of water and electrolytes. These conditions trigger additional hepatic glucose production, resulting in severe hyperglycemia.

Unlike DKA, HNKS doesn't involve ketoacidosis — probably because enough insulin is present to prevent lipolysis, thus averting ketone body formation and subsequent metabolic acidosis. This syndrome occurs in patients with non-insulin-dependent diabetes mellitus; they are not insulin-deficient, but lack sufficient or effective insulin.

Complications
HNKS once carried a mortality of 50% to 70%, mostly from congestive heart failure induced by too-rapid fluid replacement. Better monitoring during treatment has reduced the mortality to 15% to 20%. Typically, death results from a thromboembolytic episode, such as MI or CVA, rather than from an acute metabolic disturbance. Cerebral edema is a rare complication, but it can lead to death.

Assessment
History
Typically, an altered LOC, reported by a friend or family member, is the patient's chief symptom. Ask this person if the patient recently exhibited other changes in mental status or behavior.

Unlike DKA, HNKS rarely causes GI symptoms, such as abdominal discomfort, nausea, and vomiting. (See *Comparing signs and symptoms of DKA, HNKS, and hypoglycemia,* page 153.) If the patient does report these symptoms, suspect that HNKS was induced by an intra-abdominal event, such as a bowel obstruction or infarction, a gangrenous or infected gallbladder, a ruptured appendix, or peritonitis.

Try to determine if the patient has an underlying disease or had a recent illness or infection. If he did, ask if he changed his usual diabetes regimen during the episode. For instance, did he omit his insulin or oral antidiabetic dose or reduce the dosage?

Keep in mind that some older patients minimize their health problems, failing to seek care for seemingly minor complaints. So make sure you're specific when eliciting information about recent illnesses. For instance, ask if the patient has had a fever, a sore throat, a productive cough, burning or pain on urination, a draining or weeping wound, or a wound that took a long time to heal.

Obtain a list of the patient's current medications. This may pose a challenge, especially with an older patient who has received multiple medications from several doctors. However, a duplicate prescription for the same medication may cause HNKS, so you must explore this possibility.

Physical examination

Measure the patient's vital signs. In HNKS, body temperature usually is normal or slightly elevated, with no axillary sweating. Suspect sepsis if an older patient has a subnormal temperature or hypothermia. With concomitant cardiopulmonary disease, you may detect tachycardia when measuring the pulse. Blood pressure may be low; old age, deep coma, hypothermia, and hypotension are all poor prognostic indicators. If you suspect a pulmonary infection, auscultate the patient's lungs.

HNKS typically causes impaired consciousness. If your older patient has an altered LOC, expect to find dry oral mucous membranes,

When your patient has HNKS

For the patient with hyperosmolar nonketotic syndrome (HNKS), emergency care focuses on rapid, aggressive rehydration. This measure will start to lower his blood glucose level—even without the addition of insulin. The average fluid deficit in HNKS is 9 liters. The patient needs rapid rehydration because slow rehydration won't correct the underlying condition.

Rehydrating the patient

• As ordered, infuse 1 to 2 liters of 0.9% or 0.45% sodium chloride solution over 2 hours, followed by an additional 2 liters over the next 3 hours. However, if your patient has anuric renal failure, fluid replacement must be less aggressive and insulin will serve as the primary treatment.
• The typical patient is usually older and has underlying cardiac problems. Infusing too much fluid at once can cause fluid overload and cardiac failure. To prevent congestive heart failure from rapid rehydration, the doctor may insert a pulmonary artery catheter to monitor pulmonary artery pressure.

Monitoring urine output and blood glucose

• Monitor your patient's urine output closely. Typically, only the patient who is obtunded or stuporous needs urinary catheterization. Once urine output has been restored, he must receive electrolyte replacements, especially potassium. Expect to administer potassium at a rate of 20 mEq/hour. During the infusion, monitor his serum potassium level and observe his electrocardiogram, checking T waves in leads V_4 and V_6. These two leads show T-wave alterations that may reflect hypokalemia.
• As ordered, start an insulin infusion with regular insulin at a rate of 0.1 unit/kg/hour, piggybacking it into the infusion line used for fluids. Obtain hourly blood glucose measurements, and titrate the insulin infusion according to the established protocol.
• If the patient has gastric distention or absent bowel sounds, the doctor may insert a nasogastric tube to aid in gastric decompression and prevent accidental aspiration if vomiting occurs.

A classic case of HNKS

The patient with hyperosmolar nonketotic syndrome (HNKS) commonly fits a classic profile: He is older, has diabetes mellitus, and presents with an altered level of consciousness and signs of a fluid volume deficit.

Arthur Webb, age 72, fit this profile closely. On admission to the hospital, he was in a stupor and appeared dehydrated. Your review of his record showed that he had Type II diabetes mellitus, controlled by diet only, and a history of congestive heart failure (CHF) and hypertension.

Rapid diagnosis

When you assessed Mr. Webb, you found dry mucous membranes, poor skin turgor, and sunken eyes. The laboratory reported his blood glucose level at 1,878 mg/dl and serum osmolality at 370 mOsm. A urine dipstick test showed +4 glycosuria and negative ketone bodies. Based on Mr. Webb's history and clinical and laboratory findings, the doctor diagnosed HNKS.

Alice Webb, who accompanied her husband to the hospital, told you that he had started complaining of weakness several weeks ago and that this symptom had worsened gradually. He had been taking frequent naps and hadn't had the energy to walk the dog—something he normally did twice a day. She stated that 3 weeks ago, the family doctor increased his daily furosemide dosage from 80 to 160 mg to treat "some congestion in the heart." Since that time, diuresis had increased, and you now suspect that this diuresis precipitated HNKS.

Immediate treatment

To treat stupor and hyperglycemia, you infuse 0.45% sodium chloride solution, as ordered. Because Mr. Webb has a history of CHF, he needs a pulmonary artery (PA) catheter to monitor his PA pressure. You assist with insertion.

After 2 hours of receiving I.V. fluids only, Mr. Webb's blood glucose level falls to 1,200 mg/dl. You begin a continuous insulin infusion, as ordered, titrating it according to standing protocol. You insert an indwelling urinary catheter and send a urine specimen for culture, which later comes back negative. You also arrange for hourly blood glucose measurements.

You obtain PA pressure readings, document Mr. Webb's intake and output, measure his vital signs, and perform neurologic checks every hour. You obtain venous and arterial samples to monitor electrolyte levels and to determine complete blood count and arterial blood gas values. You also monitor Mr. Webb's electrocardiogram closely to watch for cardiac complications.

Preventive measures

After Mr. Webb is stabilized, the doctor tells him that he will need further treatment for his diabetes to help prevent future episodes of HNKS and other complications. He prescribes glyburide, 2.5 mg daily, and places him on a 1,800 calorie/day diet that conforms to American Diabetes Association guidelines.

Before discharge, you begin diabetes teaching. Mr. Webb agrees to attend outpatient diabetes education classes at a local clinic. He recuperates without complications and is discharged 6 days later.

sunken eyes, poor skin turgor, and low blood pressure. You may detect focal neurologic signs, including seizures, transient hemiparesis, extensor plantar reflexes, aphasia, and muscle fasciculations.

Perform a head-to-toe physical examination. Look for large or infected decubitus ulcers, peripheral vascular or arterial ulcers, and any other skin lesions. Be sure to remove the patient's shoes and socks and examine his feet for signs of infection. Remember that an older patient with long-standing diabetes may have peripheral sensory neuropathy as well as poor eyesight, so he may not realize he has a foot problem or infection.

Comparing signs and symptoms of DKA, HNKS, and hypoglycemia

Patients with diabetic ketoacidosis (DKA), hyperosmolar nonketotic syndrome (HNKS), or hypoglycemia typically have a history of diabetes. However, their symptoms are sometimes sufficiently similar that differentiating among these complications can be difficult. This chart can help you identify the distinctive features.

FINDINGS	D.K.A.	H.N.K.S.	HYPOGLYCEMIA
Onset	• Over several hours to days	• Over several days	• Over several minutes
Skin	• Warm, dry, flushed skin	• Warm, dry, flushed skin	• Cool, clammy skin • Sweating
Urologic and renal	• Polyuria	• Polyuria	−
Metabolic	• Polydipsia • Acetone (fruity) breath odor	• Polydipsia • No acetone breath odor	• Hunger
Musculoskeletal	• Myalgia	• Myalgia	−
GI	• Flulike symptoms • Abdominal pain • Nausea, vomiting	• Flulike symptoms • Lower incidence of abdominal discomfort, nausea, and vomiting than in DKA	−
Respiratory	• Kussmaul's respirations	−	−
Cardiac	• Orthostatic hypotension	−	• Tachycardia • Palpitations
Neurologic	• Lethargy • Hyporeflexia • Hypotonia • Stupor • Coma	• Lethargy • Hyporeflexia • Hypotonia • Stupor • Coma • Wider variety of mental status changes than in DKA (hallucinations, seizures, aphasia)	• Nervousness, agitation • Headache • Confusion • Visual disturbances (such as blurred vision) • Paresthesia • Mental dullness • Seizures • Coma

Diagnostic tests

Laboratory values that suggest HNKS include a markedly elevated blood glucose level (above 800 mg/dl, perhaps reaching 2,000 mg/dl), an elevated BUN level, an above-normal serum sodium level, and a normal to slightly elevated serum potassium level (despite total body potassium loss). The serum potassium level will be elevated as the potassium moves out of the cells and into the extracellular space, thereby depleting intracellular or total body potassium. When the cells lack potassium, severe arrhythmias can result. Expect increased serum osmolality — usually above 350 mOsm. Urine ketone bodies are absent, and arterial pH and CO_2 may be normal.

Serum calcium, magnesium, and phosphate levels usually are below normal in HNKS. Creatine kinase (CK) levels may be elevated from rhabdomyolysis (muscle disintegration brought on by hyperosmolarity).

A complete blood count (CBC) typically shows above-normal values for white blood cells (WBCs), hemoglobin, and hematocrit, reflecting dehydration.

Ongoing treatment

Once the patient is somewhat stabilized, the doctor will continue some of the treatments initiated during the emergency phase. Surgery may be a possibility for some patients.

The fluid and electrolyte replacement started during initial treatment continues. If the patient is alert and can tolerate oral intake, he may receive oral fluids as well as I.V. fluids. When his blood glucose level drops to about 250 mg/dl, the doctor will discontinue the insulin infusion initiated during emergency treatment. (The patient with HNKS doesn't require long-term insulin unless he has metabolic acidosis that requires insulin for correction.)

The doctor then reestablishes the patient's routine prior to hospitalization, including his usual diabetic diet and oral antidiabetic therapy, if appropriate. If HNKS was the presenting event in diabetes, a diabetic diet may serve as the sole therapy, monitored by close follow-up.

The patient also must receive ongoing treatment for any diagnosed infection as well as stabilizing measures, such as heparin or another anticoagulant therapy, to treat any vascular events.

Surgery

Surgery may be indicated if HNKS was caused by a surgically correctable abdominal problem, such as a bowel obstruction or bowel infarction, a gangrenous or infected gallbladder, a ruptured appendix, or peritonitis.

Ongoing nursing interventions

• Continue to monitor the patient's neurologic status, intake and output, and cardiac and renal status.
• Take appropriate measures to treat any diagnosed infection or other underlying condition.
• Begin discharge planning as soon as the patient receives initial rehydration and his blood glucose and electrolyte levels have stabilized.

With the patient and family, review the events that led to hospitalization. Teach them how to recognize signs and symptoms of hyperglycemia. Review diabetes sick-day guidelines. Teach the patient how to monitor his blood glucose levels at home, and make sure he understands his prescribed dietary and medication regimens.
• If the patient has newly diagnosed diabetes, teach him beginning management skills. These include planning meals, recognizing signs and symptoms of hyperglycemia, follow-up laboratory measurement of blood glucose values, and preventing or delaying long-term complications of diabetes (for example, eye, kidney, and vascular problems) by controlling his metabolism. Provide emotional support, and allow time for him to ask questions. Be aware that he initially may deny he has diabetes.

Thyroid storm

Thyroid storm (thyrotoxic crisis) is an acute form of severe hyperthyroidism marked by sudden and excessive release of thyroid hormones into the bloodstream. It's the most serious complication of thyroid hyperfunction.

Without immediate intervention, the patient may suffer delirium, coma, or death. Mortality from thyroid storm is roughly 20%, so make sure you know what steps to take to avert grave consequences. (See *When your patient has thyroid storm.*)

Causes

Thyroid storm typically is triggered by stressful conditions, such as trauma, surgery, infection, or emotional distress. Other precipitating factors include MI, pulmonary embolism, abrupt withdrawal of antithyroid agents, initiation of therapy with radioiodine (^{131}I) or iodine-containing agents, preeclampsia, thyroid tumor, and subtotal thyroidectomy with excessive intake of synthetic thyroid hormone.

Pathophysiology

Normally, the hypothalamus triggers the thyroid gland to release thyrotropin-releasing hor-

EMERGENCY INTERVENTIONS

When your patient has thyroid storm

For the patient with thyroid storm, immediate interventions aim to maintain the airway and tissue oxygenation, reverse hypovolemia, prevent further hypermetabolic decompensation, and decrease thyroid hyperfunction.

Maintaining the airway and oxygenation
Provide adequate ventilation to meet the patient's high metabolic demands. Administer oxygen via nasal cannula or mask, assess the patient's respiratory rate every 1 to 2 hours, and auscultate the lungs every 1 to 2 hours. Note tachypnea, dyspnea, pallor, or cyanosis. Provide chest physiotherapy and suctioning as needed.

Ensure that the patient is in a position that facilitates respiration, and turn him occasionally from side to side. If problems arise in maintaining adequate oxygenation, mechanical ventilation may be indicated.

Check his oxygenation status periodically by monitoring pulse oximetry or arterial blood gas values. (To prevent hypoventilation, the doctor will avoid sedatives or use them cautiously.)

Reversing hypovolemia
As ordered, give I.V. fluid replacement containing dextrose to reverse hypovolemia and prevent further glycogen depletion.

Reducing hypermetabolic decompensation
To lower the patient's body temperature, keep him cool with ice, fans, hypothermia blankets, and antipyretics. Give only non-aspirin-containing antipyretics, such as acetaminophen, to lower body temperature. (Aspirin further displaces thyroid hormones, worsening the hypermetabolic state.)

The doctor will order appropriate drugs to treat cardiovascular and other hypermetabolic complications. He may order a beta-adrenergic blocker to reduce sympathetic nervous system activity and relieve arrhythmias. Propranolol I.V. is preferred because it blocks further thyroid activity. The doctor also may place the patient on digoxin and diuretics to prevent or treat cardiac failure. If the patient is in shock or has adrenal insufficiency, the doctor may initiate hydrocortisone therapy.

Decreasing thyroid hyperfunction
Expect to give an antithyroid agent, as ordered, to halt the production of triiodothyronine and thyroxine. You'll probably give propylthiouracil or methimazole orally or by nasogastric tube, followed by an iodine preparation to prevent release of stored thyroid hormones. Give the iodine preparation 1 to 3 hours after administering the antithyroid agent to minimize hormone formation from the iodine.

---

mone (TRH), which in turn causes the anterior pituitary gland to secrete thyroid-stimulating hormone (TSH). This pituitary activity enhances the release of the thyroid hormones triiodothyronine (T_3) and thyroxine (T_4) into the bloodstream.

In hyperthyroid disorders, however, excessive thyroid hormones are released, causing systemic adrenergic activity. Epinephrine overproduction leads to severe hypermetabolic decompensation, which usually affects the cardiovascular, GI, and sympathetic nervous systems but may involve all body systems. (See *Understanding thyroid storm,* page 156.)

Complications
Thyroid storm may lead to heart failure, shock, hyperthermia, fatal arrhythmias, and coma.

Assessment
History
The patient's history may reveal abrupt onset of symptoms after a typical precipitating event, such as physical stress, infection, or an acute emotional shock. Check for a family history of hyperthyroidism (Graves' disease), a common finding in patients with thyroid storm. The patient or an accompanying family member may report such classic symptoms as nervousness, heat intolerance, weight loss de-

Understanding thyroid storm

Normally, the hypothalamus stimulates the release of thyrotropin-releasing hormone (TRH), which causes the anterior pituitary gland to release thyroid-stimulating hormone (TSH). The thyroid gland then secretes triiodothyronine (T_3) and thyroxine (T_4).

In thyroid storm, however, the thyroid overproduces T_3 and T_4, and systemic adrenergic activity increases. This causes epinephrine overproduction and severe hypermetabolism, leading rapidly to GI, cardiovascular, and sympathetic nervous system decompensation.

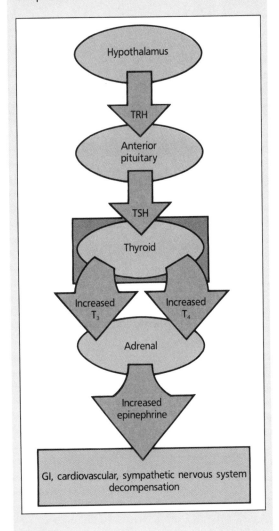

spite increased appetite, excessive sweating, diarrhea, tremor, and palpitations.

Physical examination

Measure the patient's vital signs and check for characteristic cardiovascular, GI, and sympathetic hypermetabolic activity. Expect hyperpyrexia, tachyarrhythmias, and hypermetabolic decompensation. Body temperature initially may measure 100° F (37.8° C), then rise to 106° F (41.1° C).

Obvious signs of hypermetabolic cardiovascular activity are tachyarrhythmias, starting at 130 beats/minute and increasing to 300 beats/minute; angina; palpitations; respiratory distress; and atrial fibrillation. These problems may bring on vascular collapse.

Hypermetabolic GI activity may manifest as nausea, vomiting, and diarrhea, possibly causing dehydration and hypovolemia. Hypermetabolic sympathetic activity may produce fine tremors, agitation, and restlessness progressing to manic or psychotic behavior. (Because thyroid storm may cause psychotic behavior, be sure to assess for this endocrine disorder in a patient who exhibits such behavior.)

Diagnostic tests

Emergency diagnosis relies on clinical findings and the results of serum T_3 and T_4 tests. After the acute crisis passes, the doctor may order a TSH test to identify an underlying thyroid, pituitary, or hypothalamic disorder. He also may order a ^{131}I uptake test and a thyroid scan to gauge thyroid size and help establish how much ^{131}I to prescribe later.

Ongoing treatment

After the patient is somewhat stabilized, the doctor will try to determine what caused thyroid storm. Then he'll prescribe medications or recommend surgery to treat hyperthyroidism.

Drug treatment

The doctor may prescribe antithyroid agents, iodine preparations, or [131]I.

Antithyroid agents. Thyroid hormone antagonists, such as propylthiouracil and methimazole, are used to help relieve thyrotoxicosis and prepare the patient for thyroidectomy. To become euthyroid, the patient may require relatively high doses of antithyroid agents before switching to maintenance doses.

Iodine. If the patient will undergo surgery, the doctor may prescribe an iodine agent, such as potassium iodide, Lugol's solution, or saturated solution of potassium iodide, in combination with an antithyroid agent and a beta-adrenergic blocker (such as propranolol). Iodine prevents thyroid hormone release and reduces thyroid vascularity and size, while beta-adrenergic blockers help manage tachycardia and other peripheral effects of excessive sympathetic nervous system activity.

Radioiodine. When treated with ^{131}I, the thyroid gland picks up the radioactive element as it would regular iodine. Radioactivity then destroys some of the cells that normally concentrate iodine, thus decreasing thyroid hormone production and normalizing thyroid size and function.

To restore euthyroidism and make radiation or surgery safer, the patient must receive antithyroid drugs for 6 to 18 months before starting [131]I. Hypothyroidism is a common adverse effect of ^{131}I, so the patient must be monitored closely during therapy.

Surgery

If drug therapy proves ineffective in a patient under age 40, he may undergo subtotal thyroidectomy to remove five-sixths of the thyroid gland and ensure remission of hyperthyroidism. Surgery proceeds only after the patient's basal metabolic rate returns to normal. Iodine therapy, given in advance, begins to reduce thyroid size and vascularity.

Ongoing nursing interventions

• To help prevent complications or recurrences of thyroid storm, closely monitor the patient's vital signs and weight.
• Take the patient's temperature frequently to help maintain a normal body temperature. Keep room temperature cool; the patient's increased metabolic rate and heat intolerance will make him uncomfortably warm in a room of normal temperature. Provide cool baths and offer iced fluids as needed. Also provide lightweight sheets and loose pajamas. Have the sheets changed frequently if the patient is diaphoretic. Reassure him that heat intolerance will subside as the disorder resolves.
• Use caution when administering antithyroid agents to a pregnant or breast-feeding patient. These drugs may cause goiter and cretinism in the fetus and may impair thyroid hormone production in a breast-feeding infant. Also administer these agents cautiously to a patient receiving anticoagulants because they may cause hypoprothrombinemia and subsequent bleeding problems.
• If you're administering an iodine solution, give it with milk or fruit juice to make it more palatable and provide a straw to prevent tooth staining.
• Be aware that such over-the-counter medications as antitussives, expectorants, bronchodilators, and salt substitutes may contain iodine and thus may precipitate iodine toxicity when given in conjunction with an iodine agent.
• Evaluate the patient for desired and adverse effects of drug therapy by assessing him for changes in pulse rate, blood pressure, weight, affect and mannerisms (such as euphoria, delirium, irritability, and disorientation).
• If your patient is receiving an antithyroid agent, check for drug toxicity by assessing for a sudden increase in weight, edema, depression, and cold intolerance. During high-dose therapy, the patient is also at risk for agranulocytosis, pancytopenia, and thrombocytopenia. Be sure to assess him periodically for fever, rash, sore throat, epistaxis, and unexplained bruising or bleeding.
• Assess laboratory results, checking particularly for increased levels of T_3, T_4, and blood glucose, and a decreased level of plasma cortisol.
• To counteract hypermetabolism, supply a diet high in calories, carbohydrates, proteins, vitamins, and minerals. If necessary, provide up to six full meals a day. Minimize the patient's intake of fiber and highly seasoned foods because they increase peristalsis and cause diarrhea. Also limit his intake of alcohol and such stimulants as caffeine and tobacco.

• Ensure a fluid intake of 3 to 4 liters daily (unless contraindicated by the patient's age or a preexisting cardiovascular disease) to compensate for excessive diaphoresis and to help correct hypovolemic states caused by polyuria, diarrhea, and vomiting.

• Assume a calm, reassuring manner when providing care. Provide periods of uninterrupted rest.

• Convey an accepting attitude toward changes in the patient's appearance, weight, behavior, and appetite, such as tremor, confusion, agitation, and exophthalmia. Help him develop positive coping strategies to deal with these problems. Reassure him that these changes result from hyperthyroidism and will subside with treatment. Help the patient's family cope with the patient's altered behavior and appearance.

• Provide a safe environment for the patient by reducing environmental hazards. Keep noises to a minimum, keep the room temperature cool and the lights dim, and limit procedures to counter the effects of hypermetabolism. If possible, arrange for the patient to have a private room to minimize external noise and prevent him from disturbing others. Provide safety measures, such as side rails and soft restraints, and perform frequent bed checks.

• Note if the patient has an increased appetite with an associated weight loss. Monitor his food intake and weight daily. Promote a high-calorie, high-protein, easily digested diet. Avoid fluids that cause diarrhea (such as prune and apple juice).

• Teach the patient about the importance of reporting changes in temperature, pulse rate, and weight to the doctor. Stress that he must comply with the prescribed medication regimen to help prevent recurrence of thyroid storm. Provide him with a written treatment plan, and review it with him and family members to reinforce the information. Describe potential adverse drug effects, such as fever, sore throat, and rash, and emphasize the need to report these at once. Teach the patient how to recognize signs and symptoms of hypothyroidism. Urge him to make and keep appointments for frequent follow-up medical visits.

Syndrome of inappropriate antidiuretic hormone

In this syndrome, commonly known as SIADH, excessive amounts of antidiuretic hormone (ADH) are secreted. Found in the posterior pituitary gland, ADH acts as an antidiuretic and has a pressor effect that elevates blood pressure. Too much ADH seriously disrupts fluid and electrolyte balance and leads to increased water retention, greater extracellular fluid volume, and hyponatremia. Urine output ceases.

SIADH calls for prompt treatment to avert seizures and death. (See *When your patient has SIADH.*)

Causes
SIADH may result from ectopic ADH release by a cancerous tumor, autonomous ADH release by the lungs, or ADH release from the neurohypophysis secondary to drugs or to neighboring inflammatory, neoplastic, or vascular lesions.

Cancerous tumors that may release ectopic ADH include oat cell lung carcinomas, thymomas, GI tumors, and lymphoid tumors. Autonomous ADH release by lung tissue may occur in tuberculosis, viral pneumonia, chronic obstructive pulmonary disease, and lung abscess.

Drugs that may stimulate ADH release include chlorpropamide, vincristine, clofibrate, tolbutamide, thiazide diuretics, cyclophosphamide, haloperidol, carbamazepine, nicotine, barbiturates, analgesics (such as morphine), antineoplastic drugs, anesthetics, and tricyclic antidepressants.

Various CNS disorders also may stimulate ADH release—brain tumor, head trauma, subdural hematoma, CVA, pituitary adenoma, brain abscess, meningitis, encephalitis, cerebral atrophy, acute encephalopathy, acute psychosis, and Guillain-Barré syndrome.

Other disorders, conditions, and procedures that may lead to SIADH include lupus erythematosus, emotional stress, pain, and positive-pressure mechanical ventilation.

Pathophysiology

Normally, ADH secretion is dependent on serum osmolality and blood volume. In SIADH, hypothalamic osmoreceptors can't sense changing levels of plasma solute concentrations, causing prolonged or aberrant ADH secretion. The renal tubules become more permeable, promoting water retention. Serum osmolality then drops as extracellular fluid volume expands. The glomerular filtration rate rises and aldosterone secretion falls, ultimately causing hyponatremia and hypotonicity.

Compensatory mechanisms trigger a marked drop in the serum sodium level. As the sodium concentration of extracellular fluid falls, water moves into cells. In the brain, this causes swelling that increases ICP, and chronic hyponatremia leads to sodium loss in cells. Urine osmolality rises. Although the kidneys excrete abundant sodium in the urine, elevated ADH levels cause continued water retention. (See *What happens in SIADH*, page 160.)

Complications

SIADH may cause water intoxication, overhydration, cranial nerve palsies, focal weakness, Babinski's reflex, depressed deep tendon reflexes, ataxia, Cheyne-Stokes respirations, depression, and psychosis. Ultimately, these complications may bring on seizures, irreversible brain damage, and death.

Assessment

History

A patient in the initial phase of SIADH may complain of headache, abdominal discomfort, nausea, and malaise. Sometimes nausea, vomiting, and weight gain (with or without edema) are the only initial signs and symptoms.

EMERGENCY INTERVENTIONS

When your patient has SIADH

For the patient with the syndrome of inappropriate antidiuretic hormone (SIADH), your priority is to restore normal serum osmolality without further expanding extracellular fluid volume.

If the patient has severe hyponatremia (a serum sodium level below 125 mEq/liter), expect to infuse an I.V. solution of hypertonic saline solution, 200 to 300 ml over several hours, until cerebral symptoms improve or the serum sodium level rises above 125 mEq/liter. However, use extreme caution when administering this solution because fluid overload may precipitate heart failure or circulatory collapse. If the patient has mild hyponatremia, fluid restriction may be the main treatment. I.V. furosemide will also usually be infused.

Other treatments focus on eliminating the underlying cause of SIADH. For instance, if a specific drug is the known or suspected cause, the doctor will discontinue it. If the patient has an infection, you'll give antibiotics as ordered. The doctor may place the patient on steroids to treat an underlying adrenal insufficiency. If cancer is the cause of SIADH, the patient will need appropriate treatment and follow-up care. Carefully monitor the patient's blood urea nitrogen and creatinine levels. Also, place the patient on seizure precautions, and perform frequent neurologic checks.

Try to determine if the patient has any risk factors for SIADH. If SIADH is severe, he may be unable to answer questions, so you'll need to interview family members. Check for a history of cancer, pulmonary disease, head injury, CVA, or another condition that may precipitate SIADH. Also check the patient's medication history for drugs linked with this syndrome. (See *Lack of history hampers SIADH treatment*, page 161.)

Physical examination

Physical findings depend on the severity of water retention and hyponatremia. The patient with a serum sodium level of 125 mEq/liter or

PATHOPHYSIOLOGY

What happens in SIADH

This flow chart shows the abnormal events occurring in the syndrome of inappropriate antidiuretic hormone (SIADH).

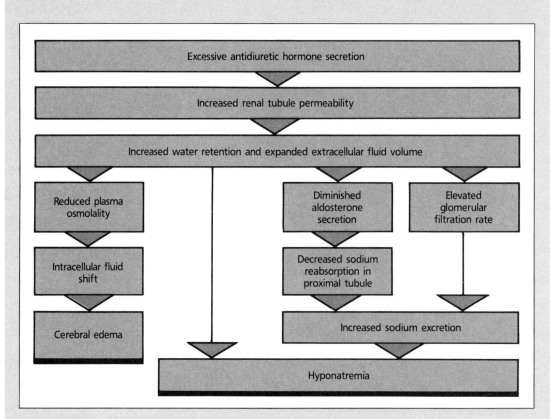

Diagnostic tests
Laboratory studies may help identify SIADH. Expect profoundly decreased serum osmolality (below 280 mOsm), elevated urine osmolality, a serum sodium level below 125 mEq/liter, (normal values range from 135 to 145 mEq/liter), a markedly increased urine sodium level, and urine specific gravity above 1.025 (1.005 to 1.020 is normal). Urine output is low, and the urine appears highly concentrated.

more usually is asymptomatic or complains only of mild GI discomfort. With acute hyponatremia (a serum sodium level below 125 mEq/liter), expect seizures and signs of diffuse cerebral edema, such as irritability, personality changes, and an altered LOC ranging from disorientation and confusion to coma.

Measure the patient's heart rate and blood pressure, and check for signs of altered fluid and electrolyte status. However, be aware that edema is rare, despite weight gain, because the hypotonicity of extracellular fluid causes intracellular swelling.

Lack of history hampers SIADH treatment

For the patient with the syndrome of inappropriate antidiuretic hormone (SIADH), eliminating the underlying cause is a primary treatment goal. But if the patient is unable to provide history information, pinpointing the cause of SIADH and treating him effectively can be a real challenge.

Consider the case of Anthony Granese, age 55, admitted with tonic-clonic seizures and too lethargic to give his history.

Establishing the diagnosis

Nurse Marianne James measured Mr. Granese's blood pressure at 160/90 mm Hg. She found no signs of heart failure or peripheral edema, and she recorded his skin turgor as normal. He was severely hypertensive and had no symptoms of dehydration or generalized edema. A patient with Mr. Granese's blood pressure might be expected to have cardiac symptoms associated with edema, but he had none.

Laboratory results hinted strongly at SIADH. Mr. Granese's serum sodium level was very low at 117 mEq/liter, his urine specific gravity was 1.024, and his urine sodium level was 20 mEq/liter. His serum osmolality was also low at 260 mOsm.

Based on these findings and the patient's clinical status, the doctor diagnosed SIADH. Marianne infused 100 ml of 5% sodium chloride solution over 2 hours and then monitored the patient's response closely. She also restricted his fluids and monitored his intake and output to evaluate his fluid status. With this patient, a satisfactory urine output would be an increase to at least 30 ml/hour. Mr. Granese was placed on seizure precautions, and Marianne evaluated his neurologic status every 15 minutes.

Although Mr. Granese's condition improved somewhat, the health care team still didn't know why he'd developed SIADH. And unless they discovered the reason, they couldn't develop an effective treatment plan.

Establishing the history

To find out more about Mr. Granese's history, Marianne questioned the person who'd accompanied him to the hospital. Unfortunately, he didn't know the patient all that well. However, he did say that Mr. Granese once mentioned he had diabetes.

The real break came later that day when Mr. Granese's daughter arrived. She told Marianne her father had been taking 500 mg of chlorpropamide twice daily for years to treat his diabetes. A few days earlier, he'd called his doctor's office complaining that he felt tired all the time. The office staff told him to simply double his chlorpropamide doses.

Recalling that chlorpropamide is one of many drugs that may stimulate antidiuretic hormone release, Marianne suspected she'd uncovered the cause of her patient's SIADH. She reported the daughter's revelation to the doctor. Having already ruled out other causes of hyponatremia, he now concluded that the increased chlorpropamide dosage had precipitated SIADH.

Eliminating the problem

On doctor's orders, Marianne discontinued chlorpropamide and started administering glyburide, 5 mg/day. Mr. Granese didn't have another seizure during his hospital stay. This can be attributed to a return to normal serum sodium levels after infusion of the 5% sodium chloride solution.

Before discharge, Marianne taught Mr. Granese to weigh himself every day to detect any future recurrences of SIADH. She also told him to report any significant weight gain (5 lb or more over 2 days) and to measure liquid consumed as well as urine voided to ensure that his urine output was close to the amount of fluid consumed. Decreased urine output could mean that fluid was being retained and that SIADH could recur.

She instructed him to continue taking glyburide instead of chlorpropamide. She made sure he could identify the warning signs of an SIADH recurrence or worsening diabetes and told him to notify his doctor at once if he had these signs.

The doctor diagnoses SIADH by ruling out other possible causes of hyponatremia — such as hyperglycemia, hypertriglyceridemia, and hyperproteinemia — and cardiac, renal, and hepatic factors.

Ongoing treatment

Medical measures aim to treat the underlying cause of SIADH and to halt water retention. If drug use is the cause, the doctor will discontinue the offending drug.

To treat acute SIADH, the doctor may order hypertonic saline solution (infused by I.V. pump) to replace lost sodium. Using small I.V. bottles reduces the risk of inadvertent overadministration. To prevent fluid and cardiac overload and enhance free water loss, the doctor may place the patient on I.V. furosemide along with hypertonic saline solution.

Be aware that administering 0.9% sodium chloride solution doesn't adequately correct hyponatremia in a patient with SIADH — and may even worsen the condition. A rapid serum sodium rise may cause central pontine myelinolysis, a neurologic disorder involving loss of myelin and supporting structures in the pons and possibly in other brain areas. Cranial nerve deficits, coma, and quadriplegia may result.

Drug treatment

To counter the renal action of ADH, expect to administer demeclocycline, 1 to 2 g/day by mouth. This drug causes a reversible form of diabetes insipidus and may induce azotemia, so be sure to monitor the patient's BUN and serum creatinine levels. Demeclocycline is used mainly in long-term management of SIADH in cancer patients.

Lithium also impedes the renal response to ADH. This drug causes polyuria, which disappears when the drug is discontinued. However, lithium is usually considered too toxic to use in SIADH.

Ongoing nursing interventions

• Closely monitor your patient's vital signs and perform frequent neurologic checks. Evaluate him for increasing irritability, restlessness, seizures, and unresponsiveness — possible signs of worsening cerebral edema and water intoxication.
• As ordered, restrict the patient's water intake to normalize his serum osmolality and serum sodium level.
• Measure and record hourly fluid output. Carefully document all infused fluids as well as those given orally — especially if the doctor has ordered strict fluid restriction.
• Monitor the serum sodium level and measure urine specific gravity.
• Weigh the patient daily while he's wearing the same type of clothing.
• Perform frequent oral hygiene and provide nutritional support as needed.
• Provide emotional support to the patient and family.
• Teach the patient and family about the need for continued fluid restriction. Explain how to measure daily weight, maintain fluid balance, and monitor fluid intake and output after discharge. Provide thorough instruction about prescribed medications and explain the importance of taking these exactly as ordered. Make sure they know how to recognize signs and symptoms of disease exacerbation.

Adrenal crisis

Adrenal crisis (also called addisonian crisis or acute adrenal insufficiency) is the rapid and severe onset of adrenal hypofunction or insufficiency. The patient experiences metabolic and endocrine imbalances (hyponatremia, hypoglycemia, and hyperkalemia), his blood pressure falls severely, and his fluid volume drops profoundly.

Adrenal crisis is the most serious complication of adrenocortical insufficiency. Left untreated, the condition is fatal. (See *When your patient is in adrenal crisis.*)

Causes

Adrenal crisis typically occurs when a patient doesn't respond to hormone replacement therapy or undergoes pronounced stress (such as from infection, trauma, or surgery) without sufficient glucocorticoid replacement. In a patient who has been receiving high or chronic glucocorticoid doses, this emergency may occur after abrupt drug withdrawal. (See *Adrenal crisis caused by steroid withdrawal,* page 164.)

Other precipitating factors include adrenal tumor, burns, hemorrhage associated with anticoagulant therapy, hypermetabolic states, bilateral adrenalectomy, sudden cessation of antineoplastic therapy, hypopituitarism, and hypothalamic suppression.

Pathophysiology

Normally, the hypothalamus secretes corticotropin-releasing factor, which triggers the anterior pituitary gland to secrete corticotropin. This, in turn, induces cortisol production by the adrenal cortex. Meanwhile, renin secreted by the kidneys is converted to angiotensin I, which is then converted to angiotensin II. This latter substance stimulates the adrenal cortex to release aldosterone, which helps the kidneys conserve sodium and water and promotes potassium excretion.

In adrenal crisis, these mechanisms are disrupted. Insufficient production of cortisol causes hypotension and hypoglycemia; insufficient release of aldosterone leads to hyponatremia, hypovolemia, and hyperkalemia.

Complications

Adrenal crisis may lead to hypoglycemia, hypotension, hyponatremia, hypovolemia, and hyperkalemia. (See *Effects of adrenal crisis,* page 165.)

Assessment

History

A history of adrenal insufficiency is a strong indicator of adrenal crisis when the patient exhibits signs and symptoms of this disorder. Find out if the patient has been receiving steroid

EMERGENCY INTERVENTIONS

When your patient is in adrenal crisis

Emergency treatment for the patient in adrenal crisis has three primary goals: reversing shock, replacing fluids, and replacing cortisol. As soon as blood is drawn for laboratory studies, the doctor will order dextrose 5% in 0.9% sodium chloride solution for rapid fluid replacement—up to 3 liters over the first few hours. He will order diagnostic tests—cultures, abdominal magnetic resonance imaging scans, or skin testing—to investigate the underlying cause.

As ordered, replace cortisol by administering hydrocortisone, 100 mg I.V. As needed and ordered, administer plasma, oxygen, and short-term vasopressor therapy. If the patient has an infection, give antibiotics as ordered.

Most of the metabolic and electrolyte abnormalities that accompany adrenal crisis resolve without further treatment. Because high-dose cortisol therapy has a mineralocorticoid effect, the patient probably won't need aldosterone replacement.

therapy, has undergone adrenal surgery, or has recently had an infection or suffered pronounced physical or emotional stress. Obtain a medication history and ask if the patient has complied with his drug regimen.

Note any recent history of nausea, vomiting, diarrhea, abdominal pain, anxiety, irritability, fatigue, anorexia, muscle cramps, excessive thirst, headache, fever, or progressive muscle weakness. These symptoms reflect hyponatremia, hyperkalemia, and hypoglycemia from adrenal crisis. Also ask about reduced urine output, which reflects hypovolemia.

Physical examination

Measure the patient's vital signs, which may reveal an elevated temperature, low blood pressure, a weak and irregular pulse, and an increased respiratory rate. Check for signs of de-

Adrenal crisis caused by steroid withdrawal

A patient who suddenly discontinues his steroid regimen may suffer adrenal crisis during an illness, when the added stress combines with adrenal insufficiency to cause acute symptoms. That's what happened to Carlos Junto, age 70, who came to the emergency department 3 days ago with shortness of breath and was later admitted to your unit with pneumonia.

Establishing the background
According to his history, Mr. Junto is a widower with no relatives. His memory is poor and he's confused about his medical and medication history. He remembers having a breathing problem and taking drugs for it—but cannot remember their names. He does know that he smokes cigarettes.

The doctor has placed Mr. Junto on oxygen at 2 liters/minute through a nasal cannula and ordered an I.V. infusion of aminophylline at 30 mg/ hour to treat Mr. Junto's chronic obstructive pulmonary disease (COPD). A heparin lock has been placed, and he is receiving ampicillin at 500 mg every 6 hours for his pneumonia. Mr. Junto's blood cultures indicate gram-positive cocci. Laboratory results also show a triad of problems: hyponatremia, hyperkalemia, and hypoglycemia.

Assessing the patient
Mr. Junto's condition seems stable, but then one morning you enter his room and find him vomiting and lethargic. You immediately assess his vital signs: pulse, 120 beats/minute and thready; respiratory rate, 36 breaths/minute; blood pressure, 80/56 mm Hg; and rectal temperature, 103° F (39.4° C). His skin turgor is poor, his axillary and mucous membranes dry, his neck veins flat.

Given his history and current signs and symptoms, you begin to suspect that Mr. Junto was previously on long-term steroid therapy for COPD. Steroid withdrawal coupled with the stress of pneumonia and septicemia could have caused acute adrenal insufficiency—an adrenal crisis. Signs and symptoms of this condition include profound weakness, nausea, vomiting, dehydration, electrolyte imbalances, tachycardia, and hypotension.

Although you know Mr. Junto's signs and symptoms could be related to his underlying illness, blood glucose levels are usually higher, not lower, during times of physical stress.

Responding to the crisis
First, you lower the head of the bed and position Mr. Junto on his side to prevent aspiration of vomitus. You check his heparin lock for patency. You ask another nurse to inform the doctor of Mr. Junto's deteriorating condition and to bring you a bag of dextrose 5% in 0.9% sodium chloride solution to restore his glucose and sodium levels and circulating fluid volume.

Next, you place Mr. Junto on a cardiac monitor. Because hyperkalemia can cause dangerous arrhythmias, you look for tall, peaked T waves on the rhythm strip. You have a crash cart ready with suction equipment and emergency drugs, and you place an automatic blood pressure cuff on Mr. Junto's arm for continuous monitoring.

Waiting for the doctor, you prepare to insert a nasogastric tube to decompress the patient's stomach and an indwelling urinary catheter to monitor fluid output. You continue the oxygen and aminophylline as ordered. Meanwhile, call the laboratory to draw blood for serum cortisol level as ordered.

After examining Mr. Junto, the doctor confirms your assessment, and you promptly administer a 100-mg I.V. bolus of hydrocortisone. You're prepared to give vasopressors if Mr. Junto's blood pressure doesn't respond to hydrocortisone and fluid replacement. You then help the doctor place a central line for rapid fluid administration and central venous pressure readings.

Promoting recovery
You monitor Mr. Junto continuously. Because his adrenal crisis resulted from the stress of his illness coupled with adrenal insufficiency related to steroid withdrawal, he'll require supplemental steroids (either 100 mg I.V. every 8 hours or a continuous infusion after a bolus dose) until acute symptoms subside. Oral doses will be increased once Mr. Junto can tolerate food.

His mental status is questionable, so you'll need to assess his ability to care for himself after discharge. Alert the hospital social worker to his case. You also recommend that he carry a medical identification card or wear a medical identification bracelet to inform future caregivers of his condition, drug regimen, and doctor's name.

Effects of adrenal crisis

As this flow chart shows, adrenal crisis may lead to a group of complications known as the five H's: hypoglycemia, hypotension, hyponatremia, hyperkalemia, and hypovolemia.

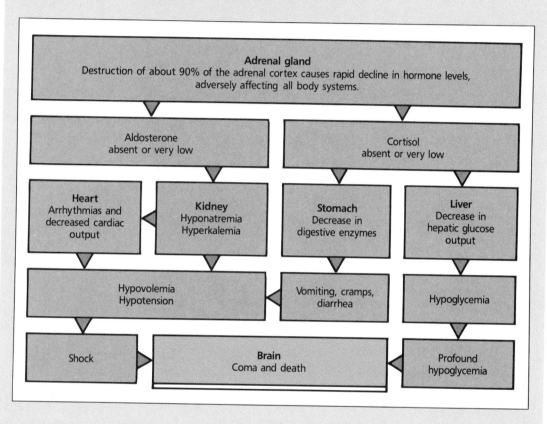

hydration (such as dry skin and mucous membranes), flaccid extremities, lethargy, confusion, restlessness, or a progressively diminishing LOC. You also may detect coordination problems.

If the patient has a long-standing history of chronic adrenal insufficiency, you may see a bronze coloration similar to deep suntan on his elbows, knees, and knuckles and possibly on his lips, buccal mucosa, and scars. Vitiligo (depigmented skin patches) or abnormal hyperpigmentation may be evident. Hyperpigmentation results from excessive secretion of melanocyte-stimulating hormone and corticotropin (an effect of reduced cortisol secretion).

Diagnostic tests
The diagnosis of adrenal crisis is confirmed by laboratory studies — but treatment shouldn't be delayed until laboratory results arrive. Laboratory indicators of adrenal crisis include:
• above-normal serum potassium and calcium levels
• increased BUN levels
• elevated hematocrit and hemoglobin levels
• above-normal lymphocyte, eosinophil, and WBC counts

• below-normal serum sodium and glucose levels

• below-normal serum and urine cortisol levels.

The patient with adrenal insufficiency also has a decreased corticotropin level. Electrocardiogram (ECG) abnormalities may include tall, peaked T waves; wide QRS complexes; and ST-segment depression. Caused by hyperkalemia, these changes predispose the patient to dangerous arrhythmias.

Ongoing treatment
After adrenal crisis subsides (usually within a few hours), treatment focuses on identifying and correcting the underlying cause.

Drug treatment
The doctor will order maintenance hydrocortisone (100 mg I.V. every 8 hours or as a continuous infusion) until acute symptoms subside. When the patient can tolerate oral intake, oral doses will begin on an 8-hour schedule. Ideally, glucocorticoid administration should mimic the body's natural cortisol secretion pattern. For this reason, the doctor probably will direct you to give two-thirds of the total daily dose in the early morning and the remainder in the afternoon. The large morning dose suppresses the adrenal gland when it's most active and allows the body to compensate in the late afternoon when the serum cortisol level normally drops. This prevents cushingoid effects, such as stimulation of appetite, mobilization of fat from peripheral to central sites, moon face, buffalo hump, muscle weakness, thinning of skin, depression, sleep disturbances, hypokalemia, and menstrual irregularities in women.

To maintain normal electrolyte levels and blood pressure, the doctor may place the patient on fludrocortisone, an oral mineralocorticoid. The typical dosage is 0.1 to 0.2 mg/day.

If the patient fails to regain normal adrenal function, he'll need lifelong replacement therapy on cortisone or fluorohydrocortisone and additional salt intake during periods of GI upset. If he does regain normal adrenal function, the doctor will taper drug administration gradually to prevent steroid-induced adrenal crisis. The patient will continue to be at risk for adrenal crisis for 1 year or more after receiving cor-

ticosteroids, because this condition causes a sudden, marked decrease in hormones. If surgery is anticipated during this time, he'll need I.V. corticosteroid therapy.

Ongoing nursing interventions
Focus your care on ensuring fluid balance, reducing stress, increasing the patient's activities, preventing complications, and teaching him how to cope with adrenal insufficiency. Give oral glucocorticoid doses with meals or antacids to reduce gastric irritation and help prevent peptic ulcer formation.

Ensuring an adequate fluid balance
• Monitor fluid and electrolyte balance carefully. Weigh the patient daily and routinely assess his skin turgor, mucous membranes, and urine output.

• Watch for cushingoid signs caused by adverse effects of glucocorticoids.

• Observe the patient for excessive thirst; he may crave salty foods.

• Measure blood pressure frequently. If systolic pressure drops 20 mm Hg or more, suspect fluid volume deficit. Also, assess laboratory results to monitor fluid and electrolyte balances, such as sodium, potassium, calcium, BUN, and cortisol levels.

Reducing stress
• Maintain a quiet, calm environment to prevent recurrence of adrenal crisis. Urge family members and others to minimize stress when visiting.

• Encourage the patient to use relaxation techniques to reduce stress.

• Explain all procedures and treatments in advance to decrease anxiety.

Increasing the patient's activity tolerance
• Initially, you'll need to perform all activities of daily living for the patient for at least 24 hours, gradually adding activities according to the patient's tolerance.

• Provide frequent rest periods to prevent fatigue.

Preventing complications
• Take steps to prevent infection and protect the patient against exposure to potential sources of infection.
• To help prevent pressure ulcers, turn and reposition the patient every 2 hours, avoiding pressure over bony prominences.
• Encourage the patient to dress in layers to retain body heat because he will have a decreased tolerance for cold. Urge him to adjust room temperature, if possible.

Providing patient teaching
• Supply explicit verbal and written instructions to promote compliance with therapy. Make sure the patient understands why he may need lifelong steroid replacement therapy. Instruct him to check with the doctor during periods of stress because his dosage may need to be increased then. Caution him not to stop taking his medication suddenly.
• Warn the patient that infection, injury, or profuse sweating may trigger adrenal crisis.
• Instruct the patient to take steroids with antacids or meals to minimize gastric irritation.
• Advise the patient to carry a medical identification card describing his condition and his drug therapy and listing his doctor's name.
• Advise the patient and his family to keep an emergency kit available with a prepared syringe of hydrocortisone in case of an unexpected trauma or resurgence of adrenal crisis. Teach them how to give the injection.
• Explain that adrenal insufficiency causes mood swings and mental status changes, but reassure the patient and family that these symptoms will abate with steroid replacement therapy.

Metabolic acidosis

Metabolic acidosis is an acid-base disturbance marked by an abnormally low pH (increased hydrogen ion concentration) and a low plasma bicarbonate concentration. It accompanies or complicates an underlying disorder. Clinical manifestations result from the body's attempt to correct acidosis through compensatory mechanisms of the lungs, kidneys, and cells.

Metabolic acidosis is more common among children, whose faster metabolic rates and lower ratios of water to total body weight make them more vulnerable to acid-base imbalance. Severe or untreated metabolic acidosis can be fatal. (See *When your patient has metabolic acidosis,* page 168.)

Causes
Metabolic acidosis may develop through two separate mechanisms — acid accumulation or ingestion, or bicarbonate (base) loss.

Acid accumulation or ingestion usually occurs when proteins and fats are burned for energy instead of carbohydrates. Ketones then accumulate, producing acidosis. Underlying causes include DKA; chronic alcoholism; lactic acidosis (for example, from pulmonary and cardiac disorders, anemia, and shock); tissue hypoxia; salicylate, ethanol, or methanol intoxication; starvation; a high-fat, low-carbohydrate diet; overproduction of metabolically produced acids (for example, from hyperthyroidism, infection, trauma, and major surgery); and prolonged or inappropriate use of such drugs as ammonium chloride, ferrous sulfate, and paraldehyde.

Bicarbonate loss may stem from a wide range of conditions. When the kidneys lose the ability to excrete acids or conserve bicarbonate, acids accumulate and bicarbonates decrease. This may happen with diarrhea or prolonged vomiting, both of which cause depletion of pancreatic, biliary, and lower GI tract secretions containing bicarbonate. Other causes of bicarbonate loss include total parenteral nutrition, pancreatic fistulas, uterosigmoidostomy, ileal conduit, increased extracellular fluid volume, administration of chloride-containing acids (such as ammonium chloride), use of anion exchange resins, and rapid I.V. infusion.

Pathophysiology
The balance of hydrogen ions in the body depends on normal functioning of the kidneys, lungs, and cells. Exposure to unusually heavy acids or bicarbonates may interfere with hydrogen ion regulation, causing an acid-base im-

When your patient has metabolic acidosis

If your patient has metabolic acidosis, act immediately to replace his body fluids, restore normal serum osmolality, correct his bicarbonate deficit, and prevent further acid-base imbalances. Untreated, metabolic acidosis may lead to arrhythmias, cardiac arrest, and coma.

Rehydrating the patient
• To replace fluids and restore serum osmolality, give 0.9% sodium chloride solution or lactated Ringer's solution, as ordered. However, if the patient developed metabolic acidosis from excessive chloride intake, the doctor will use an alternative solution.
• Expect to add insulin to the regimen if the acidosis arose secondarily to diabetic ketoacidosis. For a patient with severe respiratory compromise, the doctor may institute mechanical ventilation to ensure adequate ventilation and oxygenation.

Correcting bicarbonate deficit
• To correct the bicarbonate deficit in acute metabolic acidosis (especially when the pH is below 7.2), the doctor may order I.V. sodium bicarbonate. During the infusion, be sure to monitor arterial blood gas values closely to prevent bicarbonate excess.

Preventing further imbalances
• To prevent hyperkalemia—a common finding with metabolic acidosis—make sure the patient is adequately hydrated. Monitor his serum potassium level continually to help avert arrhythmias and cardiac arrest.
• As acidosis resolves and the patient's body fluids become more alkaline, his ionized calcium level may drop, causing muscle irritability and tetany. Be sure to monitor laboratory values and calcium replacement therapy carefully.

balance. Metabolic acidosis occurs when the disturbance affects primarily the kidneys, which can't excrete enough hydrogen ions to keep blood pH in a normal range.

Complications
Unless treated promptly, metabolic acidosis may lead to coma, arrhythmias, and cardiac arrest.

Assessment
History
Check the patient's history for an underlying disorder (such as diabetes) that may predispose him to acidosis. Ask what medications he's taking, including over-the-counter (OTC) preparations, because some agents can cause lactic acidosis. Stay alert for a history of arthritis: A patient who takes salicylates to treat arthritis may suffer salicylate intoxication leading to metabolic acidosis.

Find out if the patient recently lost or gained weight, changed his diet, or altered his fluid intake. Note generalized complaints, such as apathy, drowsiness, lethargy, weakness, anorexia, nausea, vomiting, or abdominal pain.

Physical examination
Observe for hyperventilation, which indicates the patient is trying to compensate for metabolic acidosis by eliminating excess carbon dioxide. In this breathing pattern (Kussmaul's respirations), respiratory rate and depth increase.

Observe the patient for mentation changes, which may range from lethargy and drowsiness to confusion, stupor, or coma. As the pH decreases, CNS depression occurs.

Inspect the patient's skin, which may change from cold and clammy to warm and dry as metabolic acidosis worsens. You may detect a fruity breath odor if the patient is diabetic. This indicates burning of fats and proteins for energy and excretion of accumulated ketones by the lungs.

Hypotension and arrhythmias may occur as acidosis affects the heart. Neuromuscular assessment may reveal decreased muscle tone and deep tendon reflexes.

Comparing ABG values in acid-base disorders

Metabolic acidosis is an acid-base disturbance marked by an abnormally low pH (increased hydrogen ion concentration) and a low plasma bicarbonate concentration. Arterial blood gas (ABG) values, the primary assessment tool used to identify metabolic acidosis and alkalosis, indicate the body's attempt to correct acidosis using the lungs as a compensatory mechanism. When analyzing your patient's pH, partial pressure of arterial carbon dioxide ($PaCO_2$), and bicarbonate (HCO_3^-) values, keep in mind the following normal values:
• pH: 7.35 to 7.45
• $PaCO_2$: 35 to 45 mm Hg
• HCO_3^-: 21 to 25 mEq/liter.
    If the patient isn't compensating for the disorder, the $PaCO_2$ value will be normal.

METABOLIC DISORDER	pH	$PaCO_2$ IF COMPENSATED	HCO_3^-
Metabolic acidosis	Below 7.35	Below 35 mm Hg	Below 21 mEq/liter
Metabolic alkalosis	Above 7.45	Above 45 mm Hg	Above 25 mEq/liter

Diagnostic tests

ABG values are the primary diagnostic tool. In *uncompensated* metabolic acidosis, expect a pH below 7.35, a bicarbonate value below 21 mEq/liter, and a normal partial pressure of arterial carbon dioxide ($PaCO_2$) value. In *partially compensated* metabolic acidosis, $PaCO_2$ drops below 35 mm Hg. (See *Comparing ABG values in acid-base disorders.*)

Other tests used to diagnose metabolic acidosis include:
• serum potassium level, which usually rises as hydrogen moves into cells and potassium moves out of cells to maintain electroneutrality
• blood glucose level, which rises if the patient has diabetes
• number of serum ketone bodies, which increases in diabetes
• serum lactic acid level, which increases in lactic acidosis.

Measuring the anion gap helps establish the cause of acidosis. The anion gap is the difference between the serum sodium level and the sum of the bicarbonate and serum chloride values. Normally, the difference is 10 to 12 mEq/liter.

For example, suppose a patient has these normal values: serum sodium level, 140 mEq/liter; serum chloride level, 104 mEq/liter; and bicarbonate level, 24 mEq/liter. You'd calculate his anion gap to be 12 mEq/liter, as follows:

$$140 - (104 + 24) = 140 - 128$$
$$= 12 \text{ mEq/liter}$$

When metabolic acidosis results from direct bicarbonate loss (as from diarrhea, intestinal fistulas, or excessive chloride administration), the anion gap remains normal. A high anion gap (above 14 mEq/liter) occurs when metabolic acidosis is caused by an accumulation of organic acids—for example, in lactic acidosis, ketoacidosis, salicylate toxicity, or ethanol, methanol, or paraldehyde poisoning.

Ongoing treatment

Medical measures used to treat metabolic acidosis vary with the underlying cause. For instance, if the patient has DKA, expect the doctor to order insulin, sodium chloride, potassium, and water. To treat alcoholic ketoacidosis, he typically orders 0.9% sodium chloride solution and glucose. A patient with lactic acidosis usually receives sodium bicarbonate; one with renal failure will receive sodium bicarbonate and may undergo dialysis to eliminate accumulated acid waste.

If metabolic acidosis results from ingestion of acidic agents, such as salicylates or ethanol, these agents will be discontinued. If acid loss stems from severe diarrhea or intestinal fistula, expect to replace lost fluids and electrolytes.

Ongoing nursing interventions

Focus your care on monitoring the patient's vital signs and laboratory results, assessing his response to medication, and protecting him from injury.
• Assess vital signs frequently — at least every 30 minutes during the acute phase of metabolic acidosis. Watch for changes in the pulse rate, decreased blood pressure, and shallow respirations — possible signs that the patient is overcorrected to hypokalemia.
• Keep an emergency cart nearby with sodium bicarbonate ampules ready for administration in case of bicarbonate deficiency; use cautiously because bicarbonate administration may cause rebound metabolic alkalosis.
• Position the patient on his side to maintain an open airway and to prevent aspiration. Reposition him at least every 2 hours to avoid hypoxia, hyperkalemia, and lowered pH, which may in turn cause decreased mentation.
• Monitor laboratory results and report even slight changes that may indicate overcorrection, which may cause hypokalemia or metabolic alkalosis.
• Carefully measure and record intake and output to monitor renal function. Watch for signs of hyperkalemia (weakness, flaccid paralysis, and arrhythmias) and hypocalcemia (tremor and muscle spasms).
• Provide oral care at least every 2 hours, and lubricate the patient's lips with petroleum jelly; deep, rapid respirations may cause marked dehydration.
• Frequently orient the patient to the environment. Minimize environmental stimulation. If he's delirious, never leave him unattended.
• Keep the bed in a low position with the side rails up to guard against falls.

Metabolic alkalosis

Metabolic alkalosis is an acid-base disturbance marked by decreased acid and increased bicarbonate (base) in the blood. The blood pH is abnormally high, above 7.45.

Like metabolic acidosis, metabolic alkalosis accompanies or complicates an underlying disorder. Unless treated, the patient may die. (See *When your patient has metabolic alkalosis*.)

Causes

Metabolic alkalosis may result from conditions that cause hydrogen ion loss, bicarbonate gain, or potassium or chloride depletion.

Causes of hydrogen ion loss include severe diarrhea, prolonged vomiting or gastric suctioning leading to loss of large amounts of hydrochloric acid, hyperaldosteronism, laxative abuse, hypokalemia (which causes the kidneys to conserve potassium and excrete hydrogen ions), and diuretic therapy.

Bicarbonate gain may result from excessive alkali ingestion (such as from baking soda or bicarbonate-containing antacids), excessive sodium bicarbonate administration, excessive I.V. fluids with high lactate or bicarbonate concentrations, massive blood transfusions, and respiratory insufficiency.

Causes of potassium or chloride depletion include Cushing's syndrome (caused by excess production of corticotropin and consequent hyperplasia of the adrenal cortex), tumors that secrete corticotropin, potassium-losing diuretics, and increased use of adrenocorticoid hormones to treat hyperadrenocorticism or Cushing's syndrome.

Severe metabolic alkalosis (a pH above 7.6) usually results from a mixed metabolic and respiratory alkalosis.

Pathophysiology

In metabolic alkalosis, the proportion of base to acid increases by 20 to 1, indicating the presence of 20 bicarbonate ions for every hydrogen ion. A deficit of hydrogen ions and an excess of bicarbonate occurs because of excessive intake of sodium bicarbonate, gastric or intestinal loss of acid, renal excretion of hydrogen and chloride, or prolonged hypercalcemia. The normal compensatory mechanism is slow, shallow respirations that increase carbon dioxide levels and increase bicarbonate excretion and hydrogen reabsorption by the kidneys.

Complications
Untreated metabolic alkalosis may cause coma, atrioventricular arrhythmias, and death.

Assessment
History
Obtain the history from the patient or, if necessary, a family member. Stay alert for history data that suggest volume depletion (such as vomiting) or increased alkali ingestion (such as baking soda intake). Ask which medications the patient is taking, including OTC preparations. Find out if he has a history of endocrine problems. Note any recent CNS changes, as suggested by reports of irritability, disorientation, belligerence, or paresthesia.

Physical examination
Assess the patient's respiratory rate and depth. You may detect periods of apnea as the lungs try to compensate for the acid-base disturbance. Neuromuscular irritability and tetany may occur if the patient is hypocalcemic.

Evaluate the patient's LOC, which may range from apathy and confusion to stupor or coma as alkalosis worsens. Check for signs of hypokalemia — muscle weakness, arrhythmias, and decreased blood pressure.

Diagnostic tests
ABG values are the primary diagnostic tool. In *uncompensated* metabolic alkalosis, the pH rises above 7.45, the bicarbonate value exceeds 25 mEq/liter, and $PaCO_2$ is a normal 35 to 45 mm Hg. In *partially compensated* metabolic alkalosis, $PaCO_2$ exceeds 45 mm Hg. (See *Identifying the correct acid-base disturbance,* page 172.)

Serum electrolyte studies typically show abnormally low potassium, calcium, and chloride levels. An ECG may disclose a low T wave

EMERGENCY INTERVENTIONS

When your patient has metabolic alkalosis

Immediate interventions focus on correcting the underlying cause of metabolic alkalosis. Except in a patient with heart failure, the doctor will order sufficient I.V. infusion of 0.9% sodium chloride solution or lactated Ringer's solution so that the kidney can absorb sodium and chloride and excrete excess bicarbonate.

As ordered, administer electrolyte replacements with potassium chloride to treat hypokalemia and to enhance bicarbonate absorption. Discontinue diuretics if diuretic therapy caused the patient's metabolic alkalosis.

If rapid volume expansion is contraindicated, as in a patient with congestive heart failure, you may need to give oral or I.V. acetazolamide. However, acetazolamide may cause renal bicarbonate excretion and promote potassium depletion, so potassium supplementation should start before acetazolamide therapy begins.

Provide a safe environment, institute seizure precautions, and ensure the patient's comfort. Medicate for diarrhea and vomiting, if necessary.

merging with a P wave, along with atrial or sinus tachycardia.

Ongoing treatment
Medical measures focus on treating the underlying cause of metabolic alkalosis and restoring normal fluid and electrolyte balance. The doctor may order 0.9% sodium chloride solution to replace lost chloride, a carbonic anhydrase inhibitor to promote bicarbonate excretion, chloride or potassium chloride to treat electrolyte imbalances, and lactated Ringer's solution or 0.9% sodium chloride solution to treat hypokalemia. If the patient has renal dysfunction, dialysis may prevent bicarbonate clearance.

Identifying the correct acid-base disturbance

When assessing your patient for a possible acid-base disturbance, you must evaluate all pertinent factors—pH, partial pressure of arterial carbon dioxide ($Paco_2$), and bicarbonate (HCO_3^-) concentration. Otherwise, you may reach the wrong conclusion and carry out interventions that are ineffective—or even dangerous.

An acid-base imbalance triggers compensatory mechanisms that minimize pH changes and maintain a normal ratio of HCO_3^- to $Paco_2$. To return the pH to a normal or near-normal value, changes take place in the component (metabolic or respiratory) that's not primarily affected by the imbalance.

When Eileen Bickel, age 44, arrived in the emergency department, nurse Heather Springfield had to consider all of these factors when trying to identify her patient's problem.

Collecting the data
Ms. Bickel had a 3-day history of nausea, malaise, headache, and a fever of 101° F (38.3° C). She'd been vomiting for the last 12 hours and had been unable to eat or drink anything for at least 24 hours. Her mucous membranes were dry and she had poor skin turgor. Heather obtained the following vital signs:
• blood pressure, 94/62 mm Hg (supine) and 80/60 mm Hg (sitting)
• heart rate, 118 beats/minute and irregular
• respirations, 8 breaths/minute, unlabored and shallow.

When reviewing Ms. Bickel's arterial blood gas electrolyte values, Heather noted the partial pressure of arterial oxygen and oxygen saturation levels, and then homed in on the abnormal values:
• elevated pH (7.51)
• above-normal $Paco_2$ (49 mm Hg)

• markedly elevated HCO_3^- level (38 mEq/liter)
• below-normal serum sodium level (130 mEq/liter)
• below-normal serum chloride level (95 mEq/liter)
• below-normal serum potassium level (3 mEq/liter).

Based on these results (especially the pH, $Paco_2$, and HCO_3^- values), Heather knew her patient had an acid-base disturbance. The next step was to determine which one.

Piecing together the puzzle
She recognized that Ms. Bickel's elevated pH indicated alkalosis. But was it respiratory or metabolic alkalosis? She knew that $Paco_2$ represents the acid component of acid-base balance, and Ms. Bickel's $Paco_2$ was elevated. But so was her HCO_3^- concentration, representing the base component. The increased $Paco_2$ corresponded with the increased pH.

Heather knew the HCO_3^- elevation could be a compensatory response to the increased $Paco_2$. However, she also was aware that an elevated pH reflects alkalosis rather than acidosis—and in respiratory alkalosis, the pH would be increased. So she concluded that Ms. Bickel had partially compensated metabolic alkalosis.

Gathering supportive evidence
Heather reviewed other findings that supported her conclusion. She thought about the effects of Ms. Bickel's persistent vomiting—most likely, it had caused loss of gastric secretions rich in hydrochloric acid. The loss of hydrogen ions presumably had led to the excess HCO_3^-, resulting in metabolic alkalosis. She also recalled that the patient was dehydrated and had below-normal serum chloride and potassium levels—findings consistent with metabolic alkalosis.

Ongoing nursing interventions
• Monitor the patient's vital signs at least every 30 minutes during the acute phase of metabolic alkalosis.
• Observe respirations carefully and maintain the patient in a position, generally on his side, that protects his airway. Reposition him at least every 2 hours. He may be hyperventilating and therefore at risk for hypoxemia and respiratory failure.
• Watch the ECG monitor for arrhythmias and tachycardia linked with hypokalemia.

• Carefully monitor fluid and electrolyte replacement therapy. Potassium may irritate the veins, causing phlebitis and severe arrhythmias if infused too rapidly. Use a volume-control I.V. pump at all times.

• Irrigate the nasogastric tube with 0.9% sodium chloride solution instead of plain water to prevent further loss of gastric secretions.

• Observe for tremor and muscle irritability.

• Institute seizure precautions. The patient is at risk for seizures because of CNS hyperirritability (increased alkalinity of the CNS fluid).

• Record intake and output to help evaluate fluid and electrolyte status.

• Monitor serum electrolyte and other laboratory values and report any changes.

• Evaluate the patient's response to therapy and notify the doctor if you detect poor tolerance.

• Assess the patient's LOC frequently. Never leave him unattended if he's delirious.

• Frequently orient the patient to the environment.

• To help ensure patient safety, keep the bed in a low position with the side rails up.

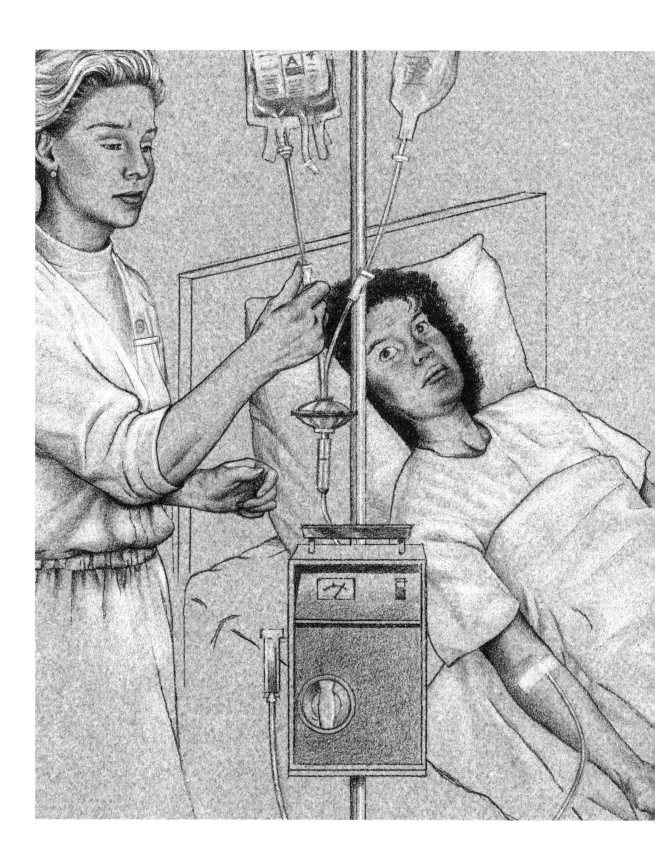

CHAPTER 6

Hematologic crises

Blood performs several vital functions within the body. The most important of these is transporting oxygen from the lungs to tissues and returning carbon dioxide from these same tissues to the lungs. Blood also produces and delivers antibodies, protects the body against viruses and cancer cells through sensitized lymphocytes, and supplies complement—a group of immunologically important protein substances in plasma.

Given the importance of blood, any disruption in its circulation or the structure of its components can have severe consequences and may cause a hematologic crisis—a life-threatening condition that requires prompt medical treatment.

This chapter focuses on two of the more common hematologic crises you're likely to encounter: sickle-cell crisis and disseminated intravascular coagulation (DIC). A red blood cell (RBC) disorder, sickle-cell crisis is a periodic exacerbation of a chronic condition. DIC, a coagulation disorder that arises as a complication of a preexisting condition or treatment, tends to develop insidiously in critically ill patients, with subtle signs and symptoms that may make it difficult to diagnose.

Besides describing the possible causes, emergency interventions, and complications of sickle-cell crisis and DIC, this chapter explains the underlying pathophysiology of these disorders. It also describes assessment—patient history, physical examination, and related diagnostic tests—and details ongoing treatment and nursing interventions that must follow to ensure the best possible outcome for your patient.

Sickle-cell crisis

Sickle-cell crisis is an acute, periodic exacerbation occurring in people with sickle cell anemia. In this inherited, incurable form of anemia, hemoglobin structure is abnormal. The defective hemoglobin molecule (hemoglobin S) reduces the oxygen-carrying capacity of RBCs and induces intravascular removal of mutant RBCs.

During a sickle-cell crisis, RBCs become sickle shaped, causing vessel obstruction and serious clinical complications. Types of sickle-cell crises include vaso-occlusive (the most common), anemic, aplastic, acute sequestration, and hemolytic.

Sickle-cell crisis can be fatal if sufficient RBCs are dysfunctional and can't carry adequate oxygen—or when major thromboses occur. To cope with this emergency, you must take rapid action. (See *When your patient suffers a sickle-cell crisis.*)

Causes
Sickle-cell *crisis* results from severe RBC sickling and obstruction of the vascular tree. Sickle cell *anemia* results from homozygous inheritance of the hemoglobin S—producing gene, which causes substitution of the amino acid valine for glutamic acid in the beta hemoglobin chain. In homozygous inheritance, the patient inherits the gene positive for the trait from both parents. Heterozygous inheritance (one normal gene from one parent and one sickle-cell gene from the other parent) leads to sickle-cell *trait,* a condition that usually shows no (or minimal) symptoms or causes minor health problems. The patient with sickle-cell trait is a carrier.

Sickle-cell disease is most common in people of African, southern European, and Middle Eastern descent, and may be endemic in areas where the heterozygous sickle-cell trait provides natural protection against malaria. Roughly 10% of African-Americans carry the sickle-cell gene, and 1 in every 400 to 600 African-American children has sickle cell anemia. If two carriers have offspring, each of their children has a 1 in 4 chance of inheriting the disease.

In a patient with sickle cell anemia, a crisis may result from the following conditions:
• decreased oxygen tension of the blood
• reduced arterial hydrogen ion concentration (decreased pH)
• increased plasma osmolarity
• diminished plasma volume.

Specific precipitators of *vaso-occlusive crisis* include extreme cold, hemorrhage, dehydration, excessive exercise, infection, respiratory disorders (including asthma and upper or lower respiratory tract infections), and tissue hypoxia (for example, from myocardial infarction, peripheral vascular disease, and trauma). (See *Common causes of sickle-cell crisis,* page 178.)

Anemic crisis results from bone marrow aplasia, increased hemolysis (cell destruction), folate deficiency, or splenic sequestration of RBCs. *Aplastic (megaloblastic) crisis* stems from bone marrow depression associated with infection (usually viral) or rapid RBC turnover. Such depression occurs because sickle cell anemia reduces the RBC life span to 10 to 20 days from the usual 100 to 120 days. Normal compensatory responses replenish the RBC supply through accelerated erythropoiesis but can become exhausted by the constant challenge.

In *acute sequestration crisis,* which typically occurs in infants ages 8 months to 2 years, massive numbers of RBCs suddenly become entrapped in the spleen and liver, and infarction develops rapidly. Acute abdominal symptoms

EMERGENCY INTERVENTIONS

When your patient suffers a sickle-cell crisis

If you suspect that your patient has a sickle-cell crisis, establish I.V. access and administer oxygen immediately. You may need to do this even before the doctor evaluates the patient's oxygenation status through arterial blood gas analysis. In a severe crisis, the patient may require endotracheal intubation.

Assess the patient for signs of organ decompensation or failure before beginning any treatment. For example, a patient with chest pain may require nitrates or vasodilators, whereas one in respiratory distress may benefit more from bronchodilators. If your findings suggest life-threatening complications, you'll need to set priorities for interventions quickly.

Fluid resuscitation

Focus on fluid resuscitation – the top priority for managing sickle-cell crisis. Blood hyperviscosity and sickling worsen the hypoxia that stimulated the crisis initially. For this reason, fluid resuscitation is the key intervention. Besides diluting sickled cells, volume expansion enhances tissue perfusion and counteracts tissue hypoxia.

Expect to give an isotonic solution, such as 0.9% sodium chloride solution, at an initial rate of 200 to 500 ml/hour. As the patient's volume status normalizes, taper the infusion as ordered. Be sure to monitor fluid administration carefully because sickle-cell crisis may lead to heart failure.

RBC transfusions

To improve the patient's oxygenation status, you may need to transfuse red blood cells (RBCs) after fluid resuscitation, although this rarely is done initially. Transfusions are especially important if the patient has lost RBC volume through sickling and removal by the liver or spleen.

Other measures

Try to anticipate and monitor the patient for disease progression and evaluate his response to treatment.

Be sure to provide emotional support throughout your interventions. Take measures to reduce pain, anxiety, and stress – conditions that worsen hypoxia and sickling and increase the work of breathing.

To manage pain and anxiety, give prescribed narcotics and anxiolytics (such as benzodiazepines). Enforce complete bed rest and give antipyretics, as ordered. You also may use nonpharmacologic methods, such as relaxation exercises, deep breathing, and music.

---

also arise. This crisis nearly always occurs with a sickling crisis and may be fatal if unrecognized. It carries a 50% mortality from cardiovascular collapse related to acute loss of blood.

Hemolytic crisis, which is rare, occurs in patients with glucose-6-phosphate dehydrogenase deficiency. It probably results from complications of sickle cell anemia, such as infection, rather than from the disease itself.

Pathophysiology

During hypoxia, the abnormal hemoglobin S molecule becomes insoluble. RBCs then become rigid, rough, and elongated, forming a crescent or sickle shape. Sickled RBCs can't travel through the microcirculation and tend to plug the vessels, causing occlusion, pain, and tissue ischemia beyond the occlusion site. Sickling also may cause hemolysis.

The degree of hypoxia inducing this response, the percentage of sickled RBCs, and sickling reversibility differ from one person to another. Patients with severe disease may have sickling when the partial pressure of arterial oxygen (PaO_2) is 60 mm Hg, whereas others require a PaO_2 of 45 mm Hg. In some patients, many circulating RBCs sickle, whereas in others, only a few do. Sickling reversibility may depend partly on the degree and duration of hypoxia as well as on individual physiologic differences.

Sickled cells have the potential to revert to a normal state when oxygenation is restored.

Common causes of sickle-cell crisis

In a patient with sickle cell anemia, a crisis may result from conditions or precipitating factors that decrease arterial pH or oxygen tension, impair tissue perfusion, increase plasma osmolarity, or reduce plasma volume. This chart lists specific factors.

CAUSE	PRECIPITATING FACTORS
Decreased arterial oxygen tension	• High altitude • Respiratory infections • Chronic obstructive pulmonary disease • Pulmonary embolism • Anemia
Poor tissue perfusion	• Peripheral vascular disease • Cardiac disease (angina, myocardial infarction) • Hypotension • Vasoconstrictive drugs
Decreased arterial pH	• Septic shock • Drug overdose causing decreased respirations with hypercarbia • Obstructive lung disease • Neurologic disease resulting in reduced respiratory drive and hypoventilation with hypercarbia
Increased plasma osmolarity	• Dehydration • Excessive exercise • Diabetes insipidus • Hyperglycemia
Reduced plasma volume	• Hemorrhage • Excessive diuretics • Excessive heat

However, those with irreversible plasma membrane damage can't return to normal and subsequently are transported to the spleen and hemolyzed. Abnormal and excessive RBC hemolysis leads to anemia and hyperbilirubinemia. Reduced PaO_2 causes cellular hypoxia, stagnant blood flow, and blood hyperviscosity, resulting in the circulation of sickled RBCs. Cellular hypoxia triggers cellular acidosis and, finally, tissue ischemia. Pain occurs from tissue ischemia and blood hyperviscosity.

During initial sickling episodes (usually in childhood), the spleen is enlarged and tender. However, nearly all victims eventually suffer autosplenectomy, in which frequent splenic infarctions with thrombosis cause such extensive splenic damage and scarring that the spleen progressively shrinks, becoming nontender, nonpalpable, and nonfunctional. If splenic infarction occurs gradually, the body can adjust to diminished spleen function and avoid acute decompensation.

Complications

Sickle-cell crisis may lead to life-threatening thrombosis, hemorrhagic diathesis, uncontrolled infection (from circulatory stasis), and multisystem effects.

Cerebral infarction with hemiplegia is the most common complication, although myocardial infarction, pulmonary embolism, and cerebrovascular accident are more dangerous. Thrombosis in the bowel, joints, and peripheral vessels may cause serious tissue necrosis, severe pain, and an increased risk of infection. Hemorrhagic diathesis results from ruptured vessels secondary to thromboses or coagulopathy related to hyperbilirubinemia.

Multisystem infections are common because autosplenectomy makes the patient prone to infection with encapsulated organisms. To prevent these infections, most patients with sickle cell anemia must receive immunizations against pneumococcus, tuberculosis, and *Haemophilus influenza*. Many also require prophylactic penicillin to prevent potentially fatal streptococcal infections.

Less severe complications of sickle-cell crisis include frequent retinal thromboses, which may cause retinal hemorrhage or detachment and blindness, and chronic hemolysis, which leads to gallstones with cholecystitis. In a child, frequent sickling episodes may result in painful, swollen joints. With age, joint infarction and arthritic changes eventually occur. Later, the patient may suffer aseptic necrosis (particularly of the head of the femur) or salmonella osteomyelitis of the joint, necessitating joint replacement surgery.

Assessment
History
The patient who suffers a sickle-cell crisis typically reports a sudden, severe pain in the chest, abdomen, back, hand, or foot; headache and optical problems; aching joint pain; in-

creased weakness; and dyspnea. Ask if he experienced a typical precipitating event, such as a recent infection or illness, exposure to cold, or generalized life stress. Suspect sickle-cell crisis if the patient complains of shortness of breath, a symptom of hypoxia brought on by a decrease in RBCs.

To help evaluate sickle-cell crisis, ask if the patient or family has a history of sickle-cell disease or trait. When investigating a suspected crisis episode, ask the patient or family to describe other crises the patient has experienced, the treatment he received, and the outcome. Some diagnosed patients have had extensive testing and can identify their threshold PaO_2 for sickling or know which situations typically cause a crisis.

If the patient has no known history of sickle-cell crises, ask about a history of protracted abdominal pain, joint pain with swelling, jaundice, and chronic respiratory infections. Investigate the family history for childhood and young adult deaths, and ask if any young family members have had joint swelling or heart or lung problems.

Physical examination
Suspect sickle-cell crisis if you detect typical signs and symptoms of cardiopulmonary compromise in a patient with suggestive history data. Usually, a patient in crisis has yellow sclerae and pallor evident in the lips, tongue, palms, or nail beds. He seems lethargic, irritable, or sleepy. With infection (which may have precipitated the crisis), you may detect a fever, productive cough, dyspnea, and tachypnea.

Assess the patient's vital signs, staying alert for an altered breathing pattern and a temperature above 104° F (40° C). A fever that persists for 2 days or longer also suggests infection. Palpate for an enlarged liver or spleen.

Distinct physical findings are associated with certain types of sickle-cell crisis. For example, with vaso-occlusive crisis, you may detect jaundice, dark urine, and a low-grade fever. After the crisis subsides (4 days to several weeks), infection may develop, causing lethargy, sleepiness, fever, or apathy. Aplastic crisis (usually associated with infection) may cause pallor, lethargy, sleepiness, dyspnea, and possibly coma. With acute sequestration crisis, expect lethargy and pallor; with hemolytic crisis, expect increased jaundice and hepatomegaly.

Between crises, patients with sickle cell anemia may seem to lead a normal life-style. However, nearly all are susceptible to heart failure, respiratory compromise, and infections. Adults usually have complications stemming from organ infarction, such as retinopathy and nephropathy. To assess the degree of organ damage caused by the underlying disease, perform a complete examination of all body systems.

Evaluate the patient's cardiovascular status by checking for heart gallops or murmurs, abnormal heart rate or rhythm, elevated blood pressure, lateral shifting of the point of maximal impulse from the fifth intercostal space to the midclavicular line, elevated jugular vein pulsations (more than 3/4″ [2 cm] above the clavicle), peripheral edema, and pulmonary crackles at end-inspiration. These findings signal heart failure and may become severe during sickle-cell crisis. They also may occur in patients with repeated minor sickling episodes.

To assess the patient's respiratory status, analyze his respiratory effort, auscultate breath sounds, and inspect the skin and mucous membranes for cyanosis. Use pulse oximetry to measure oxygen saturation.

Inspect the patient's build. A child with sickle cell anemia typically is small for his age and has delayed puberty. If he reaches adulthood, his body tends to be spiderlike with narrow shoulders and hips, long arms and legs, a curved spine, a barrel chest, and an elongated skull.

Diagnostic tests
Definitive diagnosis of sickle-cell crisis is usually confirmed by a stained blood smear showing sickled RBCs. In a patient who hasn't been previously diagnosed, the doctor orders hemoglobin electrophoresis and arterial blood gas (ABG) analysis to evaluate oxygenation. (Pulse oximetry may yield inaccurate results because of the abnormal hemoglobin structure, circulat-

Diagnostic findings in sickle-cell crisis

This chart lists abnormal diagnostic findings in patients with sickle-cell crisis and describes the cause of each abnormality.

TEST	RESULT	CAUSE
ABG analysis		
pH	Low	Microthrombi block circulation, promoting anaerobic metabolism and acidosis.
Partial pressure of arterial oxygen	Low	Abnormal hemoglobin causes red blood cell (RBC) lysis, decreasing oxygen-carrying capacity; microthrombi reduce oxygen circulation and gas exchange.
Bicarbonate	Low	Microthrombi block circulation, promoting anaerobic metabolism and acidosis.
Blood chemistry		
Bilirubin (indirect)	Increased	Excessive indirect bilirubin (an RBC breakdown product) overwhelms the liver's conjugating mechanism.
Blood urea nitrogen	Elevated	Serum levels increase when RBCs (protein molecules) are lysed.
Creatinine	Elevated	Microthrombi block renal circulation, causing nephron damage and inability to clear creatinine.
Blood count		
Hematocrit and hemoglobin counts	Decreased	RBCs are sickled or permanently destroyed.
Mean corpuscular hemoglobin	Decreased	Abnormal hemoglobin reduces hemoglobin concentration in RBCs.
Platelet count	Decreased	Platelets are destroyed by microthrombi in the microvasculature.
RBC count	Decreased	RBCs are sickled or permanently destroyed.
Reticulocyte count	Increased	Reticulocytes (early RBC precursors) are released from bone marrow early to compensate for RBC loss.
Other tests		
Erythrocyte sedimentation rate	Increased	Sickled cells don't settle in a column as rapidly as normal RBCs.
Total serum iron	Increased	RBC hemolysis causes increased RBC turnover with resulting increases in free iron.

ing sickled cells, and tissue hypoxia.)

Serum lactate analysis also helps measure tissue oxygenation. Lactic acid forms during anaerobic metabolism in conditions of tissue hypoxia, such as RBC sickling. *Note:* Although arterial pH and bicarbonate values can identify acidosis, they won't reflect lactic acidosis caused by anaerobic metabolism.

A complete blood count (CBC) helps determine the severity of the crisis by evaluating hemoglobin levels, hematocrit, white blood cell count, RBC count, RBC morphology, and RBC indices.

Other tests used for this purpose include a reticulocyte count and an erythrocyte sedimentation rate.

To investigate for organ damage, the doctor may measure levels of serum bilirubin, serum electrolytes (especially potassium, phosphate, and uric acid, which are all released from lysed cells), blood urea nitrogen, and creatinine and may test liver function. The serum bilirubin level commonly is elevated in sickle-cell crisis, reflecting accelerated RBC turnover that exceeds the liver's ability to conjugate and remove bilirubin. Even patients without bilirubin elevations or visible jaundice may have increased urobilinogen in the urine and dark stools. Electrocardiography and chest X-ray also aid diagnosis of organ damage.

Because sickle-cell crisis causes a wide spectrum of abnormal diagnostic results, assessing the severity of a crisis may pose a challenge. (See *Diagnostic findings in sickle-cell crisis*.) Yet the range of diagnostic abnormalities and the severity of the patient's pain don't necessarily reflect the severity of the crisis. Observing the patient for organ failure, thromboses, and hemorrhage is the best method of determining the severity of the crisis.

Ongoing treatment

Oxygen is the most important pharmacologic agent used to manage sickle-cell crisis: Unless tissue oxygenation improves, sickling will persist. Oxygen therapy, initiated during emergency treatment, will continue during the recuperative phase until the patient's oxygen saturation exceeds 97%. (PaO_2 may vary with the acid-base status, partial pressure of arterial carbon dioxide, and body temperature. Therefore, PaO_2 isn't the major factor in determining how much oxygen to administer.) Some patients will return home with oxygen to use periodically or to have on standby.

After the patient is somewhat stabilized, medical treatment involves careful management of fluid and circulatory status. Achieving normal fluid volume may pose a particular challenge if the patient has heart failure.

Expect the doctor to order crystalloid solutions. RBC transfusions usually aren't given until the sickling has been stabilized because they may increase blood viscosity and osmolarity, increasing sickling. However, the patient with significant RBC hemolysis or anemia (from loss of RBC mass) will require RBC transfusions. The doctor will augment transfusions with oral iron and folic acid supplements to enhance growth of functional RBCs, as needed. Physical findings and liver function tests must be monitored daily for 1 to 7 days to assess whether the patient can manage the excess cellular wastes.

Drug treatment
During treatment, rapid RBC turnover may lead to elevated bilirubin levels, hyperkalemia, hyperphosphatemia, and signs of liver failure. To treat hyperkalemia, the doctor may prescribe sodium polystyrene sulfonate; to treat hyperphosphatemia, he may order phosphate-binding agents. To prevent infection caused by stagnant blood flow and thromboses within organs, he may order broad-spectrum antibiotics.

The patient also requires analgesics to reduce the severe, prolonged pain of sickle-cell crisis. Narcotics are preferred because they are highly effective against somatic pain. However, a patient with mild thromboses and coagulopathy may receive nonsteroidal anti-inflammatory drugs. These agents interfere with clotting and thus pose some risk of spontaneous bleeding. Expect the doctor to order acetaminophen rather than aspirin, which may promote acidosis and worsen sickling. Some patients benefit from patient-controlled analgesia.

Antisickling agents are still in the experimental stage. Drugs currently under investigation for this use include carbamylphosphate, sodium cyanate, and urea. Vasodilatory agents eventually may be used to treat sickle-cell crisis because they enhance blood flow through the microvasculature. However, experts haven't made specific recommendations for their use.

Surgery
The patient with acute sequestration crisis or an enlarged, tender liver accompanied by coagulopathy or thrombocytopenia usually benefits from a therapeutic splenectomy. Removing the spleen eliminates the organ that sensitizes and removes both normal and abnormal RBC components. However, this procedure is performed only if the patient has significant refractory symptoms, such as acute abdominal sepsis or refractory thrombocytopenia.

Before surgery, the patient needs extensive preparation because the procedure and the anesthetic may precipitate a sickle-cell crisis. The doctor may order a series of preoperative exchange transfusions to replace defective RBCs. He'll also order additional oxygen and carefully regulate the patient's vascular volume status.

Ongoing nursing interventions
Nursing responsibilities for the patient who is stabilized and recovering from sickle-cell crisis include ensuring adequate fluid balance and oxygenation, monitoring for complications, avoiding disease exacerbation, and evaluating the patient's response to therapy.

As the patient recovers, ask him and his family to help you devise a plan that balances care with rest and individualized activities. To enhance his well-being, encourage family members to participate in the patient's care, such as by bringing favorite foods from home.

Ensuring fluid balance and oxygenation
• To assess the patient's fluid status, closely monitor hematologic and serum electrolyte tests, intake and output, and daily weight. If a central venous line is in place, obtain central venous pressure measurements.
• To avoid hypoxia and consequent sickling, monitor the patient's arterial and tissue oxygenation status frequently through ABG analysis, pulse oximetry, serum lactate levels, and

Monitoring your patient during sickle-cell crisis

During a sickle-cell crisis, your patient is at risk for many potentially fatal complications. In the earliest hours, when sickling is worst, you must assess your patient thoroughly to uncover early signs and symptoms of complications. The following chart covers the body systems at risk, and how often you should check vital indicators within each.

BODY SYSTEM	ASSESSMENT FREQUENCY
Cardiovascular	
Vital signs	Hourly
Skin color and capillary refill	Every 1 to 2 hours
Pulses	Every 4 to 8 hours
Heart sounds	Every 4 to 8 hours
Fluid balance indicators, such as intake and output and central venous pressure	Every 4 to 8 hours
GI	
Abdominal size and tenderness	Every 4 to 8 hours
Bowel sounds	Every 4 to 8 hours
Neurologic	
Orientation	Every 1 to 2 hours
Ability to move all body parts on command	Every 1 to 2 hours
Cognitive functioning, such as counting, memory, and calculating	Every 2 to 4 hours
Pupillary response	Every 4 to 8 hours
Renal	
Urine output	Every 1 to 2 hours
Respiratory	
Oxygenation indicators, such as dyspnea, skin color, and mentation	Every 1 to 2 hours
Breath sounds	Every 4 to 8 hours
Skin and mucous membranes	
Total body, checking for decreased perfusion	Every 8 hours
Extremities, checking color, capillary refill, and integrity	Every 4 to 8 hours

cardiopulmonary assessment.
• To promote tissue oxygenation, use such measures as early mobility, coughing and deep breathing, frequent position changes, adequate rest periods, and optimal nutrition. If ordered and appropriate, continue to administer oxygen.
• Assess all body systems frequently for signs and symptoms of reduced oxygenation or circulatory impairment.

Monitoring for complications
• Frequently assess all body systems to help detect complications early. (See *Monitoring your patient during sickle-cell crisis*.)
• Take appropriate measures to prevent infection. Monitor the patient continuously for signs and symptoms of infection.

Avoiding disease exacerbation
• Avoid known precipitators and risk factors for sickle-cell crisis. For instance, manage continuous oxygen administration, enforce bed rest, instruct the patient to avoid exertion, ensure adequate I.V. fluids, control environmental temperature, and administer prescribed anxiolytics, pain medication, and antibiotics.
• Investigate and treat all complaints of pain. The physiologic and emotional stress brought on by pain exacerbates physical stress-related responses—tachycardia, chest tightness, dyspnea, and vasoconstriction. These, in turn, may increase the risk of sickling.
   Be aware that pain may occur separately from other clinical evidence of sickling. It is uncertain whether the pain associated with sickle-cell crisis is unrelated to the sickling of RBCs or if the pain indicates a low-level crisis.
• Titrate analgesic dosages to the patient's reported pain level to reduce or eliminate pain, which may worsen the sickling process.

Evaluating the response to therapy
• Monitor the patient's renal function closely and adjust antibiotic dosages as needed and ordered.
• Monitor potassium levels closely, since hyperkalemia may occur during a sickle-cell crisis. To assess the response to therapy, monitor diagnostic tests that reveal continued sickling, such

as reticulocyte count, RBC morphology, bilirubin measurement, and ABG analysis.

Providing patient teaching
• To compensate for abnormal hemoglobin production, the patient may need lifelong RBC precursor nutrients, such as B vitamins and iron. To promote compliance with therapy, explain the rationale for these medications and how to avoid adverse reactions. For instance, if the patient must take iron supplements, teach him how to avoid constipation by following a high-fiber diet and how to offset their unpleasant taste by taking them with food.
• Inform the patient that he'll require periodic CBCs with RBC monitoring even after the crisis ends. Emphasize that these tests will help identify such conditions as slow, continuous sickling, nutrition-related anemias, and altered fluid status.
• Teach the patient how to prevent infection as he performs his activities of daily living. Instruct him to wear gloves when gardening, avoid tight clothing, always wear shoes to prevent inadvertent injury, get vaccinations as recommended, abstain from smoking, and seek prompt medical attention for respiratory and oropharyngeal infections.
• To help prevent future crises, teach the patient to avoid both obvious and subtle conditions that may trigger sickle-cell crisis. For example, caution him to avoid temperature extremes, excessive exercise, dehydration, unpressurized aircraft, and high altitudes.

Disseminated intravascular coagulation

An acquired coagulation disorder causing life-threatening ischemia and bleeding, DIC represents dysfunctional compensation by the body. Abnormal activation of the coagulation cascade and accelerated fibrinolysis cause thrombosis and hemorrhage at the same time.

This extremely complex multisystem disorder carries a high mortality (50% to 80%). Many patients who survive the immediate crisis remain ill for a prolonged period. Be sure you know which actions to take to avert a crisis. (See *When your patient has DIC,* page 184.)

Causes
DIC occurs secondarily to other disorders and conditions that accelerate clotting. The most common precipitators are tissue or vessel injuries, or a foreign body in the patient's bloodstream. Tissue injuries include trauma, burns, major surgery (such as bowel surgery), organ failure (liver, kidney, or heart), adult respiratory distress syndrome, neoplastic disease, placenta previa, and graft-versus-host disease. Vessel injuries include sepsis, vasculitis, and diabetic ketoacidosis. Foreign body precipitators include amniotic fluid embolism, gram-negative endotoxins, pulmonary embolism, sickle cell anemia (sickled RBCs), snake and insect venom, and transfusion reactions (hemolyzed RBCs). (See *How DIC affects blood clots,* page 185.)

Pathophysiology
In DIC, the typical accelerated clotting leads to generalized activation of prothrombin and a resulting excess of thrombin. Excessive thrombin causes conversion of fibrinogen to fibrin, producing fibrin clots in the microcirculation. This process consumes exorbitant amounts of coagulation factors (especially fibrinogen, prothrombin, platelets, and factors V and VIII), causing hypofibrinogenemia, hypoprothrombinemia, thrombocytopenia, and deficiencies in factors V and VIII. Circulating thrombin activates the fibrinolytic system, which lyses fibrin clots into fibrin degradation products (FDPs). Hemorrhage results mainly from the anticoagulant activity of FDPs as well as from depletion of coagulation factors.

Excessive clotting in the microcirculation also causes vessel thrombosis with tissue ischemia, which leads to vascular damage and results in hypoxia and shock. Clotting continues even as clots are lysed, resulting in thrombi and hemorrhage at the same time in different parts of the body.

(Text continues on page 186.)

When your patient has DIC

The first priority in treating a patient with disseminated intravascular coagulation (DIC) is preserving organ function during acute thrombosis or hemorrhage. Both thrombosis and hemorrhage are potentially fatal and require different treatment strategies.

Restoring vascular volume

The doctor will order measures aimed at restoring adequate vascular volume, which will promote perfusion beyond the clots and replace volume lost through bleeding. Be prepared to administer blood products, including red blood cells (RBCs), to improve tissue oxygenation and fluid volume. To further enhance tissue oxygenation and reduce necrosis, he'll probably order oxygen therapy.

However, the doctor won't order such volume expanders without concomitant coagulation products, such as fresh frozen plasma or platelets, if your patient has abnormal coagulation. If a coagulopathy exists when RBCs are given, the patient will continue to bleed from susceptible sites. A few doctors suspect that administering platelets, fresh frozen plasma, or cryoprecipitate may feed the clotting disorder. However, most doctors advocate administering these agents while correcting the underlying disorder.

Caring for the patient with DIC is extremely challenging even for the most experienced nurse. You may have difficulty monitoring and regulating the multiple I.V. fluids and blood products the patient needs. Nursing priorities include monitoring the patient's fluid volume status through central venous pressure or pulmonary artery pressure monitoring, measuring intake and output, obtaining vital signs, and assessing his cardiopulmonary status.

Before giving a blood product transfusion, always verify that it has been typed and cross-matched. Also be sure to use the appropriate filter. Carefully coordinate administration of blood products with that of other I.V. fluids and drugs.

Stay alert for transfusion reactions, and plan for premedication with antihistamines (such as diphenhydramine) and antipyretics (such as acetaminophen) to prevent minor febrile or allergic reactions. If you've administered large amounts of blood products, be sure to monitor for signs of congestive heart failure and respiratory failure.

Treating clotting abnormalities

If your patient receives multiple RBC transfusions, he's likely to suffer clotting abnormalities and will need platelets, fresh frozen plasma, and cryoprecipitate. The doctor will also consider treating adverse effects of banked blood, such as hyperkalemia, hypocalcemia, acidosis, and hypothermia.

Treating the underlying cause

Another medical priority is to identify and treat the underlying cause of the disorder. If it goes untreated, the clotting stimulus will continue despite supportive therapy and replacement of RBCs and clotting factors.

A thrombin inhibitor may be used to impede the pathophysiologic mechanisms responsible for microvascular clotting and clotting factor consumption. Heparin, the most commonly used thrombin inhibitor, also reduces platelet agglutination. Although its use in managing DIC is controversial, it remains a logical therapeutic option when the disorder is still in a thrombotic stage. Closely monitor your patient during administration of a thrombin inhibitor. And remember that heparin doesn't lyse existing clots, so its benefits won't be evident for several days.

Managing bleeding sites

You may be able to control bleeding at least partially by applying local pressure or a topical hemostatic agent (such as topical thrombin).

Avoid ice and vasoconstrictive agents because they potentiate the circulatory impairment caused by clotting.

How DIC affects blood clots

In disseminated intravascular coagulation (DIC), overabundant anticoagulant factors destroy red blood cells (RBCs) and dissolve a stable clot in an arteriole.

Normal clotting

In a normal clot, a group of substances known as prothrombin activator is formed in response to vessel rupture. Prothrombin activator converts prothrombin into thrombin, and thrombin converts fibrinogen to fibrin to form a clot of platelets, RBCs, and plasma.

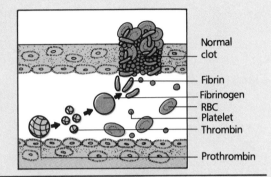

Normal clot
Fibrin
Fibrinogen
RBC
Platelet
Thrombin
Prothrombin

Clotting in DIC

In typical accelerated clotting, prothrombin activation results in an excess of thrombin. Excessive thrombin converts fibrinogen to fibrin, producing fibrin clots in the microcirculation.

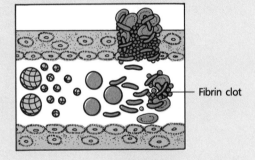

Fibrin clot

The circulating thrombin activates the fibrinolytic system, which lyses fibrin clots into fibrin degradation products (FDPs), causing hemorrhage.

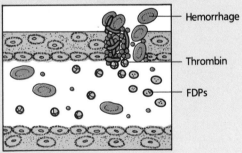

Hemorrhage

Thrombin

FDPs

Excessive clotting in the microcirculation also causes vessel thrombosis with tissue ischemia. Clotting continues as clots are lysed, resulting in thrombi and hemorrhage.

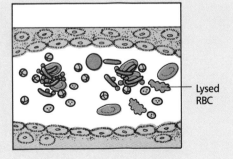

Lysed RBC

Complications

Because DIC involves simultaneous thrombosis and hemorrhage, it may cause a wide range of complications. Although recent advances in treatment have increased the survival rate after the acute life-threatening event, many patients later die of multisystem organ failure. (See Chapter 7, Multisystem crises.)

Thrombotic complications typically stem from tissue ischemia and organ damage. They include hypoxemia, pulmonary embolism, cerebral infarction, myocardial infarction, bowel infarction, splenic infarction, acute renal failure, peripheral thrombi or emboli, and tissue necrosis or gangrene. If microcirculatory clots don't resolve before significant cell death occurs, shock ensues, followed by organ failure.

Clot lysis and the anticoagulant effects of FDPs predispose the patient to bleeding from breaks in barrier integrity or physiologically weak areas. For example, a patient with an existing peptic ulcer may have acute GI hemorrhage when clot lysis occurs. Other bleeding complications include cerebral hemorrhage (the most common cause of death in patients with DIC), retinal or scleral hemorrhage, pulmonary hemorrhage, pericardial tamponade, hypovolemic shock, and hemorrhagic cystitis.

The severity of bleeding symptoms varies widely, as does the reversibility of the effects. Some patients who survive DIC are plagued by complications related to thromboses, such as chronic renal failure requiring dialysis treatments or even amputation of extremities due to tissue necrosis or gangrene.

Assessment

History

DIC occurs mainly in acutely ill patients, so the medical record is a prime source of information. Check for a history of multiple physiologic injuries with the potential to trigger clotting. Also look for other precipitating conditions as well as disorders that may increase the risk of organ failure or hemorrhage in a specific body region.

Thrombotic complications of DIC tend to exacerbate existing or borderline organ dysfunction, causing ischemic tissue death followed by organ failure. Conditions likely to present as a hemorrhagic event when DIC occurs include previous head injury, arteriovenous malformation, aneurysm, diabetic retinopathy, sinusitis, cavitating pulmonary lesions, peptic ulcers, colitis, liver disease, and low platelet count.

Review the patient's health and medication history for disorders or drugs whose effects may mimic signs of DIC. Such disorders include liver disease, severe renal failure, bone marrow disease, and immune thrombocytopenia. Such drugs include antibiotics, anti-inflammatory agents, antiarrhythmics, and histamine blockers.

Physical examination

DIC causes a wide variety of signs and symptoms. Physical findings may range from subtle changes reflecting small-vessel thrombosis or hemorrhage to organ failure or acute hemorrhage with shock. Because clotting and bleeding are simultaneous, be sure to examine all body systems for changes reflecting bleeding and impaired circulation. (See *Physical findings in DIC*.)

Usually, you'll first detect skin and soft-tissue ischemia or bleeding. Coolness and mottling of the extremities or peripheral soft tissue, such as the earlobes and genitalia, may be among the first notable changes. You also may detect acrocyanosis — a clear demarcation between cool, cyanotic skin and normal warm, perfused skin. Scattered petechiae signal small-vessel damage, especially in dependent areas (such as the back and buttocks) or in places where pressure has been applied (for instance, under a blood pressure cuff). (See *Identifying DIC*, page 188.)

Because blood vessels are close to the external surface of mucous membranes, occult blood or minor bleeding from these surfaces in the oropharynx, GI tract, renal system, and vagina may occur early in DIC.

Early signs of DIC typically involve the neurologic, renal, and GI systems because blood shunts to these organs when blood flow diminishes. The brain is highly sensitive to hypoxia, producing symptoms even with relatively small reductions in blood flow. Check for

Physical findings in DIC

You may detect the following clinical abnormalities when assessing a patient with disseminated intravascular coagulation (DIC).

Skin
- Cool and moist
- Petechiae
- Ecchymoses
- Mottling

Eyes
- Blurred vision
- Intraocular hemorrhage

Nose and mouth
- Epistaxis
- Gangrene on tip of nose
- Bleeding gums

Ears
- Gangrene on earlobes
- Inner ear bleeding

Brain
- Confusion
- Irritability
- Headache
- Dizziness
- Fever
- Seizures
- Signs of increased intracranial pressure
- Hemiplegia
- Flat electroencephalogram (brain death)

Spinal cord
- Muscle weakness
- Diminished tendon reflex
- Fasciculations
- Diminished pain sensation
- Tremor

Heart
- Decreased blood return to heart (preload), as determined by pulmonary artery pressure (PAP) monitoring
- Increased pressure needed to pump against capillary clots (afterload), as determined by PAP monitoring
- Tachycardia
- Chest pain, irregular heartbeat, and decreased blood pressure from myocardial infarction or ischemia

Venous system
- Decreased blood pressure
- Bleeding from venipuncture sites or around I.V. insertion sites

Arterial system
- Absent or irregular pulse
- Bleeding from needles inserted into an artery

Lungs
- Hemoptysis
- Diffuse infiltrate on X-ray
- Chest pain (possibly indicating pulmonary embolism)
- Hypoxia
- Crackles
- Dyspnea
- Hemorrhage

GI system
- Occult blood in stool
- Severe pain and high-pitched bowel sounds, indicating mesenteric artery infarction
- Pain
- Nausea
- Vomiting

Kidneys
- Progressive oliguria
- Hematuria
- Failure

Genitalia
- Bleeding around indwelling catheters
- In a female, abnormally severe bleeding during menstruation and bleeding from vaginal mucous membranes

Fingers
- Cool, mottled skin
- Gangrene on fingertips
- Cyanosis

Legs
- Severe mottling of skin on lower legs
- Absent popliteal, posterior tibial, or pedal pulses
- Calf swelling
- Pain on foot dorsiflexion
- Blood pooling
- Acrocyanosis

Toes
- Cool, mottled skin
- Gangrene on tips of toes

Identifying DIC

An acquired disorder that causes ischemia and bleeding, disseminated intravascular coagulation (DIC) proves fatal at least half of the time. It can result from a wide range of conditions, and its signs and symptoms can be confusing and difficult to discern. Nevertheless, the health care team must identify DIC quickly and treat it appropriately to ensure the best possible outcome for the patient.

Consider, for example, the case of Marsha Ames, age 45, whose medical history made diagnosis particularly difficult.

Assessing the patient

Ms. Ames was admitted to the hospital with respiratory distress and a fever and placed in your care. You take her history and find that the respiratory distress began 3 days ago and has worsened. You also discover that Ms. Ames had a kidney transplant 8 months ago and has been receiving immunosuppressive therapy (azathioprine and cyclosporine) since the operation. Until now, she's had no problems; the kidney seems to have engrafted well and the patient hasn't required dialysis.

You obtain Ms. Ames's vital signs:
• temperature: 102.2° F (39° C)
• heart rate: 130 beats/minute
• respiratory rate: 36 breaths/minute
• blood pressure: 98/42 mm Hg.

Then you auscultate fine crackles and note that the patient is oriented but sleepy. When performing a head-to-toe assessment, you discover petechiae on the chest and abdomen and mottling and coolness of both feet to a well-marked line at midshin—classic signs of DIC. You also find mild gum bleeding and flushed skin.

After drawing blood for hematology, chemistry, and coagulation tests, you have trouble achieving hemostasis, and the laboratory report returns with the following results:
• white blood cell count: 12,200/mm³
• red blood cell (RBC) smear: fragmented platelets
• hematocrit: 32%
• hemoglobin: 10 mg/dl
• platelet count: 98,000/mm³
• prothrombin time (PT): 24 seconds
• partial thromboplastin time (PTT): 56 seconds
• fibrinogen: 178 mg/dl
• serum sodium: 148 mEq/liter
• serum chloride: 104 mEq/liter
• serum potassium: 4.4 mEq/liter
• serum glucose: 144 mg/dl
• blood urea nitrogen: 19 mg/dl
• creatinine: 1.2 mg/dl.

Establishing a diagnosis of DIC

You immediately alert the doctor to Ms. Ames's laboratory results and physical findings because you suspect that the patient is suffering not only from overwhelming infection due to transplant rejection but also from DIC. The doctor confirms your diagnosis of DIC.

To treat her condition, you begin by inserting an I.V. line and starting fluid volume resuscitation. You give her 5,000 units of heparin by I.V. bolus, followed by 1,000 units/hour of heparin I.V., and initiate oxygen therapy—3 liters/minute through a nasal cannula, as ordered. You also need to treat the underlying cause of DIC with antimicrobials.

Maintaining a close vigil

Over the next 3 days, you monitor Ms. Ames closely for signs and symptoms of bleeding or clotting complications. As ordered, you administer two units of packed RBCs and two units of fresh frozen plasma; then you monitor for therapeutic effects and transfusion reactions.

By the fourth day, Ms. Ames shows a good response to therapy. Her blood test results have returned to normal, with PT slowing to 14 seconds, PTT decreasing to 30 seconds, and the fibrinogen level dropping to 167 mg/dl.

You find her afebrile and note that all mottling and petechiae have disappeared and that her gum bleeding has stopped. As ordered, you wean her off heparin and begin discharge planning. Seven days after admission, Ms. Ames is discharged.

Conclusion

Luckily for Ms. Ames, your skillful nursing assessment uncovered the fact that although her history and physical findings suggested kidney rejection complications, she was also suffering from DIC. This assessment helped ensure expert treatment and the best possible prognosis for her.

subtle neurologic symptoms, such as sleepiness and changes in personality, attention span, and short-term memory.

Renal and GI signs of DIC include oliguria, reduced bowel sounds, abdominal distention, constipation, and bowel ischemia with abdominal pain. If circulatory impairment is prolonged, you may detect signs of acute renal failure, bowel infarction, and shock liver.

Hemorrhage and tissue ischemia may arise late in DIC. Once the disorder progresses to the point of massive hemorrhage refractory to blood transfusions, the patient is likely to die from bleeding.

Diagnostic tests
If clinical findings suggest DIC, the doctor will order laboratory coagulation tests, especially FDPs. To definitively diagnose DIC, he may test for d-dimer, a fibrin monomer whose presence indicates DIC. However, some hospitals lack the facilities to perform this new test.

A CBC may detect loss of platelets and RBC mass, possibly signaling consumption during clotting or bleeding. Platelets are the first cells to respond to injury when a clotting stimulus occurs, so a decrease in their circulating numbers may indicate DIC. However, the doctor usually rules out other possible causes of thrombocytopenia — sepsis, invasive lines, drugs, bone marrow suppression, and postviral syndrome — before diagnosing DIC based on the platelet count.

Routine coagulation tests, including prothrombin time (PT), partial thromboplastin time (PTT), and fibrinogen level, help assess deficiencies of coagulation factors made in the liver. In DIC, PT and PTT are prolonged as fewer clotting factors take a longer time to produce a clot. The fibrinogen level falls as fibrinogen is used to make clots. Thrombin time becomes prolonged, although this test is seldom used to help diagnose DIC because of its excessive sensitivity to circulating anticoagulants. The FDP level typically increases, indicating excessive clotting or diminished clot clearance by the liver. (See *Test findings in DIC.*)

To rule out other causes of abnormal coagulation test results, the doctor will investigate

Test findings in DIC

In disseminated intravascular coagulation (DIC), the laboratory tests listed here usually yield abnormal results.

TEST	NORMAL RESULT	RESULT IN D.I.C.
Antithrombin III	100%	Less than 70%
D-dimer	Positive at less than 1:8 dilution	Positive at greater than 1:8 dilution
Ethanol	Negative	Positive
Fibrin degradation products (FDPs)	Less than 10 mcg/ml or FDPs present at less than 1:100 dilution	Higher than 45 mcg/ml or FDPs present at greater than 1:100 dilution
Fibrinogen	170 to 400 mg/dl	Less than 170 mg/dl
Partial thromboplastin time	16 to 42 seconds	More than 42 seconds
Platelet count	150,000 to 400,000/mm³	Less than 150,000/mm³
Prothrombin time	16 to 19 seconds	More than 19 seconds
Red blood cell (RBC) morphology	Normal	Schistocytes
RBC count	4 to 8 million/mm³	Below normal
Reticulocytes	0% to 2% RBC count	Higher than 4% RBC count
Thrombin time	10 to 15 seconds	More than 19 seconds

for possible liver disease, vitamin K deficiency, and drug toxicity.

Ongoing treatment
After the patient has been somewhat stabilized, he'll require supportive care aimed at preventing life-threatening impairment of organ perfusion. Oxygen and fluids are administered to maintain tissue circulation, and all blood components (RBCs, platelets, fresh frozen plasma, cryoprecipitate) are given to replace consumed products. Careful monitoring of fluid volume, oxygenation, and hematologic and coagulatory stability must continue for at least 72 hours after initial treatment begins. Usually, some changes take place during this time.

To help ensure a complete recovery, the doctor will strive to prevent major thrombotic

Detecting transfusion reactions

If your patient is receiving blood product transfusions, stay alert for possible reactions. This table lists signs and symptoms of possible transfusion reactions.

REACTION	SIGNS AND SYMPTOMS
Acidosis	Bradycardia, heart block
Allergic reaction	Rash, itching, wheezing
Febrile reaction	Fever, chills, flushing
Hemolytic reaction	Pain at transfusion site, hypotension, dyspnea, chest pain
Hyperammonemia	Confusion, lethargy, combativeness
Hyperkalemia	Flaccid muscles, hyperactive bowel sounds, abdominal cramps, peaked T waves on electrocardiogram, ventricular arrhythmias
Hypocalcemia	Bradycardia, ventricular arrhythmias, tetany
Hypothermia	Decreased temperature, chills

or hemorrhagic complications. A patient with serious complications, such as cerebral hemorrhage, acute renal failure, or liver failure, requires additional medical consultations and reevaluation of treatment goals.

Drug treatment
The most common pharmacologic treatments for DIC are blood components and thrombin inhibitors, which are initiated during emergency intervention. The doctor also may prescribe drugs to prevent GI bleeding, such as histamine blockers, which reduce gastric acidity and decrease the risk of gastric ulcer. However, he'll choose a histamine blocker carefully because some of these agents interfere with platelet production.

Reduced immunoglobulin levels have been associated with poor platelet quality. To boost these levels, the doctor may prescribe I.V. immunoglobulin G. To increase levels of vitamin K, which promotes prothrombin synthesis by the liver, he may order vitamin K supplements. To promote RBC regeneration, he may order multivitamin and iron supplements.

The doctor also will evaluate the patient's medication history and discontinue any nonessential drugs that may have contributed to DIC.

Ongoing nursing interventions
Ongoing care for the patient with DIC primarily involves continuing emergency interventions, monitoring closely for complications, and evaluating his response to therapy. As the patient's condition improves, fewer blood products and fluids may need to be administered, giving you more time to focus on specific sites of ischemia or hematoma and resulting rehabilitation problems. Examples include hemorrhages causing blindness or limited joint motion and thromboses causing stroke or requiring amputation of extremities.
• To manage tissue ischemia (indicated by black, necrotic-appearing extremities), keep the patient warm and avoid vasoconstrictive agents and I.M. and S.C. injections.
• As ordered, administer prescribed drugs to prevent other bleeding complications, and monitor for adverse and desired drug effects.
• Focus on limiting tissue injury and preventing further insults.
• To prevent injury, enforce complete bed rest during bleeding episodes.
• To avoid dislodging clots and causing fresh bleeding, don't scrub bleeding areas. Use pressure, cold compresses, and topical hemostatic agents to control bleeding. Perform mouth care gently so as not to trigger fresh bleeding from the gums.
• Check I.V. and venipuncture sites for bleeding. Apply pressure to injection sites for at least 20 minutes. Alert other personnel to the patient's tendency to hemorrhage.
• To improve circulation, change the patient's position and perform range-of-motion exercises frequently. Use tape cautiously to prevent skin tearing and bleeding during its removal.
• Monitor intake and output hourly in acute

DIC, especially when administering blood products. Watch for transfusion reactions and signs of fluid overload. (See *Detecting transfusion reactions.*) To measure the amount of blood lost, weigh dressings and bed linen and record drainage. Weigh the patient daily, particularly if there is renal involvement.

• Watch for bleeding from the GI and genitourinary tracts. If you suspect intra-abdominal bleeding, measure the patient's abdominal girth at least every 4 hours and monitor closely for signs of shock.

• Monitor the results of serial blood studies, especially hematocrit, hemoglobin levels, and coagulation times.

• Explain all diagnostic tests and procedures. Allow time for questions.

• Provide emotional support to the patient and family. As needed, enlist the aid of a social worker and other members of the health care team in providing such support.

• As the patient gradually recovers and resumes his normal roles and responsibilities, schedule thorough follow-up assessment to check for residual effects of DIC, such as altered cognitive functioning, reduced visual acuity or blindness, and impotence.

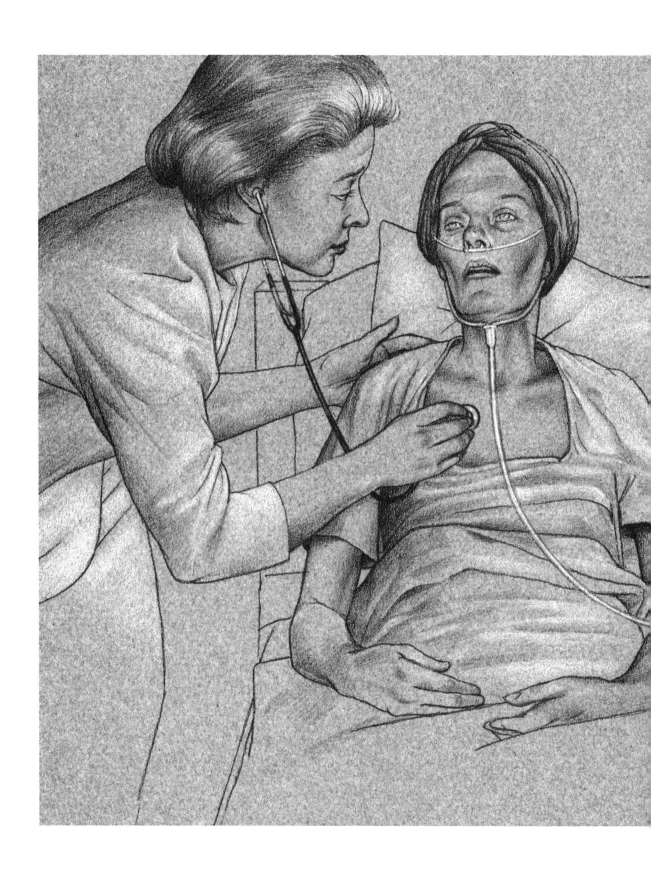

CHAPTER 7

Multisystem crises

The progressive failure of two or more organ systems, a multisystem crisis is a severe, life-threatening condition triggered by a mediator-driven response to critical injury or illness. Also called multisystem organ failure, it occurs in patients with perfusion deficits, persistent inflammation, and sepsis, and can therefore affect any patient with a critical illness or injury.

Multisystem organ failure is difficult to reverse and can be deadly. As a result, you must take all possible steps to prevent it in patients at risk. If it occurs despite the best efforts by you and the health care team, you'll need to provide intensive nursing care to save the patient's life.

This chapter can help you improve your patient's chances for surviving a multisystem crisis. It reviews multisystem organ failure in general and then as it occurs in patients with anaphylactic shock, septic shock, and cancer. Each of these conditions takes a different path to multisystem organ failure. You'll find out what causes multisystem organ failure, become familiar with the pathophysiology of these disorders, and learn how to provide appropriate care in an emergency and on an ongoing basis.

Multisystem organ failure

Multisystem organ failure occurs when such conditions as burns, multiple trauma, myocardial infarction (MI), and cancer cause injury leading to:
• stimulation of the sympathetic nervous system response
• damage to the endothelial lining of blood vessels
• activation of the inflammatory response.

These events trigger the release of substances called mediators into the bloodstream and tissues. In sepsis and multisystem organ failure, the key mediators are endotoxins, tumor necrosis factor, and interleukin-1.

Normally, mediators help the body withstand and recover from an injury. But after massive injury, their responses may go unchecked, with potentially disastrous consequences. (See *What happens in multisystem organ failure.*)

Pathophysiology

Regardless of the original illness, sepsis must be present for multisystem organ failure to occur. Endotoxins released by bacterial, viral, and fungal pathogens commonly cause adverse biochemical changes that indirectly affect vascular tissues and cellular metabolism. Each of these mediator types may potentiate inflammation by causing selective vasodilation and vasoconstriction. Besides damaging organs directly, a pathologic mediator response promotes organ dysfunction by inducing three major changes:
• maldistribution of circulating blood volume
• imbalance of oxygen supply and demand
• metabolic disturbances.

Maldistribution of circulating volume

Capillary permeability and vasodilation increase, causing vascular fluid to leak into tissues and pool in the periphery. As the body attempts to increase cardiac and cerebral perfusion, blood vessels in the pulmonary, renal, and splanchnic beds constrict in response to sympathetic nervous system activation (caused by catecholamines and certain other mediators). Pulmonary vascular resistance rises, causing pulmonary hypertension. Renal blood flow, glomerular filtration, and urine formation then diminish, with tubular necrosis a likely consequence.

Splanchnic vasoconstriction reduces blood flow to GI organs and exacerbates hepatic and pancreatic ischemia. Vasoconstriction and thrombus formation (caused by mediators activating the clotting system and aggregation of neutrophils and platelets) reduce oxygen and blood flow to tissues.

Progressive cellular dysfunction and release of myocardial depressant factor from pancreatic cells severely depress myocardial contractility and reduce the heart's ejection fraction. Cardiac output then declines, and systemic vascular resistance progressively increases. As multisystem organ failure reaches it terminal stage, hypotension becomes unresponsive to volume replacement or inotropic drugs.

Imbalance of oxygen supply and demand

This imbalance occurs when the body can't supply organs with enough oxygen to meet the demands of a higher metabolic rate, tissue damage, and fever. The sustained reduction in pulmonary capillary blood flow impedes gas exchange. Partial pressure of arterial oxygen (PaO_2) decreases, while partial pressure of arterial carbon dioxide ($PaCO_2$) rises.

To make matters worse, tissues can't effectively use the oxygen they receive because anaerobic metabolism begins and lactic acid accumulates. Pulmonary capillaries leak, causing excess fluid to move into lung tissue and alveoli. Collapsed alveoli, pulmonary edema, and

PATHOPHYSIOLOGY

What happens in multisystem organ failure

In an inflammatory response, mediators are released in response to trauma, infection, and other insults. These mediators may potentiate the inflammatory response by causing selective vasodilation and vasoconstriction. An out-of-control mediator response promotes organ dysfunction by inducing three major changes: maldistribution of circulating volume, imbalance of oxygen supply and demand, and metabolic disturbances. These conditions eventually cause tissue damage, ischemia, and exhaustion of metabolic stores. This degeneration leads to organ dysfunction and, eventually, multisystem organ failure.

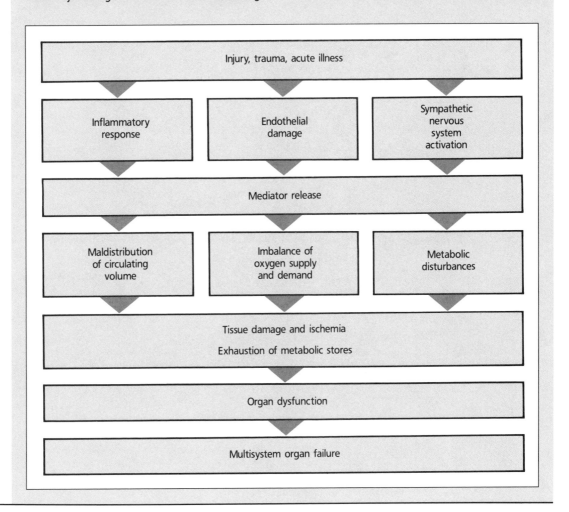

thick secretions further hinder gas exchange.

Adult respiratory distress syndrome signals the onset of pulmonary insufficiency and hypoxia—conditions that resist oxygen therapy, mechanical ventilation, and positive end-expiratory pressure. Hypotension impairs coronary artery perfusion, and the resulting imbalance between myocardial oxygen supply and demand induces arrhythmias, myocardial ischemia, and MI.

Assessing for signs of organ failure

The following physical and laboratory findings indicate the failure of specific organ systems.

BODY SYSTEM	PHYSICAL FINDINGS	LABORATORY FINDINGS
Cardiovascular	• Decreased cardiac output, blood pressure, ejection fraction • Increased pulmonary artery pressure, pulmonary artery wedge pressure (PAWP), central venous pressure (CVP) • Increased or decreased systemic vascular resistance, heart rate • Cold, pale skin; weak pulses; narrow pulse pressure; peripheral edema; cardiac ectopy	• Elevated serum enzyme levels (creatine kinase, lactate dehydrogenase [LD], lactate)
Gastrointestinal	• Diminished bowel sounds • Diarrhea, abdominal distention, fecal impaction, ileus, stress ulcers, mucosal erosion or atrophy, upper or lower GI bleeding	• Occult blood in stools • Enteric organisms on blood culture (from bacterial translocation) • Positive stool culture
Hematologic	• Pallor, fatigue • Bleeding from mucous membranes, bruises, thromboembolism, disseminated intravascular coagulation • Infection	• Decreased oxygen delivery indices (including arterial oxygen saturation [SaO_2] and hemoglobin), white blood cell count, red blood cell count, hemoglobin and hematocrit values, platelet count • Increased prothrombin time (PT) and partial thromboplastin time (PTT)
Hepatic	• Jaundice • Ascites • Bleeding from mucous membranes, I.V. catheter sites, or old puncture sites • Bruises	• Decreased plasma proteins, clotting factors, drug clearance • Increased liver enzyme levels (serum alkaline phosphatase, aspartate aminotransferase [AST], formerly SGOT; alanine aminotransferase [ALT], formerly SGPT; LD; total bilirubin), PT, PTT, blood ammonia level • Increased or decreased serum glucose level • Blood cultures positive for microorganisms
Neurologic	• Decreased level of consciousness, cerebral perfusion pressure, respiratory rate, tidal volume, Glasgow Coma Scale score • Increased or decreased temperature, blood pressure, heart rate	• None remarkable
Renal	• Elevated PAWP and CVP • Increased or decreased urine output • Weight gain and peripheral edema	• Reduced pH and bicarbonate levels • Elevated blood urea nitrogen and serum creatinine, potassium, and magnesium levels
Respiratory	• Reduced respiratory depth and compliance • Increased peak inspiratory pressure and ventilation-perfusion mismatch • Increased or decreased respiratory rate • Dyspnea, accessory muscle use, thick and greenish yellow sputum, intrapulmonary shunting greater than 20%, wheezes, crackles, infiltrates on chest X-ray, ventilatory dependence, diaphoresis	• Decreased pH, SaO_2, mixed venous oxygen saturation, partial pressure of arterial oxygen • Increased partial pressure of arterial carbon dioxide, serum lactate level

Metabolic disturbances

After the acute illness or trauma, the body tries to compensate for the damage, fight off the insult, and heal itself through hypermetabolism and hyperdynamic responses. High energy demands increase oxygen consumption and carbon dioxide production. To cope with this, the patient's respiratory rate and depth increase.

Hypermetabolism also causes the breakdown of protein stored in muscle tissue, leading to the conversion of amino acids to glucose. This process is wasteful because the body needs amino acids and protein for respiratory muscle strength, mobility, and tissue repair.

As multisystem organ failure progresses, liver function deteriorates and free fatty acids, ketones, amino acids, and nitrogenous waste products accumulate. Bilirubin builds up in the blood, causing jaundice. Cellular sodium and water content increase, depleting the cells of vital potassium and magnesium ions. Serum amylase and lipase levels rise as ischemic pancreatic cells release their enzymes into the blood and lymphatic circulations.

Finally, signs and symptoms of complete organ failure arise. To prevent multisystem failure and death, individual organs must receive every available support, and the health care team must intervene promptly to correct or halt these processes.

Complications

Death, of course, is the ultimate complication of multisystem organ failure. Experts suspect that the number of failing organs correlates directly with the patient's prognosis. Single-organ failure carries a mortality of 25% to 30%; two-organ failure, 50% to 60%; and three-organ failure, 75% to 85%. Failure of four or more organs carries a 100% fatality rate.

Assessment

Preventing multisystem organ failure is paramount—especially in patients with hypoperfusion and overwhelming inflammation, which set the stage for multisystem organ failure. When caring for the high-risk patient, monitor him closely for signs and symptoms of cardiovascular instability, poor organ perfusion, and inflammatory or infectious complications.

However, be aware that any patient with multisystem organ failure can present a contradictory picture. Also, he may be the victim of normal physiologic processes gone awry. In other words, responses designed to promote recovery could actually be worsening his condition. (See *Assessing for signs of organ failure*.)

Treatment

Once multisystem organ failure begins, major supportive interventions include administering antibiotics, oxygen, fluids, and cardiotropic drugs. Although specific methods for managing this complex syndrome are still under investigation, therapy is increasingly aimed at countering mediator-induced responses at the cellular level.

Monoclonal and polyclonal antibodies are being developed to neutralize acute inflammatory reactions to specific endotoxins. Nonsteroidal anti-inflammatory drugs show promise in decreasing prostaglandin and thromboxane synthesis, thereby inhibiting destructive vasoconstriction. Although these therapies may never replace current ones, they may complement them.

Nursing care

Care for the patient with multisystem organ failure includes maintaining a patent airway and promoting optimal gas exchange, minimizing further inflammation, and enhancing tissue perfusion and cardiac output. Other goals include providing adequate nutritional support, correcting the underlying problem, providing metabolic support, maintaining individual organ support (for example, by hemodialysis or mechanical ventilation), and preventing complications. (See *Nursing interventions for multisystem organ failure*, pages 198 and 199.)

For specific information on assessing for and managing multisystem organ failure in patients with anaphylactic shock, septic shock, or cancer, see the following sections.

Nursing interventions for multisystem organ failure

Nursing interventions for the patient with multisystem organ failure vary with the assessment findings and nursing diagnosis, as shown here.

ASSESSMENT FINDINGS	NURSING DIAGNOSIS	NURSING INTERVENTIONS
• Pulmonary infiltrates on chest X-ray • pH less than 7.35 or more than 7.45 • Partial pressure of arterial carbon dioxide less than 35 mm Hg or more than 45 mm Hg • Partial pressure of arterial oxygen less than 10% of baseline • Respiratory rate less than 12 breaths/minute or more than 20 breaths/minute • Dyspnea; crackles; wheezes; thick, blood-tinged or colored sputum	Impaired gas exchange related to atelectasis, secretions, pulmonary edema, pulmonary microthrombi, and vasoconstriction	• Maintain a patent airway and keep the head of the bed at a 15- to 45-degree angle. • Auscultate for breath sounds every 2 hours and as needed. • Assess respiratory rate, depth, and rhythm every 2 hours and as needed. • To help clear pulmonary secretions, turn the patient and encourage him to breathe deeply every 2 hours, and suction him as needed. (Placing the patient with the injured or congested lung up promotes ventilation-perfusion matching in the healthier lung.) • After suctioning, document the amount, color, character, and odor of pulmonary secretions. • Keep the patient well hydrated to enhance secretion removal. • Administer supplemental oxygen as ordered. • If the patient is on a mechanical ventilator, monitor ventilator settings: fraction of inspired oxygen, mode, tidal volume, and rate. Also monitor respiratory parameters: peak inspiratory pressure, compliance, and exhaled tidal volume. • Administer antibiotics as ordered. • Observe for adverse cardiopulmonary effects, such as respiratory distress, shallow respirations, decreased blood pressure, and tachycardia.
• Cardiac output less than 4 liters/minute • Cardiac index (CI) less than 2.5 liters/minute/m² • Blood pressure 20 mm Hg or more below baseline • Heart rate more than 100 beats/minute • Capillary refill more than 3 seconds • Urine output less than 0.5 ml/kg/hour • Decreased level of consciousness (LOC), weak pulses, cool skin	Decreased cardiac output related to decreased circulating volume, myocardial depression, and ventricular dysfunction	• Monitor heart rhythm and rate continuously. • Take vital signs hourly. • Obtain values for pulmonary artery pressure (PAP), pulmonary artery wedge pressure (PAWP), cardiac output, CI, systemic vascular resistance (SVR), and pulmonary vascular resistance (PVR) every 2 to 4 hours. • Administer I.V. fluids by infusion pump as ordered. Monitor for signs and symptoms of fluid overload (PAWP greater than 18 mm Hg, crackles, edema, weight gain, dyspnea, and pink, frothy sputum). • Administer vasoactive and inotropic drugs as ordered. • Document fluid intake and output accurately. • Administer sodium bicarbonate, as ordered, to treat acidosis, which can cause myocardial depression.
• Poor gas exchange (see assessment findings of Impaired gas exchange) • Decreased bowel sounds, abdominal distention, diarrhea, upper and lower GI bleeding • Urine output less than 0.5 ml/kg/hour • Increased blood urea nitrogen, creatinine, potassium, and magnesium levels • Decreased LOC, cardiac output, heart rate, and blood pressure • Increased PAWP • Increased liver enzyme levels • Albumin level less than 4 g/dl • pH less than 7.35	Altered tissue perfusion related to decreased circulating volume, microthrombi, reduced cardiac output, maldistribution of circulating volume, and altered cellular function	• Assess organ perfusion by monitoring cardiac rhythm and blood pressure continuously; evaluating LOC hourly; obtaining values for PAP, PAWP, and cardiac output every 4 hours and as needed; measuring urine output hourly; auscultating for bowel sounds every 4 hours; testing nasogastric aspirate every 4 hours; testing all stools for blood; monitoring pulses for regularity, amplitude, and rate; and checking skin for temperature, color, dryness, and turgor. • Enhance gas exchange and cardiac output. • Administer antiarrhythmic drugs and monitor for adverse effects. • Provide support for individual organ systems as necessary—for example, with mechanical ventilation, hemodialysis, or vasoactive drugs. • Administer sucralfate, antacids, and histamine₂ (H₂) blockers, as ordered, to reduce the risk of stress ulcers. • Continuously monitor mixed venous oxygen saturation (S v̄o₂) to assess whether oxygen delivery matches tissue oxygen demands.

Nursing interventions for multisystem organ failure (continued)

ASSESSMENT FINDINGS	NURSING DIAGNOSIS	NURSING INTERVENTIONS
• White blood cell (WBC) count higher than 10,000/mm³ • Temperature higher than 98.6° F (37° C) • Heart rate more than 100 beats/minute • Glucose level higher than 110 mg/dl • Cloudy urine • Crackles; wheezes; thick, colored pulmonary secretions • Purulent exudate from I.V. sites or wounds • Oral or vaginal candidiasis	High risk for infection and superinfection related to invasive lines and procedures, altered host defenses, and prolonged antibiotic therapy	• Wash your hands frequently. • Monitor temperature every 1 to 2 hours or continuously, using a rectal probe or a pulmonary artery catheter. • Secure the artificial airway to prevent aspiration and enhance oxygen delivery. • Provide frequent oral care to reduce the patient's risk of aspirating contaminated oropharyngeal secretions. • Use strict aseptic technique during placement and care of I.V. lines and urinary catheters. • Assess all catheter insertion sites and wounds daily for edema, erythema, warmth, pain, and drainage. • Monitor oral mucous membranes daily for candidiasis and other superinfections. • Monitor results of WBC count, chest X-ray, and glucose testing daily. • Observe urine, sputum, and wound drainage for changes in color and character. • Remove all potential contaminants from the area—for example, cut flowers, soil, and standing water.
• Weight loss • Muscle atrophy • Total serum protein level less than 6 g/dl • Negative nitrogen balance • Absent bowel sounds • Electrolyte imbalances	Altered nutrition (less than body requirements) related to lack of nutritional support, hypermetabolism, diarrhea, and altered GI function	• Arrange for a nutritional support consultation within 24 hours of admission. • Administer nutritional supplements enterally if possible. If total parenteral nutrition (TPN) is necessary, check solution, rate, and additives for accuracy. • Provide meticulous tube, line, and I.V. site care. Both enteral and parenteral feeding increase infection risks. • Assess bowel sounds and check for abdominal distention every 4 hours. • Record the patient's weight at the same time each day. • Monitor electrolyte levels, glucose level, laboratory values indicating nutritional status (such as total lymphocyte count, albumin level, and transferrin level) every 4 to 8 hours or as ordered. • Send a 24-hour urine specimen for urea nitrogen and nitrogen balance assessment once or twice a week. • Monitor for complications of enteral feeding: aspiration, abdominal distention, tube dislodgment, diarrhea, fluid and electrolyte imbalances. • Monitor for complications of TPN: catheter sepsis, hyperglycemia, infiltration, fluid and electrolyte imbalances.

Anaphylactic shock

An acute reaction, anaphylactic shock is characterized by immediate vascular and bronchial changes that cause profound hypovolemia and severe respiratory distress. To avert death, the patient needs immediate attention. (See *When your patient is in anaphylactic shock,* page 200.)

Causes

Anaphylactic shock results from an extreme hypersensitivity reaction to a foreign antigen. The antigen activates the immune system through immunoglobulin E (IgE) antibodies. Specific antigens that can cause anaphylactic shock include:
• antibiotics—most commonly, penicillin and its analogues, aminoglycosides, cephalosporins, sulfonamides, tetracycline, and vancomycin
• local anesthetics, including bupivacaine, lidocaine, procaine, and tetracaine

When your patient is in anaphylactic shock

If you suspect that your patient is having an ana-phylactic reaction, first assess his respiratory status. If he has a respiratory obstruction, administer oxy-gen as ordered until an endotracheal tube can be inserted. If laryngeal edema has closed off his air-way, call for assistance and have someone notify the doctor immediately. Be prepared to assist with an emergency tracheotomy.

Determining the cause
Try to determine the cause of the anaphylactic re-action—but don't waste precious moments doing this. Look for obvious causes. If the patient was stung by an insect or just had an injection, wrap a tourniquet or blood pressure cuff above the af-fected site to obstruct venous return. If he's receiv-ing an infusion of an I.V. medication, stop the infusion immediately—it's the likely cause of the reaction. Also stop a dye infusion or blood transfu-sion.

Inserting an I.V. line
Insert or maintain a patent I.V. line and expect to infuse epinephrine, the drug of choice for acute anaphylaxis. Epinephrine promptly reverses such life-threatening conditions as bronchoconstriction and hypotension. However, when administering this drug, stay alert for such adverse effects as tachy-cardia, hypertension, dyspnea, and electrocardio-gram changes. Expect to administer 0.9% sodium chloride solution or lactated Ringer's solution to re-store fluid volume, increase blood pressure and cardiac output, and reverse lactic acidosis.

• chemotherapeutic drugs, including doxorubi-cin, bleomycin, cisplatin, cyclophosphamide, as-paraginase, and melphalan
• other drugs, including corticotropin, aspirin, codeine, dextrans, diuretics, histamine, mepro-bamate, and morphine
• diagnostic agents, such as sulfobromophtha-lein sodium dye, dehydrocholic acid, iodinated radiographic contrast media, and iopanoic acid
• mismatched blood products and antisera,

such as cryoprecipitate, fresh frozen plasma, gamma globulin, packed red blood cells, and whole blood
• venom from bees, hornets, jellyfish, snakes, spiders, and wasps
• certain foods, including chocolate, eggs, grains, milk, nuts, seafood, shellfish, strawber-ries, and tomatoes
• immunotherapy. (To avoid anaphylaxis, immu-notherapy should be administered by a trained allergist. The patient receiving immunotherapy shouldn't receive beta blockers because these drugs may exacerbate an anaphylactic reac-tion.)

Pathophysiology
An anaphylactic reaction can occur only after the immune system has been sensitized to a particular antigen. Such sensitization happens if IgE antibodies specific to that antigen form on initial contact with the antigen. These antigen-specific IgE antibodies bind with mast cells, found in connective tissue surrounding the blood vessels, lungs, small intestine, and skin, as well as with basophils in the bloodstream.

The next time that particular antigen enters the body (such as through the skin or the re-spiratory or GI tract), anaphylaxis occurs. The antigen interacts with the IgE antibody on mast cells, triggering release of chemical me-diators from within mast cell granules. These mediators affect many types of tissue and or-gan systems and account for the physiologic response seen during an anaphylactic reaction. (See *What happens in an anaphylactic reaction*, pages 202 and 203.)

The onset and nature of an anaphylactic re-action depend on:
• the route by which the antigen enters the body
• the amount of antigen absorbed
• the absorption rate of the antigen
• the degree of patient hypersensitivity.

An anaphylactic reaction may develop sec-onds to minutes after the antigen is intro-duced; however, most reactions start 30 minutes after exposure. Usually, the faster the onset, the more severe the reaction.

Complications
Untreated, anaphylactic shock causes respiratory obstruction, systemic vascular collapse, and death — within minutes to hours after the first symptoms appear.

Assessment
History
If possible, find out which substances the patient has ingested or been exposed to recently. If he is coherent and can provide information, ask if he's having trouble breathing or making noises when breathing. If he can't provide information himself, ask a family member or someone who witnessed the reaction. Also find out if the patient has previously reacted to the substance in question and if so, what kind of reaction he had.

At the onset of the reaction, the patient may report uneasiness, fear, or a feeling of impending doom. He may say he feels a lump in his throat, followed by hoarseness, coughing, sneezing, dyspnea, chest tightness, and stridor. He may complain of weakness, disorientation, flushing, diaphoresis, or feeling hot all over.

Physical examination
On inspection, you may note warm, flushed skin and detect circumscribed, discrete cutaneous wheals with erythematous, raised, serpiginous borders and blanched centers. The wheals may progress to diffuse erythema, then to generalized urticaria and angioedema — especially of the eyelids, lips, and tongue.

The uvula, vocal cords, and posterior pharynx may appear swollen. On auscultation, you may hear diffuse wheezes and prolonged expirations. These sounds, brought on by upper and lower airway obstruction from laryngeal edema, may signal respiratory failure.

Assess for cardiovascular problems, which result from greatly decreased plasma volume (caused by vasodilation and intravascular fluid leakage into the extracellular space). Expect hypotension and myocardial ischemia. Later, myocardial depression may occur. Hypotension with decreased coronary artery perfusion may lead to myocardial ischemia, ventricular arrhythmias, and even MI.

Evaluate for GI problems, although these are relatively rare in anaphylaxis. Note any nausea, abdominal cramps, profuse vomiting, or severe diarrhea (from smooth-muscle spasms). Also note such neurologic signs and symptoms as dizziness, drowsiness, headache, restlessness, and seizures. Metabolic abnormalities may include lactic acidosis, whose signs and symptoms include lethargy, confusion, stupor, and other changes in the patient's level of consciousness (LOC); Kussmaul's respirations; cold, clammy skin that becomes warm and dry; arrhythmias; diminished muscle tone; and exaggerated deep tendon reflexes.

Diagnostic tests
Anaphylactic shock is diagnosed from clinical findings. If no known allergic stimulus can be identified, the doctor must rule out other possible causes of shock, such as MI, status asthmaticus, and congestive heart failure.

Skin scratch testing may help identify specific substances to which the patient is allergic. Diagnostic tests may reveal an elevated hematocrit (from hemoconcentration), increased serum histamine levels, clotting factor depletion, and electrocardiogram changes, such as tachycardia and bradycardia.

Ongoing treatment
In the early stages of anaphylaxis, give epinephrine I.M. or S.C.; in severe reactions, when the patient is unconscious and hypotensive, give epinephrine I.V. as ordered. Establish and maintain a patent airway, and watch for signs of laryngeal edema (stridor, hoarseness, and dyspnea). If cardiac arrest occurs, begin cardiopulmonary resuscitation. Watch for hypotension and shock, and maintain circulatory volume with volume expanders, as ordered.

Ongoing nursing interventions
As your patient recovers from anaphylactic shock, you'll need to monitor him closely, provide emotional support, and teach him how to avoid future anaphylactic reactions.
• Check the patient's vital signs frequently (every 15 to 30 minutes) for the first 1 to 4 hours. Watch closely for any changes in respi-

(Text continues on page 205.)

PATHOPHYSIOLOGY

What happens in an anaphylactic reaction

An anaphylactic reaction requires previous sensitization or exposure to the specific antigen. These illustrations show what happens during the reaction.

Response to the antigen
Immunoglobulin M (IgM) and IgG recognize the antigen as a foreign substance and attach themselves to it.

The antigen destruction process, called the *complement cascade,* begins but can't finish either because of insufficient amounts of protein catalyst A or because the antigen rejects certain complement destruction enzymes. At this stage, the patient has no signs or symptoms.

Release of chemical mediators
The antigen's continued presence activates IgE (attached to basophils and mast cells). The activated IgE causes degranulation (cell membrane breakdown) of basophils and mast cells, causing mediators within these cells to leak. These mediators

include histamine, serotonin, slow-reacting substance of anaphylaxis (SRS-A), eosinophil chemotactic factor of anaphylaxis (ECF-A), platelet-activating factor (PAF), prostaglandins, and bradykinins.

Histamine induces generalized vasodilation, increased vascular permeability, increased pulmonary secretions, and bronchoconstriction. *Serotonin,* found in large concentrations in the brain and GI tract, acts like histamine. *SRS-A* stimulates small-airway bronchoconstriction, vasodilation, increased vascular permeability, and wheal reactions. *ECF-A* causes cellular infiltration. *PAF* leads to decreased coronary blood flow, a negative inotropic effect, platelet aggregation and release, and pulmonary hypertension. *Prostaglandins* increase lung secretions and enhance histamine's effect on permeability. *Bradykinins* cause an increase in sweat and salivary gland secretions, bronchoconstriction, systemic vasodilation, and increased vascular permeability.

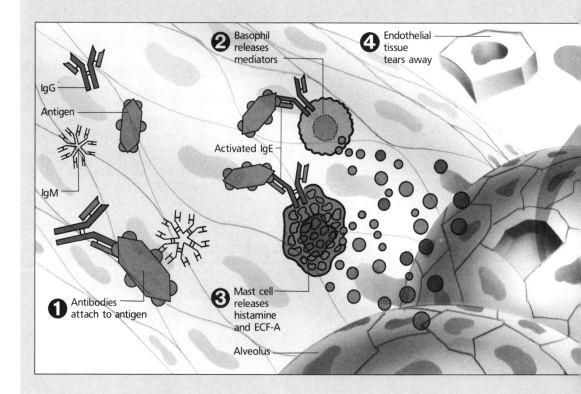

Intensification of patient response

The activated IgE also stimulates mast cells located in connective tissue along the venule walls. The mast cells release more histamine and ECF-A. These substances produce disruptive lesions, which weaken the venules.

The patient now has itchy red skin, wheals, and swelling.

Beginning of respiratory distress

In the lungs, histamine causes endothelial cells to break and endothelial tissue to tear away from surrounding tissue. Pulmonary compliance decreases as the alveoli fill with fluid and SRS-A prevents alveoli from expanding.

During this stage, expect signs of respiratory distress—tachypnea, crowing, use of accessory breathing muscles, and cyanosis. The patient also may exhibit severe anxiety, an altered level of consciousness, and possibly seizures.

Deterioration in patient's condition

Meanwhile, basophils and mast cells secrete prostaglandins and bradykinins, along with histamine and serotonin. The combination of these secretions increases vascular permeability, causing fluids to leak from vessels.

The patient may show evidence of rapid vascular collapse—shock; confusion; cool, pale skin; generalized edema; tachycardia; and hypotension.

Failure of compensatory mechanisms

Damage to endothelial cells causes basophils and mast cells to release heparin. Eosinophils release arylsulfatase B (to neutralize SRS-A), phospholipase D (to neutralize heparin), and cyclic adenosine monophosphate and prostaglandins E_1 and E_2 (to increase the metabolic rate). But this response can't reverse anaphylaxis.

The patient may experience hemorrhage, disseminated intravascular coagulation, and cardiopulmonary arrest.

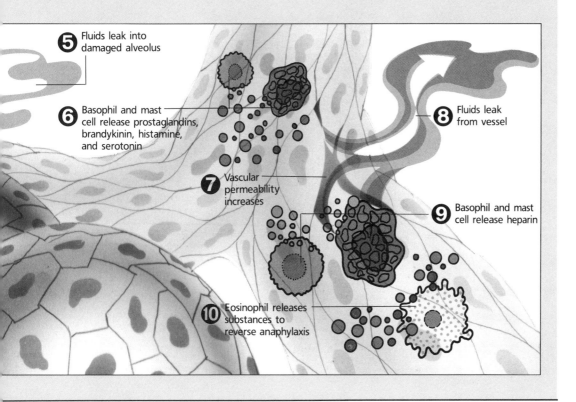

5 Fluids leak into damaged alveolus

6 Basophil and mast cell release prostaglandins, brandykinin, histamine, and serotonin

7 Vascular permeability increases

8 Fluids leak from vessel

9 Basophil and mast cell release heparin

10 Eosinophil releases substances to reverse anaphylaxis

Drugs commonly used to treat anaphylactic shock

DRUG	INDICATION	DOSAGE	ACTION	NURSING CONSIDERATIONS
Diphenhydramine Benadryl	Mild anaphylaxis	P.O.: 25 to 100 mg t.i.d. I.M. or I.V.: 25 to 50 mg q.i.d.	• An antihistamine; competes with histamine for histamine$_1$ (H$_1$) receptor sites • Prevents laryngeal edema • Controls localized itching	• Administer I.V. doses slowly to avoid hypotension. • Monitor patient for hypotension. • Caution patient about driving because drug causes drowsiness and slows reflexes. • Give oral fluids as needed. Drug causes dry mouth.
Epinephrine Adrenalin Chloride	Severe anaphylaxis (drug of choice)	*Initial infusion:* 0.2 to 0.5 mg (0.2 to 0.5 ml of 1:1,000 strength diluted in 10 ml 0.9% sodium chloride solution) given I.V. slowly over 5 to 10 minutes, followed by continuous infusion *Continuous infusion:* 1 to 4 mcg/minute. Mix 1 ml of 1:1,000 epinephrine in 250 ml of dextrose 5% in water (D$_5$W) to yield concentration of 4 mcg/ml.	*Alpha-adrenergic effects* • Increases blood pressure • Reverses peripheral vasodilation and systemic hypotension • Decreases angioedema and urticaria • Improves coronary blood flow by raising diastolic pressure • Causes peripheral vasoconstriction *Beta-adrenergic effects* • Causes bronchodilation • Causes positive inotropic and chronotropic cardiac activity • Decreases synthesis and release of chemical mediators	• Choose large vein for infusion. • Use infusion controller to regulate drip. • Check blood pressure and heart rate. • Monitor patient for arrhythmias. • Check solution strength, dosage, and label before administering. • Watch for signs of extravasation at infusion site. • Monitor intake and output. • Assess color and temperature of extremities.
Hydrocortisone Solu Cortef	Severe anaphylaxis	I.V.: 100 to 200 mg every 4 to 6 hours	• A corticosteroid; prevents neutrophil and platelet aggregation • Inhibits synthesis of mediators • Decreases capillary permeability	• Monitor fluid and electrolyte balance, intake and output, and blood pressure closely. • Maintain patient on ulcer regimen and antacids for prophylaxis.
Aminophylline Aminophyllin	Severe anaphylaxis	I.V.: 5 to 6 mg/kg as loading dose, followed by 0.4 to 0.9 mg/kg/ minute as infusion	• A xanthine derivative; causes bronchodilation • Stimulates respiratory drive • Dilates constricted pulmonary arteries • Causes diuresis • Strengthens cardiac contractions • Increases vital capacity • Causes coronary vasodilation	• Monitor blood pressure, pulse, and respirations. • Monitor intake and output, hydration status, and serum aminophylline and electrolyte levels. • Monitor patient for arrhythmias. • Use I.V. controller to reduce risk of overdose. • Maintain serum levels at 10 to 20 mcg/ml.
Cimetidine Tagamet	Severe anaphylaxis	I.V.: 600 mg diluted in D$_5$W and administered over 20 minutes	• An antihistamine; competes with histamine for histamine$_2$ (H$_2$) receptors • Prevents laryngeal edema	• Don't administer aminophylline concurrently with cimetidine. The two drugs are incompatible. • Reduce dosage for patients with impaired renal or hepatic function, as necessary and as ordered.

ratory or cardiovascular status. If hypotension persists, be ready to start a continuous epinephrine infusion or to administer plasma or vasopressors, as ordered, to raise blood pressure. (See *Drugs commonly used to treat anaphylactic shock.*)

• After a severe anaphylactic reaction, monitor the patient closely for 24 hours. Even after he's stable, he's at risk for bronchospasms, upper respiratory obstruction, tachycardia, and hypotension. Another reaction is most likely to occur within 12 to 24 hours.

• Assess the patient for signs and symptoms of fluid overload, such as crackles, dyspnea, a cough yielding frothy sputum, and a distended jugular vein.

• Monitor fluid intake and output hourly. Urine output should measure at least 30 ml/hour.

• Reassure the patient and provide continuous emotional support. Few experiences are as frightening as an anaphylactic reaction.

Providing patient teaching

• Inform the patient that he's at risk for subsequent episodes. Instruct him to avoid known allergens. If he's allergic to bee stings, advise him not to wear dark clothing (especially black) outdoors because it attracts bees.

• Instruct the patient to carry a kit containing both injectable and oral drugs to take if he's exposed to a hazardous allergen. If he's allergic to insect stings, for example, you might recommend an Ana-Kit or EpiPen Auto-Injector. The Ana-Kit includes epinephrine 1:1,000 in 1 ml (two 0.3-mg doses), one disposable sterile syringe, 2 mg of chlorpheniramine maleate (four chewable tablets), sterile alcohol pads, and a tourniquet. The EpiPen Auto-Injector delivers 0.3 mg I.M. of epinephrine 1:1,000 aqueous solution in 2-ml disposable injectors. The EpiPen Jr. Auto-Injector delivers 0.15 mg I.M. of epinephrine 1:2,000 aqueous solution in 2-ml disposable injectors.

• Instruct the patient to wear a medical identification bracelet or tag to inform rescue and health care workers of his allergies.

Preventing anaphylaxis

• Make every effort to prevent anaphylactic reactions by always asking about allergies when taking a patient's history. If he has a history of allergies, find out exactly what he's allergic to. Ask specific questions about foods, drugs, blood products, insect stings, and inhalants.

• If the patient has had a previous allergic reaction, have him describe it in detail. Document this information carefully on his chart, describing the nature and severity of the reaction. Put an allergy sticker on his chart and care plan.

• Notify the pharmacist of the patient's allergies so that he can keep a record of them.

• Before administering any drug or other agent, ask the patient if he's ever had a reaction to it. *Don't* rely on his chart alone.

• After giving any drug that can cause anaphylaxis, stay with the patient and watch for signs and symptoms of an anaphylactic reaction.

• Never administer a drug to a patient who's had a previous reaction to it. If the doctor orders a drug in the same drug family that previously caused a reaction, check with him before administering it.

• If the patient is scheduled for studies requiring contrast dye, he may need prophylactic drug therapy to avert anaphylactic shock. For instance, the doctor may order three doses of prednisone (50 mg every 8 hours) to be given before the test; 25 to 50 mg of diphenhydramine P.O. to be given 1 hour before the test (or immediately before it when administered I.M.); or 300 mg of cimetidine I.V. to be given 1 hour in advance. Be sure to hydrate the patient well before and after the test.

Septic shock

Septic shock refers to a state of impaired cellular function, decreased systemic vascular resistance, and increased cardiac output that occurs secondary to septicemia. It results in activated coagulation, cell injury, metabolic changes, and altered blood flow through the microcirculation. Septic shock signifies failure of the body's defense mechanisms.

The incidence of septic shock approaches 500,000 cases annually. Mortality is nearly 25%. To ensure early detection and intervention for this potentially lethal condition, you

When your patient is in septic shock

Locating and eliminating the source of sepsis are essential in managing septic shock. First, remove any I.V., intra-arterial, or urinary catheters and send them to the laboratory to help identify the sepsis-causing organism. Emergency treatment focuses on maintaining the patient's oxygenation, increasing his intravascular volume, and initiating antimicrobial therapy.

Oxygen therapy
Initiate oxygen therapy, as ordered, to maintain arterial oxygen saturation above 95%. If respiratory failure occurs, the patient may need mechanical ventilation. Monitor the patient's blood pressure and pulse closely. A drop in blood pressure accompanied by a thready pulse may signal inadequate cardiac output.

I.V. infusion
Start an I.V. infusion with 0.9% sodium chloride or lactated Ringer's solution. Use a large-bore (14G to 18G) catheter to ease later administration of blood transfusions. Expect the doctor to order colloid or crystalloid infusions to increase intravascular volume and raise blood pressure.

After sufficient fluid volume has been replaced, he'll probably order a diuretic (such as furosemide) to maintain urine output above 25 ml/hour. If fluid resuscitation fails to increase blood pressure, you may give a vasopressor, such as dopamine, if ordered.

Antimicrobial therapy
As ordered, begin aggressive antimicrobial therapy appropriate for the causative organism, as determined by culture and sensitivity testing. In a patient with immunosuppression secondary to drug therapy, discontinue or reduce the dosage of the offending drug. The doctor may order granulocyte transfusions if the patient has severe neutropenia.

must be familiar with its pathophysiology and clinical signs. Treatment and care are complex, and the patient will need monitoring in the intensive care unit. (See *When your patient is in septic shock.*)

Causes
Septic shock usually occurs as a complication of another disorder or of an invasive procedure that allows entry of a pathogenic microorganism into the bloodstream. The microorganism produces septicemia in patients whose resistance is already compromised by an existing condition.

Any pathogen can cause septic shock. However, in about two out of three cases, septic shock results from infection with gram-negative bacteria, such as *Escherichia coli, Klebsiella, Serratia, Enterobacter,* or *Pseudomonas.* Roughly 3% of cases result from opportunistic fungi, and even fewer involve mycobacteria, viruses, or protozoa.

Septic shock can occur in anyone with impaired immunity, but neonates and elderly patients have the greatest risk. About two-thirds of the cases occur in hospitalized patients, most of whom have underlying diseases. Patients at high risk include those with burns; chronic cardiac, hepatic, or renal disorders; diabetes mellitus; immunosuppression; malnutrition; stress; and those who have used antibiotics excessively. Patients with traumatic wounds and those who've had surgery or invasive diagnostic or therapeutic procedures are also at increased risk for septic shock.

Pathophysiology
Many microorganisms are part of the normal flora of the skin and intestines. Usually, they're beneficial and pose no threat. But if they enter the bloodstream and spread throughout the body, they can cause overwhelming infection unless natural defense mechanisms destroy them. These microorganisms may gain entry through any alteration in the body's defenses; through artificial devices that penetrate the body, such as I.V., intra-arterial, and urinary catheters; or through knife or bullet wounds.

Initially, the body releases mediators in response to the invading organisms, which trigger decreased systemic vascular resistance and increased cardiac output. Blood flow is unevenly distributed in the microcirculation, and plasma leaking from capillaries causes functional hypovolemia. Eventually, cardiac output falls, resulting in poor tissue perfusion and hypotension.

Complications
Septic shock may lead to disseminated intravascular coagulation (DIC), renal failure, heart failure, GI ulcers, and abnormal liver function. Multisystem organ failure and death may ensue.

Assessment
History
The patient's history may reveal a disorder or treatment capable of causing immunosuppression or sepsis, such as chemotherapy. Or it may reveal that he's had recent invasive tests or treatments, surgery, or trauma.

At the onset of septic shock, the patient may report fever and chills. Roughly 20% of patients are hypothermic.

Physical examination
Signs and symptoms vary with the stage of shock. During the *hyperdynamic* (early, or warm) phase, expect findings that reflect increased cardiac output, peripheral vasodilation, and decreased systemic vascular resistance. The patient's skin may appear pink and flushed, and may feel warm and dry. His LOC is altered, and you may assess agitation, anxiety, irritability, and a short attention span. A change in the patient's LOC is one of the earliest signs of septicemia. Respirations become rapid and shallow, and urine output falls below normal. Palpation may reveal rapid, full, bounding peripheral pulses. Blood pressure may be normal or slightly elevated.

Uncontrolled sepsis progresses to the *hypodynamic* (late, or cold) phase of septic shock. In this phase, you can expect signs and symptoms of decreased cardiac output, peripheral vasoconstriction, increased systemic vascular resistance, and inadequate tissue perfusion. For instance, respirations become rapid and shallow. Urine output may drop below 25 ml/hour

or may stop altogether. The patient may appear cyanotic, with cold, pale, clammy skin and peripheral mottling. You may assess a severely decreased LOC—possibly even coma.

If arrhythmias are present, the pulse may be irregular. Peripheral pulses may become rapid, weak, thready, or absent. Systolic pressure may drop below 90 mm Hg, or 50 to 80 mm Hg below the patient's previous reading. If central pressures are being monitored, pulmonary artery wedge pressure (PAWP) will be reduced or normal. Lung auscultation may reveal crackles or rhonchi if pulmonary congestion is present. (See *What to expect in early and late septic shock,* page 208.)

Be aware that not all patients progress from warm to cold shock. Some initially present in cold shock. Frequent observation can detect septic shock early, increasing the patient's survival odds.

Diagnostic tests
In a septic shock patient, blood cultures are positive for the offending organism. A complete blood count usually reveals thrombocytopenia and may show anemia, leukopenia, or severe neutropenia. The serum lactate dehydrogenase level rises, reflecting metabolic acidosis. The urine sodium level drops, urine specific gravity rises above 1.020, and urine osmolarity increases. Arterial blood gas (ABG) analysis shows elevations in pH and PaO_2. In early shock, $PaCO_2$ decreases as respiratory alkalosis sets in.

Ongoing treatment
Treatment of the underlying condition is essential in treating septic shock. Remove any I.V., intra-arterial, or urinary catheters. Oxygen therapy should be initiated to maintain arterial oxygen saturation greater than 95%. Ongoing treatment goals should aim to maintain urine output above 25 ml/hour with diuretics, to increase vascular volume, and to raise blood pressure with colloid or crystalloid infusions as ordered.

Ongoing nursing interventions
Nursing care focuses on ensuring fluid balance,

What to expect in early and late septic shock

In early (hyperdynamic, or warm) septic shock, vascular resistance decreases while cardiac output and stroke volume increase. Close assessment and prompt intervention can halt the progression of early shock to late (hypodynamic, or cold) shock. Use this chart as an assessment guide.

BODY SYSTEM	ASSESSMENT	FINDINGS IN EARLY SHOCK	FINDINGS IN LATE SHOCK
Cardiovascular	• Assess pulse and blood pressure; document pulse pressure with each blood pressure reading.	• Tachycardia, normal mean arterial blood pressure, widening pulse pressure	• Tachycardia, thready pulse, severe hypotension
	• Assess peripheral pulses.	• Bounding	• Weak, thready
	• Auscultate heart sounds at four valvular sites	• No murmur or gallop	• Possible murmur or gallop
Gastrointestinal	• Check for ascites, abdominal masses, and occult blood in stools.	• Normal	• Abdominal pain
	• Ask about recent changes in bowel habits.	• Constipation or diarrhea	• Constipation or diarrhea
	• Auscultate for bowel sounds in all four quadrants.	• Bowel sounds present	• No bowel sounds
Genitourinary	• Assess for complaints of urinary burning or frequency or decreased urine output.	• Normal or below normal urine output	• Oliguria
	• Check hourly intake and output.	• Normal or below normal urine output	• Below normal output.
	• Measure specific gravity once every shift.	• Normal specific gravity	• Increased specific gravity
	• Weigh patient daily.	• Normal or increased weight	• Normal or decreased weight
	• Monitor blood urea nitrogen and serum creatinine levels.	• Increased levels	• Increased levels
	• Check fractional urines.	• Glucose in urine	• Glucose in urine
Neurologic	• Assess mental status and level of consciousness.	• Mild irritability, lethargy, slight restlessness, disorientation, inappropriate euphoria	• Extreme irritability, restlessness, and confusion
	• Take oral temperature.	• Normal, below normal, or elevated	• Below normal or elevated
Respiratory	• Assess respiratory rate, rhythm, and effort.	• Tachypnea, hyperventilation	• Rapid, shallow breathing; respiratory distress
	• Percuss and auscultate lungs, noting adventitious sounds.	• Crackles, decreased breath sounds	• Rhonchi; decreased breath sounds
	• Obtain arterial blood gas values.	• Respiratory alkalosis	• Respiratory alkalosis
Skin	• Inspect and palpate skin; note its color, turgor, vascularity, moisture, temperature, texture, thickness, and mobility.	• Warm, flushed skin; peripheral edema	• Cold and clammy skin
	• Observe for stomatitis or mucositis.	• Dry mouth	• Inflammation

oxygenation, and cardiovascular stability, and on eliminating the infection.

• Administer prescribed antimicrobial drugs I.V. to achieve effective blood levels rapidly.

• Administer oxygen by face mask or airway to ensure adequate tissue oxygenation. Monitor serial ABG values and adjust the oxygen flow rate accordingly.

• Monitor the patient's blood pressure and pulse closely. A progressive decrease in blood pressure accompanied by a thready pulse usually signals inadequate cardiac output (from reduced intravascular volume). Notify the doctor if this occurs, and increase the infusion rate as ordered. To reduce afterload and provide myocardial support, he may order a vasodilator, such as nitroprusside, in combination with a positive inotropic agent, such as dopamine or dobutamine.

• Administer fluids cautiously and perform close hemodynamic monitoring as vascular capacity increases to normal.

• Don't give I.V. infusions in the legs of a shock patient who has suffered abdominal trauma because the infused fluid may escape through the ruptured vessel into the abdomen.

• Record the patient's blood pressure, pulse and respiratory rates, and peripheral pulses every 1 to 5 minutes until he's stable. Record his hemodynamic pressure readings every 15 minutes. Monitor his cardiac rhythm continuously. If systolic blood pressure drops to less than 80 mm Hg, increase the oxygen flow rate and notify the doctor immediately. A blood pressure this low usually causes inadequate coronary artery blood flow, cardiac ischemia, and cardiac arrhythmias.

• Measure urine output hourly. If it drops below 25 ml/hour in an adult, increase the fluid infusion rate—but watch for signs of fluid overload, such as increased PAWP. Notify the doctor if urine output doesn't improve. He may order a diuretic to increase renal blood flow and urine output.

• Assess for peripheral edema, bowel sounds, crackles, and rhonchi. To prevent atelectasis, have the patient perform deep breathing and turn him frequently.

• If the patient needs a blood transfusion, explain the associated risks to him and his family.

Answer their questions about this therapy as completely as possible.

• Provide emotional support to the patient and his family. Explain all procedures in advance to ease their anxiety.

Preventing septic shock

• Identify and closely monitor high-risk patients. Assess baseline status and then observe continuously for signs and symptoms of infection.

• Check closely for a change in mental status. If the patient is confused or disoriented, eliminate environmental hazards and reorient him to time, place, and person with each contact. Document mental status changes, and report them to the doctor.

• Document any nosocomial infection, and report it to the infection-control nurse. Investigating all nosocomial infections can help identify the source and prevent future nosocomial infections, infections from outside sources, and cross-contamination from patient to patient.

• Provide ongoing education about infection prophylaxis to the patient, family, and staff. This instruction should begin with initial contact and be reinforced consistently with all individuals involved.

Multisystem organ failure in cancer

Increasing numbers of cancer patients are living longer, thanks to multiple treatments involving surgery, radiation, chemotherapy, bone marrow transplants, and immunotherapy. The extensive research efforts of the past few decades have paid off in prolonged remission, if not in a cure.

Unfortunately, many cancer patients now suffer from the adverse effects of aggressive antineoplastic regimens. Such effects can damage organ systems enough to cause multisystem organ failure. This phenomenon, seen in critically ill cancer patients, is mediator induced and involves functional loss of two or more organs. Significant damage from tumors and in-

When a cancer patient has multisystem organ failure

Preventing further infection, correcting the underlying causes, and averting recurrent insults are crucial in caring for the cancer patient with multisystem organ failure. The doctor will order treatments that support individual organ function; take care to prevent complications of critical care that could compromise your patient.

Implementing treatments
Other important treatment and care goals include:
• maintaining a patent airway and promoting optimal gas exchange
• enhancing tissue perfusion and cardiac output
• promoting GI, hepatic, and renal elimination of metabolic by-products
• providing adequate nutritional support
• administering blood and blood products to reverse the effects of antineoplastic regimens
• administering colony-stimulating factors to increase platelet counts
• administering antibiotics as ordered.

Preventing complications
Take all necessary steps to prevent complications of critical care technology. Mechanical ventilation, for example, can extend pulmonary damage from barotrauma and oxygen toxicity. Hemodialysis can cause further cardiovascular instability, rapid fluid and electrolyte shifts, and coagulopathies. Although venous access devices simplify many nutritional and treatment regimens, they also provide a direct entry route for microbes, which could result in eventual systemic colonization and subsequent sepsis.

Establishing priorities
The patient may become even more vulnerable as his deteriorating condition mandates the need for endotracheal tubes and hemodynamic monitoring devices. You must identify these risk factors and establish critical-care treatment priorities for the patient with the multidisciplinary team.

fections contributes to the cancer patient's risk for multisystem organ failure.

Regardless of the type of primary tumor, multisystem organ failure follows a common sequence of organ dysfunction in cancer patients. The pulmonary system usually fails first, followed by the GI system, liver, kidneys, cardiovascular system, and central nervous system. The organs involved in multisystem organ failure are not necessarily near the site of injury or the initiating event. This can make a diagnosis of multisystem organ failure difficult and may explain why many patients are quite ill before treatment begins.

For many cancer patients, multisystem organ failure represents a turn for the worse — unless the health care team can anticipate, recognize, understand, and treat the physiologic alterations as they occur. (See *When a cancer patient has multisystem organ failure.*)

Causes
Multisystem organ failure results from nonspecific systemic responses to abnormal intravascular inflammation — for example, from cancer treatments that alter the body's normal homeostatic balance. It's commonly the final complication of cancer or its treatment. (See *Complications of cancer therapy.*)

Pathophysiology
Multisystem organ failure is typically the end result of two clinical conditions that are oncologic emergencies — sepsis and DIC. All three processes — multisystem organ failure, sepsis, and DIC — are activated by the inflammatory response. Fueled by common mediators, these three processes involve similar risks and produce distinctive systemic changes. They form a network of dysfunctional cellular interactions among organs rather than representing isolated cases of single-organ failure.

The combination of poor baseline health and treatment-related risk factors increases the risk of septic shock, DIC, and subsequent multisystem organ failure in the cancer patient. Each of these conditions could trigger the other in a patient whose defense mechanisms have been depleted by aggressive cancer treatment. In a domino effect, immunosuppression,

Complications of cancer therapy

In the cancer patient, complications of treatment—which may lead to multisystem organ failure—vary with the specific therapy he has received.

Chemotherapy
- Immunosuppression
- Recurrent pulmonary infections
- Superinfections
- Intubation and pneumonia
- Pulmonary edema
- Chronic gastritis or enteritis
- GI bleeding
- Diarrhea
- Nausea and vomiting
- Intestinal obstruction
- Hepatotoxicity
- Nephrotoxicity
- Cardiotoxicity
- Neurotoxicity

Radiation therapy
- Interstitial pneumonitis and pulmonary fibrosis
- Pulmonary toxicity
- Chronic gastritis or enteritis
- GI bleeding
- Diarrhea
- Intractable nausea
- Vomiting
- Intestinal obstruction
- Oral complications such as stomatitis
- Myelosuppression
- Pericarditis and pericardial effusions
- Cerebral edema with an increased risk of seizures, inflammation, and increased intracranial pressure (ICP)

Surgery
- Impaired gas exchange (with lobectomy or pneumonectomy)
- Hemorrhage
- Infection
- Malabsorption
- Thrombosis
- Small-bowel obstruction and perforation
- Poor nutritional status
- Biliary fistula
- Portal hypertension
- Clotting defects
- Venous stasis
- Hematuria
- Atelectasis
- Pneumonia
- Cerebral edema with seizures, increased ICP, and residual neurologic deficits

Immunotherapy
- Intravascular fluid shifts
- Hypotension
- Peripheral edema
- Myocardial ischemia or infarction
- Myocarditis
- Arrhythmias
- Anorexia
- Nausea and vomiting
- Diarrhea
- Weight loss
- Elevated blood urea nitrogen and serum creatinine levels
- Decreased urine output
- Proteinuria
- Neutropenia
- Thrombocytopenia
- Anaphylaxis
- Neurotoxicity

Bone marrow transplant
- Life-threatening bacterial, viral, and fungal infections
- Acute or chronic graft-versus-host disease
- Hepatic veno-occlusive disease

---

antibiotic therapy, surgical wounds, and invasive lines and procedures all enhance activation of the inflammatory response and stimulation of mediators. The result is multisystem organ failure.

Sepsis. The most common precipitator of multisystem organ failure, sepsis includes a group of events ranging from bacteremia and septicemia to septic shock. Bacteremia occurs when nonmultiplying bacteria are present in the bloodstream; septicemia results from actively multiplying pathogens that release toxins into the systemic circulation. Like multisystem organ failure, septic shock is a syndrome characterized by hemodynamic instability, coagulopathy, and alterations in energy metabolism. The most serious infections are those caused by

gram-negative, endotoxin-producing bacilli.

Septic shock or any component of sepsis may manifest over several days or may overwhelm the patient within a few hours. Factors affecting its course include the reserve of the body's immune system at the time of onset, the extent of sepsis, the ability to eradicate it, and the effectiveness of resuscitative measures. The most effective tool against sepsis is early intervention initiated as soon as the patient shows subtle changes.

DIC. This disorder involves abnormal coagulation. An alteration in the coagulation cascade causes accelerated coagulation, excessive thrombin formation, consumption of clotting factors, and activation of the fibrinolytic system. Thrombosis and hemorrhage occur simul-

Signs and symptoms of multisystem organ failure in a cancer patient

In the cancer patient, manifestations of multisystem organ failure advance in four stages, becoming progressively more severe.

BODY SYSTEM	STAGE 1	STAGE 2	STAGE 3	STAGE 4
Cardiovascular	Increased volume requirements	Hyperdynamic, volume-dependent edema	Shock, decreased cardiac output	Hypervolemia
Hematologic	No obvious change	Decreased platelet count, increased or decreased white blood cell count	Continued decreased platelet count, continued increased or decreased white blood cell count	Infection
Hepatic	No obvious change	Iatrogenic jaundice	Clinical jaundice	Encephalopathy
Metabolic	Increased insulin requirements	Severe catabolism, hyperglycemia	Metabolic acidosis, increased oxygen consumption	Severe acidosis
Neurologic	Confusion	Disorientation	Disorientation, confusion	Coma
Renal	Decreased urine output	Fixed urine output, minimal azotemia	Azotemia	Oliguria
Respiratory	Mild respiratory alkalosis	Tachypnea, hypocapnia, hypoxia	Severe hypoxia, barotrauma	Hypercapnia

taneously from accelerated fibrinolysis and abnormal activation of the coagulation cascade.

Cancer can bring on DIC by accelerating clotting. Clinical manifestations of DIC reflect uncontrolled clotting followed by microvascular hemorrhage from clotting factor depletion and circulating anticoagulants. In acute DIC, clinical findings include petechiae, purpura, GI hemorrhage, and bleeding from multiple sites. Signs of chronic DIC include spontaneous bruising, increased thromboses, and gingival bleeding with bruising.

Complications

Complications of multisystem organ failure in the cancer patient are most often associated with the form of therapy that placed the already compromised patient at risk for multisystem organ failure.

The cancer itself or aggressive cancer treat-

ment may cause such problems as septic shock, DIC, malignant pleural and pericardial effusions, superior vena cava syndrome, syndrome of inappropriate antidiuretic hormone, tumor lysis syndrome, cardiac tamponade, and spinal cord compression.

Assessment

Clinical features of multisystem organ failure progress in four stages, ranging from no obvious signs of distress to terminal illness. In *stage 1*, expect slightly increased circulating volume and insulin requirements, changes in the patient's LOC, a decrease in urine output, or mild respiratory alkalosis. In *stage 2*, also called the meta-stable stage, each body system shows some evidence of dysfunction.

By *stage 3*, the patient is overtly ill. Individual organs now require active support. Unfortunately, many patients don't receive aggressive treatment until this stage. Because decompen-

sation usually is profound, the patient's response may be tenuous at best. If he has overt
signs of failure, he can't be resuscitated.

In *stage 4*, clinical deviations usually are
overwhelming — and fatal. (See *Signs and
symptoms of multisystem organ failure in a
cancer patient.*)

The prognosis for the patient with multisystem organ failure correlates directly with the
number of organ systems involved. Three factors have the greatest impact on multisystem
organ failure progression: the severity of the
initial insult, the presence of sepsis or respiratory infection, and advanced patient age.

Ongoing treatment
For a cancer patient with multisystem organ
failure, the goals of ongoing treatment are to
prevent further infection, correct the underlying condition, and prevent a recurrence of multisystem organ failure while ensuring proper
breathing, antibiotic therapy, and nutrition.

Ongoing nursing interventions
From diagnosis to treatment, recovery, and re-
lapse, the needs of the cancer patient are varied, complex, and challenging. To ensure
appropriate supportive measures, make sure
you thoroughly understand the physiology of
multisystem organ failure.
• Monitor the patient closely. Because you'll
spend more time with him than any other
health care provider, you're in the best position
to recognize the subtle changes that may signal serious complications.
• For the cancer patient who survives multisystem organ failure, a rehabilitation period follows. All organ systems need time to
recover — with careful monitoring throughout
this period. Help the patient regain muscle
strength during this time. Arrange for comprehensive outpatient education to aid early recognition of problems that warrant follow-up.
• If you provide home nursing care, make sure
you have a clear understanding of the patient's
and family's wishes regarding life-support interventions so that pending emergencies can
be dealt with properly.

Preventing multisystem organ failure
Because multisystem organ failure is so hard to
reverse, prevention is crucial. Hypoperfusion
and overwhelming inflammation predispose a
patient to multisystem organ failure. If your
cancer patient has these or other risk factors,
assess him frequently for signs and symptoms
of cardiovascular instability, poor organ perfusion, and inflammatory or infectious complications.
• To assess for cardiovascular instability, check
for hypotension, tachycardia, and weak pulses.
• To assess for poor organ perfusion, monitor
for low urine output, changes in LOC, poor
capillary refill, and GI bleeding.
• To detect infection, assess all invasive catheter
sites for signs and symptoms of inflammation
or infection, including erythema, warmth,
edema, drainage, and pain. If you detect such
findings, discontinue invasive lines and devices
as soon as possible, including indwelling urinary
catheters, NG tubes, chest tubes, biliary and
hepatic stents, gastric feeding tubes, implanted
infusion devices, and Ommaya reservoirs, as ordered.
• Minimize the risk of infection by using strict
aseptic technique.
• Remember that cancer patients with immunosuppression are particularly prone to nosocomial infections induced by various diagnostic
and therapeutic procedures. To help prevent
sepsis, minimize microbial access to the patient's body by maintaining skin integrity. Provide proper nutritional support, skin care,
positioning, and dressing techniques to keep
the skin intact. This is especially important if
your patient has had surgery or malignancies
that may metastasize, such as breast cancer,
head or neck cancer, Kaposi's sarcoma, or malignant melanoma. All of these conditions can
lead to infection or necrosis unless you take
meticulous care to prevent contamination and
promote healing.

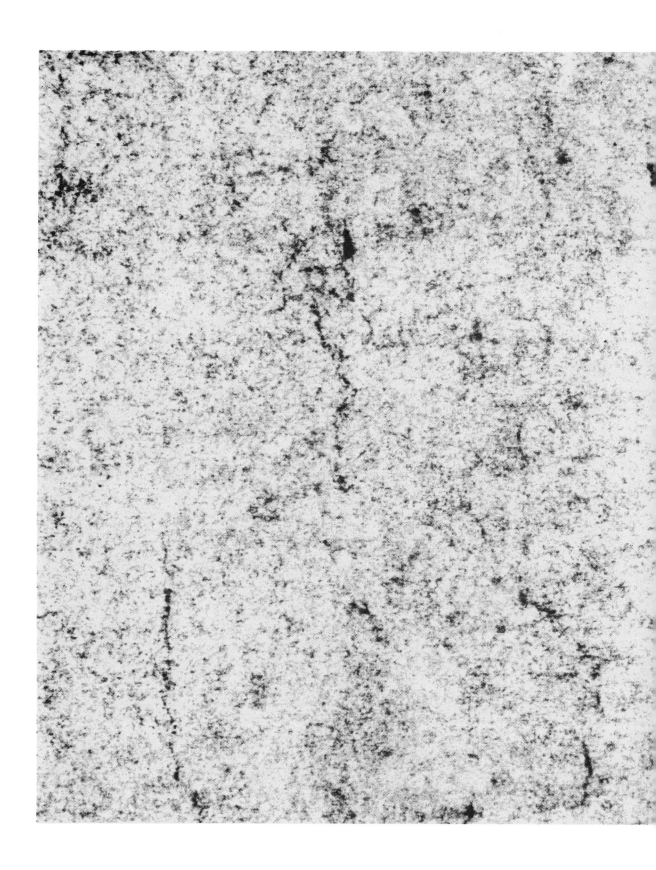

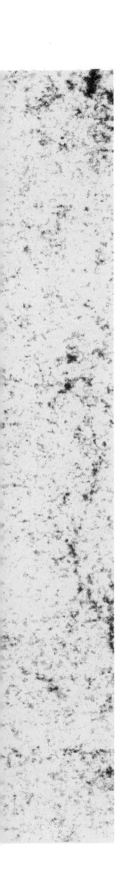

► **Suggested readings**

► **Advanced skilltest**

► **Index**

Suggested readings

Achkar, E., et al. *Clinical Gastroenterology,* 2nd ed. Philadelphia: Lea & Febiger, 1992.

Anderson, S., "ABGs: Six Easy Steps to Interpreting Blood Gas," *AJN* 90(8):42-45, August 1990.

Andrews, M., and Mooney, K.H., "Alterations in Hematologic Function in Children," in *Pathophysiology: The Biological Basis for Disease in Adults and Children.* Edited by McCance, K.L., and Huether, S.E. St. Louis: Mosby–Year Book, Inc., 1990.

Beutler, E., "Erythrocyte Disorders: Anemias Related to Abnormal Globin," in *Hematology,* 4th ed. Edited by Williams, W.J., and Beutler, E. New York: McGraw-Hill Publishing Co., 1990.

Branson, R.D., and Chatburn, R.L., "Technical Description and Classification of Modes of Ventilator Operation," *Respiratory Care* 37(9):1026-44, September 1992.

Briones, T.L., "Pressure Support Ventilation: New Ventilatory Technique," *Critical Care Nurse* 12(4):51-58, April 1992.

Carroll, P. "Nursing the Thoracotomy Patient," *RN* 55(6):34-42, June 1992.

Case, S.C., and Sabo, C.E. "Adult Respiratory Distress Syndrome: A Deadly Complication of Trauma," *Focus on Critical Care* 19(2):116-21, April 1992.

Cefalu, W. "Diabetic Ketoacidosis," *Critical Care Clinics* 7(1):89-108, January 1991.

Chatburn, R.L. "Classification of Mechanical Ventilators," *Respiratory Care* 37(9):1009-25, September 1992.

Colman, R.W., and Rubin, R.N. "Disseminated Intravascular Coagulation Due to Malignancy," *Seminars in Oncology* 17(2):172-86, April 1990.

Dettenmeier, P.A., *Pulmonary Nursing Care.* St. Louis: Mosby–Year Book, Inc., 1992.

Ehrhardt, B.S., and Graham, M. "Pulse Oximetry: An Easy Way to Check Oxygen Saturation" *Nursing90* 20(3):50-54, March 1990.

Ellstrom, K. "What's Causing your Patient's Respiratory Distress," *Nursing90* 20(11):56-61, November 1990.

Failla, S., and Radoslovich, N. "Ask the OR," *AJN* 93(1):76, January 1993.

Ferland, P.A. "Are You Ready for Ventilator Patients?" *Nursing91* 21(1):42-47, January 1991.

Gitnick, Gary. *Current Gastroenterology,* vol. 13. St. Louis: Mosby–Year Book, Inc., 1993.

Graves, L. "Diabetic Ketoacidosis and Hyperosomolar Hyperglycemic Nonketotic Coma," *Critical Care Nursing Quarterly* 13(3):50-61, November 1990.

Guyton, A.C. *Textbook of Medical Physiology,* 8th ed. Philadelphia: W.B. Saunders Co., 1991.

Halloran, T.H. "Nursing Responsibilities in Endocrine Emergencies," *Critical Care Nursing Quarterly* 13(3):74-81, November 1990.

Handerhan, B. "Managing the Patient with A.R.D.S.," *Nursing91* 21(10):102-03, 105, October 1991.

Handerhan, B. "Recognizing Pulmonary Embolism," *Nursing91* 21(2):107-08, 110, February 1991.

Hefti, D. "Chest Trauma," *RN* 54(5):28-33, May 1991.

Huggins, B. "Trauma Physiology," *Nursing Clinics of North America* 25(1):1-10, March 1990.

Isley, W. "Serum Sodium Concentration Abnormalities," *Critical Care Nursing Quarterly* 13(3):82-88, November 1990.

Jackson, D.C., et al. "Endoscopic Laser Cholecystectomy," *AORN Journal* 51(6):1546-52, June 1990.

Janson-Bjerklie, S. "Status Asthmaticus," *AJN* 90(9):52-55, September 1990.

Jarpe, M.B. "Nursing Care of Patients Receiving Long-Term Infusion of Neuromuscular Blocking Agents," *Critical Care Nurse* 12(7):58-63, October 1992.

Jess, L.W. "When Your Patient Has Asthma," *Nursing92* 22(4):48-51, April 1992.

Jordan, K. "Chest Trauma: How to Detect—and React to—Serious Trouble," *Nursing90* 19(9):34-41, September 1990.

Juarez, P. "Mechanical Ventilation for the Patient with Severe ARDS: PC-IRV," *Critical Care Nurse* 12(4):34-39, April 1992.

Kersten, L.D. *Comprehensive Respiratory Nursing: A Decision-Making Approach.* Philadelphia: W.B. Saunders Co., 1989.

McConnell, E.A. "Investigating Postoperative Muscular Pain," *Nursing91* 21(2):87-91, February 1991.

Mims, B.C., "Interpreting ABGs," *RN* 54(3):42-47, March 1991.

Moran, E., "Surgery Adds to Arsenal Against Gallstones," *Hospitals* 64(7):53 April 5, 1990.

Rakel, R.E., ed. *Conn's Current Therapy.* Philadelphia: W.B. Saunders Co., 1993.

Richless, C.I. "Current Trends in Mechanical Ventilation," *Critical Care Nurse* 11(3):41-50, 52-53, March 1991.

Smith, M.G. "Penetrating the Complexities of Chest Trauma," *JEMS* 14(8):50-59, August 1989.

Stiesmeyer, J.K., "What Triggers a Ventilator Alarm?" *AJN* 91(10):60-64, October 1991.

Surrat, S., et al. "Troubleshooting a Sump Tube," *AJN* 93(1):42-47, January 1993.

Teplitz, L. "ACTION STAT: Responding to an Air Embolism," *Nursing92* 22(7):33, July 1992.

Trofino, R.B., *Nursing Care of the Burn-Injured Patient.* Philadelphia: F.A. Davis Co., 1991.

Yeaw, E.M.J. "How Position Affects Oxygenation: Good Lung Down?" *AJN* 92(3):26-32, March 1992.

Young, N.A., and Gorzeman, J. "Managing Pneumothorax and Hemothorax," *Nursing91* 21(4):56-57, April 1991.

Advanced skilltest

This self-test presents case histories with related multiple-choice questions as well as general multiple-choice questions on responding to the patient in crisis. The questions begin on this page and continue to page 221. You'll find the answers along with rationales on pages 221 and 222.

Case history questions

Jack Cunningham, a postoperative cholecystectomy patient in the surgical unit, suddenly complains of crushing chest pain. He's hypotensive and diaphoretic, with sluggish capillary refill. You suspect he has reduced cardiac output.

1. One of the earliest signs of reduced cardiac output is:
   a. hypotension.
   b. diaphoresis.
   c. sluggish capillary refill.
   d. ashen skin.

2. Mr. Cunningham undergoes a 12-lead electrocardiogram (ECG). Which ECG finding reflects acute myocardial injury?
   a. Pathological Q waves
   b. Elevated ST segments
   c. Inverted T waves
   d. Depressed ST segments

3. Which intervention should you take immediately for Mr. Cunningham?
   a. Give him an analgesic to control his pain.
   b. Transfer him to the critical care unit.
   c. Administer a vasopressor to increase his blood pressure.
   d. Call an emergency code.

4. The goal of your immediate assessment of Mr. Cunningham is to:
   a. determine whether he's had a myocardial infarction.
   b. evaluate the adequacy of cardiac output.
   c. assess pain control.
   d. find out whether he has an arrhythmia.

5. To evaluate Mr. Cunningham's cardiac output, you would do all of the following *except*:
   a. palpate peripheral pulses.
   b. auscultate his heart.
   c. auscultate his lungs.
   d. evaluate his mental status.

As you make your afternoon rounds, you enter George Wright's room to find him struggling for breath, pale and apprehensive. Your assessment reveals a rapid respiratory rate (32 breaths/minute) and an irregular apical pulse (126 beats/minute). The cardiac monitor shows a normal sinus rhythm.
   Mr. Wright's blood pressure reading is 150/94 mm Hg—higher than his usual reading of about 126/88 mm Hg. His skin feels cool and clammy. When you auscultate his lungs, you hear crackles and wheezes two-thirds of the way up in both lungs. You also auscultate an S₃ gallop. His breathing is labored, he's using all accessory muscles to breathe, and his jugular veins are distended. Suddenly, Mr. Wright coughs up pink, frothy sputum.

6. Based on Mr. Wright's signs and symptoms, you'd suspect:
   a. pulmonary edema.
   b. hemoptysis.
   c. tension pneumothorax.
   d. pulmonary embolism.

7. What action would you take *first* for Mr. Wright?
   a. Call the doctor.
   b. Administer oxygen at 4 liters/minute by nasal cannula.
   c. Place the head of the bed flat.
   d. Administer a sedative, if ordered.

8. To diagnose Mr. Wright, the doctor is most likely to order all of the following tests *except:*

    a. arterial blood gas (ABG) analysis.

    b. ECG.

    c. ventilation-perfusion scan.

    d. chest X-ray.

9. The probable cause of Mr. Wright's signs and symptoms is:

    a. an undiagnosed preexisting asthmatic condition aggravated by his illness.

    b. diminished peripheral vascular resistance.

    c. decreased myocardial contractility.

    d. reduced pulmonary vascular resistance.

Paul Anderson, age 68, is recovering well 2 days after coronary artery bypass graft surgery. Because of his progress, the doctor removes the large-bore subclavian central venous catheter and replaces it with a peripheral I.V. line. After dressing the site, he orders Mr. Anderson's transfer to the cardiac step-down unit.

    Minutes after the doctor leaves the room, Mr. Anderson complains of light-headedness, weakness, shortness of breath, and palpitations. You note that he's pale, with cyanotic lips and nail beds. His pulse is weak and thready at 120 beats/minute, and his respirations are labored at 34 breaths/minute. His blood pressure reads 80/50 mm Hg. The cardiac monitor shows sinus tachycardia.

10. Based on your assessment findings for Mr. Anderson, you would suspect:

    a. myocardial infarction.

    b. pulmonary edema.

    c. air embolism.

    d. acute respiratory distress syndrome (ARDS).

11. Your *first* action for Mr. Anderson would be to:

    a. lower his head.

    b. place him in reverse Trendelenburg's position.

    c. place him on his right side, with his head down.

    d. place him on his left side, with his head down.

Dwight Gottstine, age 36, is admitted to the intensive care unit (ICU) with focal right-sided twitching and numbness of the face, followed by onset of a severe migraine. Several hours after admission, he complains of a worsening headache, nausea and vomiting, and a stiff neck. He grows more lethargic, then has another episode of right-sided twitching—this time involving his entire right side. Computed tomography (CT) scans of the head (with and without contrast dye) show a subarachnoid hemorrhage with enlarged ventricles and a moderately large area of denseness in his left parietal lobe, suggesting an arteriovenous malformation (AVM).

    The neurosurgeon inserts an intraventricular catheter to relieve acute hydrocephalus, and 3 days later a cerebral arteriogram is performed. Seven days after admission, Mr. Gottstine undergoes a craniotomy with AVM excision.

12. Which of Mr. Gottstine's initial signs and symptoms suggested that he had an AVM?

    a. Migraine

    b. Focal seizures

    c. Vomiting

    d. Migraine and focal seizures

13. Which of the following is *not* a complication of an AVM?

    a. Seizure

    b. Cerebral edema

    c. Hydrocephalus

    d. Increased intracranial pressure (ICP)

14. All of these tests help to diagnose an AVM *except:*

    a. CT scan without enhancement.

    b. CT scan with enhancement.

    c. cerebral angiography.

    d. magnetic resonance imaging (MRI) with gadolinium enhancement.

15. Which intervention would *not* be appropriate for a postoperative AVM patient with cerebral breakthrough symptoms, such as Mr. Gottstine?

    a. Diuretic therapy

    b. Elevating the head of the bed

    c. Hyperventilation therapy

    d. Hypervolemic therapy

Maria Kotera, age 34, is admitted to the emergency department complaining of acute left-sided abdominal pain, a fever of 101.3° to 102.6° F (38.5° to 39.2° C), and intermittent diarrhea for the past 3 days. She says she's had two sickle-cell crises in the last 5 years after severe respiratory infections; both episodes required hospitalization.

Your initial assessment reveals warm, dry skin with poor turgor and cyanotic nail beds, a heart rate of 122 beats/minute sitting and 100 beats/minute lying down, blood pressure of 148/90 mm Hg, full bounding pulses, and a diffusely tender abdomen. You note that Ms. Kotera is dehydrated and has signs of sickle-cell crisis.

As ordered, you establish an I.V. line, start infusing 0.9% sodium chloride solution at 250 ml/hour, and administer oxygen at 2 liters/minute. Then you give 1 mg of morphine, as ordered, to relieve pain. Before transferring Ms. Kotera to a telemetry unit, where she can be monitored for arrhythmias and heart failure, you draw blood for a complete blood count, ABG analysis, a coagulation profile, and liver function tests.

16. Ms. Kotera's sickle-cell crisis was probably precipitated by:

    a. anxiety.

    b. dehydration.

    c. bowel obstruction.

    d. heart failure.

17. The doctor orders 0.9% sodium chloride to:

    a. increase volume and improve cardiac performance.

    b. temporarily replace volume loss caused by red blood cell (RBC) sickling.

    c. restore circulation and reduce RBC sickling.

    d. enhance blood flow to the abdomen, a possible microthrombi site.

18. Which hematologic findings would you expect in a patient with sickle-cell crisis?

    a. Increased reticulocyte count

    b. Increased hematocrit count

    c. Increased platelet count

    d. Reduced erythrocyte sedimentation rate

General questions

19. The most dangerous complication of bleeding esophageal varices is:

    a. hepatic failure.

    b. hemorrhagic shock.

    c. perforated ulcer.

    d. splenic rupture.

20. The drug most commonly used to treat ruptured esophageal varices is:

    a. ranitidine.

    b. cimetidine.

    c. vitamin K_1.

    d. vasopressin.

21. All of the following drugs can cause stress ulcers *except:*

    a. corticosteroids.

    b. nicotine.

    c. digoxin.

    d. aspirin.

22. A rising blood ammonia level, as occurs in a patient with hepatic failure, can result from all of the following *except:*

    a. dehydration.

    b. cirrhosis.

    c. portal hypertension.

    d. excessive protein intake.

23. Which neurologic problem can occur as a complication of hepatic failure?

    a. Delirium

    b. Encephalopathy

    c. Alcohol withdrawal delirium

    d. Organic brain syndrome

24. In a patient with thyroid storm, you would expect to see the symptom triad of:

    a. hyperpyrexia, irritability, and delirium.

    b. hyperpyrexia, tachyarrhythmia, and hypermetabolic decompensation.

    c. hypotension, tachycardia, and agitation.

    d. nausea, vomiting, and diarrhea.

25. During thyroid storm, which laboratory tests usually show increases?

    a. Hemoglobin, hematocrit, and serum glucose, calcium, triiodothyronine (T_3), and thyroxine (T_4)

    b. Hemoglobin, hematocrit, serum magnesium, and serum potassium

    c. Serum glucose, leukocyte count, and serum salicylates

    d. Serum T_3, T_4, lactate dehydrogenase, and aspartate aminotransferase (formerly SGOT)

26. If the doctor prescribed a sedative for a patient with thyroid storm, you would stay alert for:

    a. increased agitation.

    b. masking of other symptoms.

    c. hypoventilation.

    d. arrhythmias.

27. The hyperthyroid patient should be placed on which diet?

    a. An 1,800-calorie/day diet that conforms to American Dietary Association standards

    b. A 3,000-calorie/day diet low in protein

    c. A 2,000-calorie/day diet consisting of 60 g protein, 2 g sodium, and no more than 1 liter of fluid

    d. A 3,000-calorie/day diet high in protein, with at least 3 liters of fluid

28. Which statement about the patient with hyperosmolar nonketotic syndrome (HNKS) is true?

    a. He has ketonuria and a slightly elevated blood glucose level.

    b. He requires insulin during the acute treatment phase and after discharge.

    c. He's mildly dehydrated.

    d. He has enough circulating insulin to prevent lipolysis and ketonuria.

29. Which statement about the syndrome of inappropriate antidiuretic hormone is true?

    a. It may result from malignant tumors or from drugs that cause unchecked antidiuretic hormone (ADH) secretion.

    b. It doesn't alter water balance within the body.

    c. It causes low urine output and low specific gravity.

    d. It leads to weight gain and generalized edema.

30. Which condition is essential in the initiation and progression of multisystem organ failure?

    a. Trauma

    b. Sepsis

    c. Cancer

    d. ARDS

31. In multisystem organ failure, which of the following is *not* among the major changes caused by an out-of-control mediator response?

    a. Maldistribution of circulating volume

    b. Imbalance between oxygen supply and demand

    c. Metabolic disturbances

    d. Slowing of feedback mechanisms

Answers and rationales

1. c. Sluggish capillary refill, a sign of poor perfusion, occurs early when cardiac output decreases. Hypotension, diaphoresis, and ashen color occur only after compensatory mechanisms fail.

2. b. ST-segment elevation reflects acute injury. Pathological Q waves indicate necrosis or infarction, whereas inverted T waves and depressed ST segments reflect ischemia.

3. a. Pain is a sign of myocardial injury. Controlling pain reduces catecholamine release and sympathetic stimulation, thus decreasing oxygen demand.

4. b. Evaluating if the patient has adequate cardiac output is the goal of immediate assessment. Reduced cardiac output can quickly make myocardial infarction life-threatening.

5. c. Lung auscultation has no value in determining cardiac output. To evaluate cardiac output, you'd palpate the patient's peripheral pulses, auscultate his heart, evaluate his mental status, observe his color, and measure his urine output.

6. a. The patient's signs and symptoms point to pulmonary edema. Pulmonary embolism is associated with sudden dyspnea and chest pain and usually causes a heart rhythm change such as atrial fibrillation.

7. b. The correct first step is to administer oxygen to reduce the work of breathing and promote oxygenation. Then you'd elevate the head of the bed to ease the patient's breathing and call the doctor, who might order a sedative. You'd also stay with the patient to help reduce his anxiety.

8. c. The ventilation-perfusion scan is used to detect pulmonary embolism, which isn't suspected in this case. ABG analysis, ECG, and chest X-ray help distinguish cardiogenic pulmonary edema from noncardiogenic pulmonary edema.

9. c. Pulmonary edema causes decreased myocardial contractility. This, in turn, reduces cardiac output and causes blood to back up in the pulmonary circulation.

10. c. Mr. Anderson's signs and symptoms suggest air embolism, a complication of central venous catheter removal.

11. d. The patient should be placed on his left side with his head down to divert air in the right ventricular outflow tract to the right atrium and away from the pulmonary artery. This, in turn, would reduce the risk of air bubbles entering the pulmonary circulation.

12. d. An episodic headache, such as a migraine, in conjunction with focal seizures suggests an AVM. Vomiting may be related to the headache and meningeal signs but isn't necessarily associated with an AVM.

13. a. A seizure is a sign, not a complication, of an AVM. Cerebral edema (caused by ischemia), hydrocephalus (caused by hemorrhage), and increased ICP (caused by compression) are potential complications of an AVM.

14. a. A CT scan without enhancement may show a bleed, but it won't reveal a potential vascular lesion such as an AVM. A CT scan with enhancement, cerebral angiography, and MRI with gadolinium enhancement would all be done to diagnose an AVM.

15. d. Hypervolemic therapy is contraindicated once the vessels surrounding an excised AVM lose their autoregulating ability. Diuretic therapy, elevating the head of the bed, and hyperventilation therapy are methods used to manage the patient with cerebral breakthrough symptoms.

16. b. Common precipitators of sickle-cell crisis include dehydration, extreme cold, hemorrhage, strenuous exercise, infection, respiratory compromise, and tissue hypoxia.

17. c. Fluid restoration is the highest-priority intervention in suspected sickle-cell crisis. Hyperviscosity and RBC sickling worsen the hypoxia that initiated the crisis; hemodilution is needed to reverse these conditions.

18. a. The reticulocyte count increases in sickle-cell crisis because reticulocytes are RBC precursors released from the bone marrow early to compensate for RBC loss.

19. b. When bleeding varices rupture, they cause massive hematemesis, which requires emergency treatment to control hemorrhage and prevent the progression to shock.

20. d. Vasopressin has a powerful vasoconstrictive effect that reduces portal hypertension and constricts mesenteric blood flow by causing constriction of arterioles.

21. c. Digoxin doesn't fall into any classification of drugs known to cause stress ulcers. Three classes of drugs can produce such ulcers: those that impair renewal of the gastric mucosa, such as corticosteroids and phenylbutazone; those that stimulate acidity, such as nicotine and caffeine; and those that alter the mucosal barrier, such as aspirin and alcohol.

22. a. Dehydration doesn't cause the blood ammonia level to rise. An increased blood ammonia level signals impaired hepatic synthesis of urea, as occurs in advanced liver disease and hepatic failure.

23. b. Encephalopathy occurs in patients with hepatic failure and advanced cirrhosis. This syndrome, which causes a decreased level of consciousness, is related to ammonia in the blood. Ammonia acts as a direct toxin to brain cells, inhibiting neurotransmission and cerebral metabolism. Ultimately, encephalopathy leads to coma.

24. b. Thyroid storm causes hyperpyrexia, tachyarrhythmia, and hypermetabolic decompensation. Body temperature may rise as high as 106° F (41.1° C), and tachyarrhythmias may

speed the heart rate to 300 beats/minute. Hypermetabolic decompensation affects the GI, cardiovascular, and central nervous systems.

25. a. Hemoglobin and hematocrit levels rise from dehydration, the serum glucose level increases from glycogenolysis or decreased insulin production or secretion, the serum calcium level rises from increased bone metabolism, and T_3 and T_4 levels increase from hyperthyroidism. The serum magnesium level may be low from decreased cardiac contractility. Serum salicylates shouldn't be measurable because aspirin is contraindicated in thyroid storm (it further displaces thyroid hormone and worsens hypermetabolism).

26. c. Sedatives calm the patient and allay his anxiety, but they should be used with extreme caution in thyroid storm because they may cause hypoventilation.

27. d. The hyperthyroid patient needs a diet high in calories (at least 3,000 daily), carbohydrates, protein, vitamins, and minerals. He may need to eat six full meals a day. His fluid intake should be increased to 3 or 4 liters a day to prevent dehydration and compensate for diaphoresis.

28. d. HNKS occurs in patients with Type II diabetes mellitus, who have at least some endogenous insulin production. Signs and symptoms of HNKS resemble those of diabetic ketoacidosis, including catabolism of proteins and carbohydrates, which ultimately causes dehydration and electrolyte imbalance. The patient produces enough insulin to avoid fat catabolism, thereby preventing the development of ketone bodies with resultant metabolic acidosis.

29. a. Vasopressin and certain other drugs release ADH, and some malignant tumors cause ectopic release of vasopressin.

30. b. Sepsis is the essential focus for the initiation and progression of multisystem organ failure.

31. d. Feedback mechanisms aren't slowed by an out-of-control mediator response in multisystem organ failure. The three major changes caused by such a mediator response are maldistribution of circulating volume, an imbalance between oxygen supply and demand, and metabolic disturbances.

Index

i refers to illustration; t refers to a table

i refers to illustration; t refers to a table

i refers to illustration; t refers to a table

i refers to illustration; t refers to a table

i refers to illustration; t refers to a table